Slimming
EATS
Made Simple

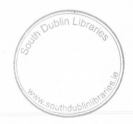

Slimming
EATS
Made Simple

Delicious & easy recipes –
100+ under 500 calories

Siobhan Wightman

Photography by Haarala Hamilton

yellow
kite

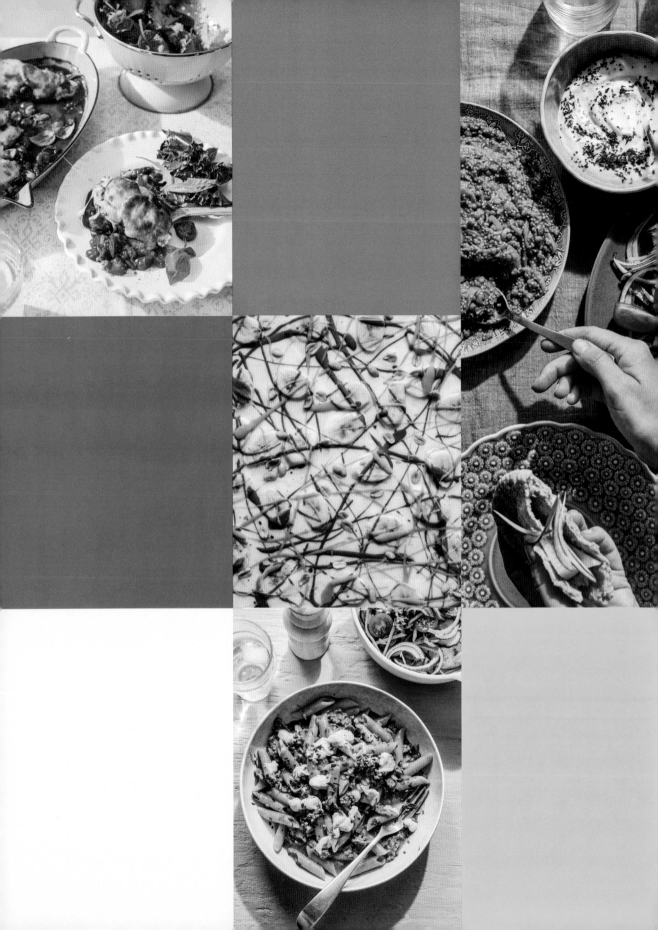

Introduction 6

1. Simple Stovetop 28

2. Sheet-pan Meals
   Made Simple 64

3. Made Simple in the Oven 102

4. Slow Cooker Recipes 136

5. Delicious Bowls 166

6. Blog Favourites 202

7. Desserts Made Simple 234

8. Simple Extras 256

Index 282

Recipe Index 286

Acknowledgements 287

Introduction

I never for a moment thought I would write one cookbook, let alone a second, but here it is – and it's all thanks to you, my incredible readers. In fact, your support has been so amazing that you made my first book, *Slimming Eats*, a *Sunday Times* bestseller. For me, that was an amazing accomplishment, and something I could never have imagined. I still can't quite believe my name is printed on a cookbook in an actual bookshop. It's quite a surreal thing to see, and I don't think it will ever not feel strange to me.

In case you are venturing into this book without having seen my first one, let me introduce myself. My name is Siobhan. I'm married and the mum of two children – who are growing up too fast, might I add. If you're unfamiliar with me or my blog, then you're probably wondering what these recipes are all about. When I first started Slimming Eats, all I really intended to do was share the recipes I had written online and keep a record of my creations. I quickly discovered that these recipes were proving very popular. I had set out to create healthier, 'slimming' versions of favourite dishes, aiming to do this without compromising on flavour, which can often be the first thing to go when it comes to healthy recipes. Fast-forward over a decade, and now I have one of the most popular healthy recipe websites – and a bestselling cookbook. Millions of people have found my recipes useful, which is mind-blowing considering how it all started. I've never trained as a chef, so I still find it a bit of a shock to this day that so many of you love the recipes I share. I am just a home cook who loves creating healthy food for my family, and I'm thrilled that this resonates with so many of you.

I am originally from the UK, but now reside in Ontario, Canada. We moved here back in 2008, when my oldest had just turned two. It was quite a change in many ways, but Canada has definitely become home. I still feel a little homesick every time I go back to London though; that city will always have a special place in my heart, as it holds so many memories from my childhood.

Finding Joy in Cooking Real Food

The last few years have been a bit hard on my mental health: with ongoing health issues, severe anxiety and then being thrown into a pandemic, I have struggled in many ways. The world has changed in recent years, and we have many challenges still ahead of us, but cooking and providing recipes that people enjoy is one small thing I can do to make people's lives just a little better and happier.

My first book gave me something to keep myself busy with during this challenging time, and it was all a bit surreal. In normal circumstances, I would have travelled to London to be with the amazing team through the recipe photoshoot, but we were on strict lockdown at that time here in Canada, so it was all done remotely. I would join the team over Zoom each day to see them in action and watch all my creations come to life with their amazing food styling and photography. I am so lucky to have a fantastic publisher and team; I couldn't ask for a better group of people to bring my vision and recipes to life.

Even with such an amazing team supporting me, writing a cookbook can be quite nerve-racking, and I must admit there are times when I have struggled with my anxiety. It's definitely something that takes me completely out of my comfort zone, but I think it's a good thing to push ourselves, and it has given me something really positive to focus on.

About This Book

One of the trickiest things can be choosing which recipes to include! With my website, I can just add a new recipe when I feel like it, as there is enough choice there that I can be sure there's something for everyone. With a cookbook, you have to be really selective, as there is only space for a certain number of recipes, and you have to ensure there is enough variety.

For this book, I wanted to create recipes that were simple to make, whether that meant a one-pot recipe, a sheet-pan meal, an easy oven bake, or something made in a slow cooker. And with that came the name: *Slimming Eats Made Simple*.

We begin with *Simple Stovetop*, a selection of easy-to-make, delicious meals that can all be cooked on the stove, with plenty of one-pot dishes so you get all the flavour and none of the washing-up. Next comes *Sheet-pan Meals Made Simple*, where all the recipes use just one or two sheet pans, with the occasional bit of stovetop action to help things cook faster. This chapter is full of tasty traybakes and treats your whole family will love. *Made Simple in the Oven* brings together all my favourite roasts, bakes and casseroles, with healthy swaps and time-saving tips. *Slow Cooker Recipes* is all about minimal prep and maximum flavour, with simple meals cooked low and slow for comfort food without all the calories.

One of my favourite chapters is *Delicious Bowls*, as this is my family's favourite kind of meal. While some of them may not seem quite so 'simple', containing quite a few ingredients, they have all been created with the idea that you get a complete meal in a bowl. Often, recipes just give you the main element of a dish, and when you are tired and exhausted after a long day at work, trying to come up with ideas for side dishes can be just too much. So I thought these bowls would be great to include, as they really do offer an entire meal in one recipe. In addition, I've included some soup recipes, because who doesn't love a nice filling bowl of soup?

As with my last book, I've included some **Blog Favourites** as bonus extras. This means that as well as the new recipes here, there are some of those much-loved top choices you all go back to again and again. Obviously, it's not possible to include everyone's favourites, as they can be so different from one person to the next, but I chose the recipes based on the ones my blog visitors view the most. I hope there are plenty of tasty recipes here that you will all love.

Desserts Made Simple is sure to be a popular chapter with everyone in your house, with yummy treats to satisfy the sweetest of tooths, with cakes, cookies and desserts all created with a lighter touch so you can enjoy them to your heart's content.

And there's more! In **Simple Extras** I have put together a selection of my go-to sides and salads so you can turn any meal into a Slimming Eats feast. I've also shared some of my favourite spice blends, too, which you can make up and keep in an airtight jar so they're ready whenever you need them. These can be used again and again, both in my recipes and in your own creations; they're great for adding flavour to any protein you are using for a traybake or one-pot dish.

Over the last couple of years, I have been trying to teach myself lots of different cuisines. We are very lucky to have a big international supermarket where I live that has aisles and aisles of ingredients from all over the world, including China, Korea, Japan, Thailand, India and the Caribbean. It's an amazing place for sourcing things that I may not get at the usual grocery store, and I love discovering new ingredients I haven't cooked with before. Korean food has become one of my favourite cuisines to experiment with in the last couple of years, and you will see some of that influence in this book.

Explore Your Own Creations

I always try to encourage my readers to use my recipes as a base that you can build on to come up with some of your own creations. The more you cook, the more you will get used to what does and doesn't work together. That was exactly the way I taught myself, by recreating all my favourite foods at home. You can easily vary a simple recipe by just swapping a few ingredients, and I have tried to include some tips for how to do that as I know many of you are keen to get creative in your kitchens. That was something I really loved about the first book; not only were many of you telling me you were enjoying cooking again, but you were also using my recipes as a basis for your own creations, swapping ingredients and trying out different flavour combinations. There is nothing more rewarding than seeing my recipes inspiring you all to cook.

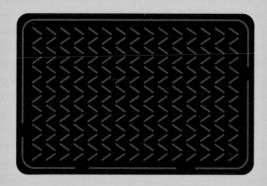

If you think you just won't get much use out of a slow cooker and so don't want to waste money by purchasing one, you can easily convert a slow-cooker recipe to be cooked in the oven. Here's a rough guide, but bear in mind that ovens do vary, so you may have to adjust slightly to suit yours.

Slow Cooker to Oven Conversion:

- Use a large lidded casserole pot or Dutch oven.

- If the recipe calls for the slow cooker to be set to low, cook in the oven at 160°C/140°C fan/325°F/gas 4 and divide the cooking time by four.

- If the recipe calls for the slow cooker to be set to high, cook in the oven at 160°C/140°C fan/325°F/gas 4 and divide the cooking time by two.

BAKING TRAYS AND DISHES

For sheet-pan meals and traybakes, a variety of different-sized baking trays is a must. When you're making a traybake, it's important that all the ingredients fit on the tray in a thin, even layer so that the heat circulates around the food evenly. If you have it all piled high in a too-small dish, the cooking will be uneven, and the food tends to steam instead of bake, so you will end up with soggy, mushy vegetables.

You can get baking trays and sheet pans with non-stick coating, or just aluminium. I go for the latter, personally; they clean up easily as long as you wash up as soon as you can. I also recommend lining them with baking paper or foil for some items, to ensure food doesn't stick and for ease of clean-up afterwards.

SLOW COOKER

Slow cookers are perfect for those days when you are rushed for time and need a filling, hearty meal waiting for you at the end of the day. I use mine for things like soups, chillies, stews, casseroles and curries. Sometimes I prefer to make these on the stove or in the oven, but for tender meat and dishes that are best slow-cooked, a slow cooker is a great gadget to have.

If you are investing in one for the first time, opt for one that has a sear function, or one where you can remove the insert dish and use it on the stove. This will mean you can easily brown anything that needs browning first, with minimal clean-up afterwards. You don't have to brown your meat and base ingredients first if you are rushed for time, but I always recommend doing so if you can, as it gives the dish a better flavour overall.

FOOD CONTAINERS

If you like to prepare meals in advance or are cooking a recipe that serves four for just two people, then having some handy food containers to freeze leftovers is a great option. I try to avoid using plastic ones and have swapped all mine for glass. They are more expensive, but will last a long time and most are microwave- and oven-safe, which means you don't need to transfer to another container.

You can also get some with different-sized compartments, which is handy for freezing a complete meal with sides and vegetables.

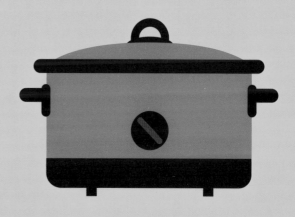

Building Up Your Store Cupboard Ingredients

When first starting out with healthy eating and cooking your own food, it can be all too tempting to go and buy everything at once, but this is really not necessary. Just plan your meals each week, and only buy what you need as you go along. It's much more budget-friendly to do it this way. Once you have been doing this for a few weeks, you will find your spices and store cupboard ingredients are well stocked.

STORE CUPBOARD INGREDIENTS

Once you have built up a well-stocked store cupboard, you will always have plenty of ingredients on hand to create delicious healthy meals, even when you're running low on fresh produce before a grocery shop. Many of these don't even need to be refrigerated or frozen once opened, especially things like pasta and grains.

- RICE
  long-grain, arborio, basmati, jasmine, brown

- PASTA
  various shapes (but most shapes will work in any recipe)

- COUSCOUS
  regular and giant
  (pearl or Israeli)

- QUINOA

- WHOLE GRAINS
  barley, bulgur wheat, oats

- DRIED AND CANNED PULSES/LEGUMES
  lentils, beans, chickpeas

- CANNED TOMATOES
  chopped or whole

- TOMATO PURÉE (paste)

- PASSATA

- CANNED FISH
  tuna, salmon, sardines

- COOKING OILS
  ghee, olive, avocado, coconut, sesame, etc.

- COOKING OIL SPRAY
  I prefer to use ones without emulsifiers

- STOCK
  cartons of broth, stock cubes, bouillon, etc.

- SAUCES/CONDIMENTS
  soy sauce, oyster sauce, hoisin sauce, fish sauce, sriracha, mirin, Shaoxing wine, Worcestershire sauce, gochujang, etc. (most of these can be kept in the cupboard; some will require refrigeration once opened)

- VINEGARS
  balsamic, apple cider, etc.

- SWEETENERS
  maple syrup, honey, brown sugar, granulated sweetener (I use erythritol – brown and white varieties)

- BAKING ESSENTIALS
  flour, bicarbonate of soda (baking soda), baking powder, vanilla extract, etc.

- THICKENING AGENTS
  cornflour (cornstarch), arrowroot or tapioca flour (see page 17)

HERBS AND SPICES

My collection of herbs and spices, as you can probably imagine, is huge. As I have explained, you certainly don't need to go and buy them all at once; just gather them as you go along, and you will soon build up a great collection. I've also included my own spice mixes on pages 280–281.

- SEA SALT
  both coarse and fine
  (see page 16)

- BLACK PEPPER
  (whole peppercorns in
  a pepper grinder are best)
  (see page 16)

- ITALIAN SEASONING
  (mixed herbs)

- HERBES DE PROVENCE

- GROUND CUMIN

- GROUND CORIANDER

- CHILLI POWDER
  mild and hot

- CURRY POWDER

- PAPRIKA
  sweet and smoked

- GARLIC POWDER OR GRANULES

- ONION POWDER OR GRANULES

- DRIED HERBS
  basil, oregano, thyme, rosemary,
  parsley, mint, dill, chives

- CAYENNE PEPPER

- GARAM MASALA

- GROUND TURMERIC

- GROUND GINGER

- CLOVES

- GREEN CARDAMOM PODS

- CINNAMON
  ground and whole

- BAY LEAVES

- MUSTARD POWDER

Slimming Eats Tips

The price of groceries has really gone up in the last couple of years, so trying to reduce costs can be really important for many who are on a low budget.

Meal planning is vital if you want to save money, as you can plan your week and only buy the items you need. Impulse buys are the things that will really bump up your shopping bill, and may also end up being less healthy choices. If you can order your groceries online, this is a great option, as it means you avoid those end-of-aisle deals that often tempt you into buying things you don't really need.

Fresh ingredients are great, but can sometimes spoil a lot quicker, which is something you want to avoid if you are on a budget. I always grab a few bags of different frozen vegetables and fruits, as they are great for bulking out meals.

For dry ingredients, like rice, pasta and pulses, I suggest you buy in bulk where you can if you have the space to store them, as this usually works out much cheaper. Canned beans and pulses are great, too, but often have lots of sodium added, so check the labels and choose those with no added salt where possible.

If you have a weekly farmers' market nearby, those are sometimes great options for picking up cheaper produce. You could also explore budget grocery stores that don't sell lots of different brands of the same item.

I often check out the reduced-items area too, as there are normally some great deals to be found. These items do usually need to be used quickly, though, so are not always ideal for everyone.

Wholesale stores like Costco can be a great option for some items if you are lucky enough to have a membership, but as the items tend to come in larger amounts, this may not be suitable for you if you don't have lots of storage space.

Choose cheaper cuts of meat where possible, too. While the occasional steak or roast is yummy, you don't want to be eating that every day, or your weekly food bill will be excessive. I try to balance things out with occasional meat-free meals, as pulses and beans are so much cheaper. A big tray of chicken thighs is often much cheaper than a pack of boneless, skinless chicken breasts, and if you invest in some good kitchen scissors, it's so easy to remove the skin and bone yourself. Although I know not everyone likes thigh meat, I find it has much more flavour, especially in things like curries and casseroles.

SOURCING HARD-TO-FIND INGREDIENTS

Luckily, there not any very unusual ingredients in this book. I try to ensure the ingredients I use in my recipes are easy to source, bar the odd few, that are needed for that authentic flavour. Where you may have to buy something a little more unusual, I have tried to create more than one recipe using that ingredient, so you will get enough use out of it, for example gochujang.

If there is a swap that can be made, I will usually recommend one within the recipe, but sometimes there is no replacement for that particular flavour.

Most less-common ingredients can be bought online nowadays, so if you are struggling to find something at your local grocery store, try a quick online search.

It's also a great idea to seek out Chinese or Indian grocery stores in your area, as these will be your best place to find certain ingredients, especially spices. I usually find they are much cheaper, too. European and Caribbean markets are also good places to explore.

I am lucky enough to live in a town that has some great food shops and markets, including the huge international supermarket I mentioned earlier, which has almost every ingredient you can imagine from all over the world. So if I need something in particular, that is where I go, especially now I am venturing into teaching myself different cuisines.

SCALING DOWN

You will notice most of the recipes in this book serve four; that's because we are a family of four. Occasionally, if I am doing a lunch recipe when the kids are at school, it may be a recipe for two; or if I want some extra portions, I might make a recipe for six or eight (this is usually when I am doing something in the slow cooker).

If you are cooking for fewer people, most recipes in this book can be scaled down. For example, if a recipe serves four, just halve all the ingredients to make it serve two. This may not work for every recipe, though, especially one-pot recipes, where simply halving everything might mean the end result is not quite the same. As you grow in confidence with your cooking, you will develop a knack for knowing how to adjust quantities to suit your needs.

PORTION SIZES

The nutritional information given for each recipe in this book is per portion (serving) and includes only the items listed in the ingredients of the recipe; it doesn't include any additional sides or 'to serve' items, unless stated.

The portions in the book are, of course, a guideline. We all have different appetites, and so while a recipe may serve my family of four, some of you may find the portions are not enough, while others might find them too generous. It all really depends on your own calorie goal and appetite. If your goal is to lose weight, then of course, you need to ensure you are not going over your daily calorie goal.

I always try to stick to recommend serving sizes and bulk meals out with healthy vegetables if I am feeling really hungry. This is a really healthy habit to get into: adding some extra vegetables to your plate can help you feel satisfied and stop you going back for seconds. As well as bulking out your plate with some low-calorie, nutrient-dense vegetables, you can also try reducing the amount of carbs by swapping them for things like cauliflower rice, spiralized veggies, vegetable mash or roasted vegetables. I also love to serve a big bowl of salad in the middle of the table so everyone can help themselves.

LEAN MEATS/PROTEIN

The nutritional information in this book is always using the leanest cuts of meat. This ensures calories are kept low. I always trim any visible fat, even if the packaging advertises the meat as lean. Some meats, like boneless chicken thighs, can still have quite a bit of fat attached. The best tool for trimming meat (as I've mentioned previously) is a pair of kitchen scissors.

If you are removing skin from chicken yourself, the easiest way to do this is by gripping it with a piece of paper towel; it should come away easily.

When I'm using minced (ground) meats, I always go for 5% fat. I don't tend to go any leaner than this, especially if I'm making things like burgers or meatballs, as it can become a bit dry.

You will notice I tend to prefer chicken thighs rather than breasts in dishes like curries, stews and casseroles. This is because thighs are much more flavoursome, and also stay tender. Chicken breast cooks really quickly, and can become a bit dry in these types of recipes.

If you want to occasionally enjoy a little bit of crispy skin on some roast chicken, or a piece of streaky crispy bacon, you can totally do this; it's all about balance. As long as it fits into your daily calorie goal, that's all that really matters.

OIL SPRAYS AND COOKING FATS

Eating healthily is a lifestyle change, and in order to make it sustainable, I strongly believe in using real ingredients in recipes. While I do use cooking oil sprays, if I feel a recipe needs a little bit of olive oil or butter, then I will always use it in a recipe. If you are cooking for a family of four, a little bit of olive oil in a recipe is not going to be that much calorie-wise, and is well worth it in terms of flavour. So don't be afraid to use olive oil or butter where I've suggested it.

DAIRY PRODUCTS

When it comes to solid cheeses, like Cheddar and mozzarella, I always buy the regular kind, never the reduced-fat varieties. I just find the regular kind has much more flavour and melts better.

For cream cheese, though, I do opt for the light or reduced-fat versions, although it's worth noting there really isn't a great deal of difference in calories for some of these. Don't mistake cream cheese for quark, by the way – these are not the same thing. Cream cheese can withstand heat and melts to a creamy sauce without splitting, whereas quark tends to split in sauces if heated and is more sour-tasting than creamy.

For yogurt, I use fat-free Greek or natural yogurt in my recipes. However, for unflavoured varieties, there is not a huge difference in calories if you want to use 2% fat instead.

For milk, I like to include dairy-free options like cashew or oat, but if I use dairy milk, I always go for semi-skimmed or whole. I personally don't care for skimmed milk. That's just my preference, if you prefer to use skimmed milk in your tea or coffee, for example, then go for it. However, if one of my recipes calls for semi-skimmed milk, I do recommend sticking to that, as otherwise the final result may not quite be the same.

STOCK

Did you know that not all stock cubes etc. are equal? This is one of the biggest mistakes I see when a certain measurement of stock is called for in a recipe.

I love to make my own stock from scratch and freeze it, but sometimes I don't have any on hand, or just don't have the time to make my own, and that's when bouillon, stock pots or stock cubes are handy.

However, different brands require different ratios of liquid, so always check the packaging of the one you are using. For example, some stock cubes are mixed with just 180ml (6fl oz) water, which makes 180ml stock. So if you are only using one of those stock cubes for, say, 500ml (18fl oz) of stock, it's going to be very bland and watery in taste, which can then affect the taste of the whole recipe. There are also some brands where one stock cube makes over 500ml (18fl oz) of stock, so if you used one of those and only mixed it with 240ml (8½ fl oz) water, the result would be quite salty and could overpower the recipe. So, always check the packaging to ensure you get the ratios correct.

You will sometimes see me use stock as a way to soften down vegetables instead of using lots of oil. This is a great trick I discovered many years ago now, and it works really well. It will also add heaps of flavour to your dish as an added bonus. When you are cooking vegetables, just add a little bit of stock at a time, let it reduce down around the veg, and then repeat until they are lovely and softened. It's great for making things like soups, curries and more.

SALT AND PEPPER – the basic flavour enhancers

These are the most important seasonings there are and are what are called flavour enhancers.

Everyone has a different level of preferred seasoning. It's why it is very important to taste food as you go along and adjust seasoning as needed. However, if you are cooking for several people, getting the balance right for everyone is not always possible; someone on a low-sodium diet may be accustomed to far less seasoning than someone who likes their food heavily flavoured. This is why you always see salt and pepper on any dining table, and why recipes often say 'season to taste'.

If you use salt and pepper as intended, your food will never be bland. It's a misconception that to add flavour, you need to add heaps of different spices. While these do add flavour if your food is bland, all that is usually needed is a little more salt and pepper. You will be surprised how much make the flavours in a dish pop, and all it takes is an additional pinch here and there.

ADJUSTING SEASONING

Don't be scared to adjust the balance of spices and seasonings in a recipe to suit your taste. If you like your food spicier, then add more spice; if there is a spice or herb you don't like, it should be fine to omit it or replace it with another similar spice, so long as it is not a major part of the dish.

The recipes are intended for you to build from. The more you cook, the more your understanding will grow of which flavours work well together.

GRANULATED SWEETENERS

Overall, I tend to prefer to use maple syrup, honey or sugar, rather than sweeteners. But sometimes, when you want to bring the calories down, swapping for a sweetener may be your preferred option. There are so many different types of sweeteners available now, and it can be hard to know which is best to use. Over the last decade, I have probably tried every single one on the market – and most, I didn't care for. Not all sweeteners are created equal, and it's something to be aware of, especially when making baked goods.

When I do use a granulated sweetener in a recipe, the only one I will use is erythritol – it's naturally derived and is the closest thing I have found to the real deal. There are lots of different brands of erythritol out there, and you can get both white and brown varieties.

If you choose to use a different type of sweetener, then you must check the packaging to ensure you use the correct ratio, otherwise it could affect the taste or the bake. With erythritol, I generally use it like for like with sugar, but with other types of sweetener, you may need a lot less or more.

THICKENING SAUCES
There are various options available when it comes to thickening sauces.

First are the basic starches: flour, cornflour (cornstarch), tapioca flour and arrowroot. All of these, except for the flour, are generally gluten-free, and you don't always need to create a roux (by mixing with butter). Some people use xanthan gum as a thickening agent, but I don't like the final result it yields for sauces.

I usually use cornflour. Typically, you need 1 tablespoon of cornflour for every 240ml (8½fl oz) of liquid, but it will depend on the other ingredients in the recipe. Always mix it with a couple of tablespoons of cold liquid first to make a slurry, which you can then stir in. If you try and stir the powder straight into your sauce, it will go lumpy.

Another option for thickening is to stir in some blended vegetables that have been cooked in stock. This is also a great option for sneaking vegetables into any fussy eaters in your household, and works really well with pasta sauces and curries.

Tomato purée (paste) is also another great option for thickening sauces, as it's concentrated, so as your ingredients are bubbling away on the stove, the liquid will reduce and thicken the sauce.

Lentils, floury potatoes or any kind of item that releases a starch will also thicken your sauce.

STOVETOP TEMPERATURES AND REDUCING SAUCES
When frying and searing food on the stove, you generally want to place your pan over a medium–high to high heat.

When it comes to browning, frying or searing items, especially things like chicken and beef, always ensure your pan is hot enough before you add the ingredient, and don't overcrowd the pan. If your pan isn't hot enough or big enough, your ingredients will steam rather than brown, and you will lose all that flavour and colour. If you don't have a big enough pan, cook in two batches.

It's also important that you don't rush the browning process, especially when it comes to base ingredients, like onion, garlic, ginger and carrots. If you burn these, you risk ruining the whole dish. Burned garlic especially is unpleasantly bitter.

If you are making a stew, casserole or soup that has a lot of liquid in a dish and you want to reduce it, you can turn the heat right up to the highest setting so that you see vigorous bubbles in the liquid. If you want to simmer, reduce the heat to medium for a rapid simmer or medium–low for a gentle simmer.

Sauces not thickening or reducing?

This is one of the most common problems I see, and there can be numerous reasons. First, make sure you have used all the correct ingredients. For example, if maple syrup or honey is used in the recipe, make sure you are not using a sugar-free substitute instead. The sugar in maple syrup and honey will caramelize as it heats, which causes the sauce to reduce and thicken. You don't get this same caramelization with sugar-free alternatives.

Using the wrong-sized pan can also mean your sauce takes forever to reduce. Flat-based pans with a large circumference are best for reducing sauces, as the heat will penetrate evenly and quickly.

It's also good to ensure your heat is not too low to reduce a sauce; even when simmering, it still needs to be bubbling, otherwise the sauce will just sit in the pan.

OVEN TEMPERATURES
All the recipes on the Slimming Eats blog use a regular, non-fan oven, but in this book, I've included settings for fan, non-fan and gas ovens. However, these are a guideline, and I always recommend getting used to your own oven, as there are so many variables that could affect cooking times, such as low and high altitudes, older vs newer ovens, slightly different ingredients, or slightly different types of cooking vessels.

Low-carb Sides

There are so many great options for low-carb sides nowadays, and these are a great way to bulk out your plate or reduce calories in a meal if you want to enjoy more of the main part of the dish. I have offered some suggestions with each recipe where possible, but here are my favourite low-carb sides. There are plenty of other ideas on the Slimming Eats website.

CAULIFLOWER RICE

There are many quick options, such as frozen microwave bags of ready-made cauliflower rice, but I personally like to just buy a whole cauliflower and make my own; it just tastes so much better.

I line a large tray with baking paper and grate the cauliflower straight on to the tray. Alternatively, you can blitz it in a food processor until it resembles grains of rice, then transfer to the tray. Spread it out in a thin, even layer (remember to ensure your tray is big enough).

Season with salt and black pepper, spray all over with olive oil spray and bake for 30 minutes at 180°C/160°C fan/350°F/gas 4 until lightly charred on the edges (I give it a toss on the tray halfway through baking). If you prefer, you can sauté the cauliflower rice in a frying pan with some onion and garlic, and use your favourite seasonings for flavour, depending on what you are serving it with.

You can also make this with grated broccoli, although some people find the green colour a bit off-putting, and prefer the resemblance cauliflower has to real rice.

CAULIFLOWER MASH

Place a cauliflower – broken into florets – and a couple of garlic cloves into a large saucepan over a medium–high heat and cover with stock. Bring to the boil, then reduce the heat to medium–low and simmer for about 15 minutes until the cauliflower is tender.

Reserve a mugful of the stock, then drain completely. Add the cauliflower and garlic to a blender and blend until smooth, adding some of the reserved stock if needed to help it blend. Season with salt and pepper. Serve with a small knob of butter on top.

VEGGIE MASH

Any root veg makes a delicious mash, and some squashes work well, too. I like to simmer the veg until soft – I recommend you do so in stock for additional flavour – then drain and mash. Great options for a veggie mash include butternut squash, pumpkin, carrots, swede (rutabaga) and celeriac (celery root). If you can't live without potatoes, you could try a part-potato, part-veg mash for a lower-calorie version.

SPIRALIZED VEGETABLES

Courgettes (zucchini), carrots, butternut squash, swede (rutabaga) and radishes all work well for spiralizing. As long as it's not hollow or too soft, it will spiralize.

I sauté my spiralized veg in a pan with some cooking oil spray and my favourite seasonings – usually salt and black pepper, and occasionally paprika if I want some colour. They make a great replacement for pasta or noodles.

Some of these take longer to cook than others. Courgette takes no more than a couple of minutes; don't be tempted to overcook it, or it will become mushy and really wet. I prefer it to still have a slight bite.

ROASTED VEGETABLES

Pretty much any vegetable tastes great when roasted. Just make up a tray of your favourite chopped vegetables, and add some seasoning (why not use one of my seasoning blends on pages 280–281?). Don't be scared to use a little olive oil if you're doing a big tray for the whole family, as this will add much more flavour than cooking oil spray.

The oven temperature will vary depending on what vegetables you are roasting, but typically I go for about 200°C/180°C fan/400°F/gas 6; you don't really want it any lower than this for roasted vegetables.

VEGGIE FRIES/CUBES

I know this is pretty much just roasted vegetables again, but if you dice veg into cubes or slice it into fries, you can make a low-carb version of chips or a sub for roasted potatoes. My favourite vegetable to use for this is butternut squash. I like to dice it into cubes, and mix with a little diced onion (some crushed garlic is great too). I season with salt and pepper, plus some paprika for a little colour and caramelization. Roast at 200°C/180°C fan/400°F/gas 6 for 35–40 minutes.

You can also buy crinkle cutters, which are great for making veggies look interesting, especially for fussy kids.

SHREDDED VEGETABLES

These are great in all kinds of dishes, especially stir-fries, but they also make a perfect veggie side. Greens like Brussels sprouts, cabbage and kale are ideal for shredding, and they can then be pan-fried or baked/roasted. Try my Lemon and Garlic Shredded Brussels (page 90). These are so good – I can literally eat a bowl of the Brussels on their own!

VEGGIES ANY WAY

Sometimes, just some simple veggies are perfect. Vegetables are low in calories and nutrient-dense so they're a great way to bulk out your meals. Choose ones that complement the main dish. There are so many great options out there, and if you find yourself always sticking to the same ones, make it a challenge to find as many new vegetables as you can, and try different ways of cooking them. If you go to specialist grocer's, you can often find unusual vegetables to try, and autumn is great for lots of different varieties of squash.

BEANSPROUTS

Beansprouts are a great low-carb substitute for noodles, and have a lovely crunch. They're also super-quick to cook. I usually blanch them in hot water, and then just pan-fry for a couple of minutes with chopped spring onions (scallions), soy sauce, garlic, ginger, sesame oil and a little black pepper.

STALKS AND LEAVES

We often throw away broccoli stalks and the leaves of vegetables like cauliflower, but these can be used to made delicious sides. Use a julienne peeler for broccoli stalks and pan-fry them (they're also great added to stir-fries), and sauté the leaves of veggies like beetroot (beets) for a great side dish.

SALADS

Salads pair well with most dishes, and are a great way to bulk out your plate. There are so many options, too. I love a mix of lots of different veggies, and also like to add fruit for that sweet crunch and taste; plus, this often means you don't need as much dressing. If you add some roasted veg or a little cheese, like feta, goats' cheese or Cheddar (you really don't need much), you can create even more flavour. You can also add some grains or pulses like pasta, rice, quinoa, spelt, farro or chickpeas. Yes, I know these are not low-carb, but you won't need as much as you would for a plain side. If you're enjoying a salad as your main meal, add some protein to make it more filling: try cooked meats, prawns, eggs or vegetarian proteins.

Here are some of my favourite items to add to salads:

- mixture of leaves – crisp lettuce, baby leaves, spinach, rocket (arugula)
- thinly sliced raw veggies – cauliflower, broccoli, fennel, carrots, etc.
- radishes
- cucumber
- peppers
- onion
- beetroot (beets) – steamed or roasted
- roasted butternut squash cubes (or any roasted veg)
- fruit – apples, pears, grapes, berries, watermelon
- tomatoes
- cheese
- seeds/nuts – these can be quite calorific, so watch your portions
- cooked grains/pastas/beans
- pickled veg – onions, pickles, etc.
- olives

SUBSTITUTES FOR BREAD/ROLLS/BUNS

There is no reason why you can't enjoy a proper piece of bread if you want a sandwich, burger or similar. But if you do want to reduce calories, large leaves of lettuce are great for wraps or burgers.

Creating Your Own One-pot and Sheet-pan Meals

ONE-POT MEALS

If you've tried some of my one-pot meals and want to have a go at creating your own, here are my top tips for how to put together a one-pot recipe.

CHOOSE YOUR PAN
A large, deep frying pan with a lid is a must. Mine is 28cm (11in), big enough to make a meal for my family of four. If your pan is too small, as I've explained, the cooking will be uneven and the ratios may need adjusting. If you can get a pan that can be used in the oven as well as on the stove, it will be a life-saver.

CHOOSE YOUR PROTEIN
Protein is an important part of a meal. It doesn't have to be included with every meal, but it what will keep you feeling satiated for longer.

CHOOSE SOME VEGGIES
Take into account different cooking times if you can, and try to use vegetables that cook at similar rates, otherwise you can end up with some veg that is really mushy and some that is still hard.

CHOOSE YOUR SEASONINGS/SAUCES
This is where your flavour is going to come in, so choose the seasonings and sauces based on what style of dish you want to make. As you start to cook more and follow some of the recipes in this book, you will build a good understanding of what kind of flavours go well together. Make cooking fun, and don't be scared to experiment.

CHOOSE RICE OR PASTA (OPTIONAL)
These are not always part of a one-pot recipe, but tend to be the most favoured options, especially for my family. To feed a family of four, I normally go for about 180g (6½oz) uncooked rice (which is plenty when bulked out with protein and veg), or around 240g (8½oz) uncooked pasta.

ADD LIQUID
This is what will cook everything in the pot. Bear in mind that if you add tomato products, you may need to add a little more liquid, as some tomato products will thicken the sauce, which causes the cooking to slow, and may also stick to the bottom of the pan. See below for how much liquid to use.

ONE-POT RICE DISHES
If you're making a one-pot rice dish, the general rule is however much uncooked rice you use, you want twice the volume of liquid (stock). So, for example, 180g (6½oz) uncooked rice is about 1 cup, so you'll need 2 cups of stock (480ml/16fl oz). Brown the veggies and protein first, then add your chosen seasonings. Add in the rice, followed by the liquid. Stir to make sure nothing is stuck to the bottom, but then do not stir again. Bring to the boil, cover with a lid, and simmer until the liquid is just absorbed. Turn off the heat, and leave for 10–12 minutes; the steam trapped underneath the lid will cook the one-pot rice dish to perfection. Use one of the one-pot rice dishes in this book as your starting point, and try swapping the protein and/ or seasonings to create your own version.

ONE-POT PASTA DISHES
For a one-pot pasta dish, you need a bit more liquid. I usually start with 720ml (3 cups/24fl oz) liquid for 240g (8½oz) uncooked pasta. It will vary depending on what else you add. You want the liquid to bubble vigorously so that it cooks the pasta with everything else. Once the stock or liquid is absorbed, you can check the pasta, and add a little more liquid if it's still slightly undercooked. Use one of the one-pot pasta dishes in this book as your starting point and swap to different protein/ veggies/seasonings to create your own.

SHEET-PAN MEALS/TRAYBAKES

These are one of the easiest all-in-one meals to make, as you don't have to worry about getting the ratio of liquids right. It's just a case of timing things correctly and using the right-sized tray.

CHOOSE YOUR PROTEIN
As with the one-pot dishes, a protein isn't essential, but it's a great way to add flavour to your dish and make you feel full and satisfied.

CHOOSE SOME VEGGIES
Think about how long your protein needs to cook, and at what oven temperature, and try to choose vegetables that will cook in the same conditions; this will make it really easy. It doesn't really matter if they cook at different times – it just means you will need to remove the tray at the appropriate intervals to add the next ingredients.

CHOOSE YOUR SEASONING/SAUCE/MARINADE
You can use one of the homemade seasoning blends on pages 280–281, or create your own favourite blend. Seasoning, marinades and sauces are important for sheet-pan meals, as this is where a lot of your flavour will come from. If you are gravy person, make up some of the delicious onion gravy on page 135.

CHOOSE YOUR TRAY
I know I've mentioned this several times now, but I cannot overstate the importance of having the correct-sized tray. For a sheet-pan meal, everything should be in a thin, even layer, not crammed too close together, so that the heat can penetrate evenly for perfect cooking. If you don't have one tray big enough, use two smaller trays.

And as with the one-pot recipes, use the sheet-pan dishes in this book as your starting point and swap the protein/veggies/seasonings to create your own.

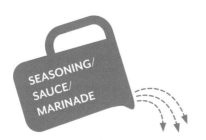

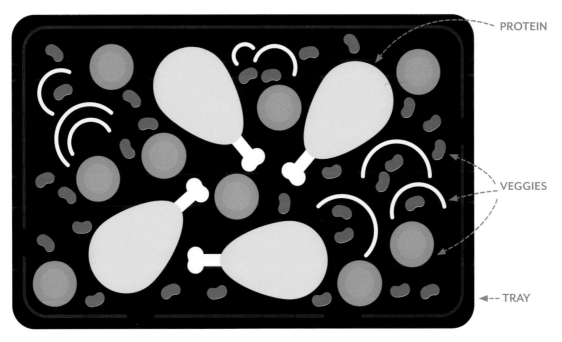

PROTEIN

VEGGIES

TRAY

Freezing Tips

All recipes that are suitable for freezing are marked with a freezer symbol. However, there really isn't much that can't be frozen; it all comes down to preference, really. Not everyone likes cooked pasta that has been frozen and reheated, and some dishes can be a bit dry after freezing if they have no sauce, especially if you've used lean protein.

RICE
People often worry about whether it's safe to freeze rice, but it's actually fine as long as you follow food safety guidelines and ensure you refrigerate or freeze it quickly, as soon as it cools down – do not leave it to sit at room temperature for any length of time. Rice should only be reheated once, and always ensure it's piping hot all the way through.

AROMATICS
I use so much garlic and ginger that I always buy it in bulk. I add whole bulbs of garlic to a tub and peel the ginger, then freeze them. That way, you can just pop out garlic cloves as you need them, and you can grate the ginger from frozen and use it straight away. You can also freeze chillies. I often used to find ones in the fridge that had been forgotten about and had gone off, so now I just freeze as soon as I buy them. It means I always have them on hand for a recipe.

DEFROSTING
While you can reheat some meals straight from frozen, I prefer to remove them from the freezer and let them defrost in the fridge before reheating them on the stove or in the oven, air fryer or microwave (depending on what type of dish it is).

CONTAINERS
As I explained on page 11, I swapped all my plastic containers for glass ones. There are so many different options nowadays. If you are low on freezer space, freezer bags might be a better option for you, as you can lie them flat; you can even buy reusable freezer bags made of silicone.

Try and use containers that are of a similar shape and size so that they're easy to stack. I also recommend freezing in portions rather than in one big container; that way, you don't need to defrost the whole lot if you only want one serving.

With things like burgers, patties and cakes, I always place a square of greaseproof paper between each one, so they don't all stick together.

Label the tub or bag clearly, noting down the contents along with the date, otherwise you forget what you've frozen! Not the end of the world if you like a freezer-meal surprise, but I have often taken something out for dinner only to discover it wasn't what I thought it was. This is why I stopped using labels, which tend to fall off, and instead write straight on the container with a marker pen.

If you have leftover coconut milk, tomato purée (paste) or canned products you don't think you will be able to use up quickly, pour them into a tub or an ice-cube tray and freeze.

Dietary Requirements

Beside each recipe, you will see these dietary symbols, which state which recipes are vegetarian, vegan, gluten-free and dairy-free, plus which are freezer-friendly.

Each recipe also features a full nutritional analysis. This is per portion, and has been made with the following ingredients (unless otherwise stated): skimmed milk, wholemeal (whole wheat) low-calorie bread, skinless and lean meat, fat-free yogurt, granulated sweetener and light cream cheese. They exclude optional items and 'to serve' items, unless specifically noted on the recipe, so bear this in mind if you're adding in optional extras.

When a recipe includes the freezer icon, it can be frozen and stored in the freezer for a maximum of 3 months.

V Vegetarian   **VG** Vegan   **GF** Gluten-free   **DF** Dairy-free   ❄ Freezer-friendly

ALLERGENS

If you or someone you are cooking for has specific dietary needs, you should always check the products or ingredients you use in any recipe to ensure they are allergen-free (gluten-free, egg-free, soy-free, dairy-free, for example) as these things can vary from brand to brand. Just because one stock cube brand is free of allergens, for example, it doesn't mean they all are. I generally use stock, spices and condiments that are free of allergens, so know which ones to look out for and avoid, but it's very important to check all the ingredients you are using carefully.

For some recipes, I've suggested swaps that you can use to make a recipe free of such allergens; please note that these will alter the final nutritional analysis.

For more general swaps, here are a few great products you may not be aware of if someone in your family or a friend has allergens.

PASTA

There are so many great gluten-free pasta options these days. Brown rice pasta is my favourite, but you can also get pasta made from quinoa, chickpeas, lentils and beans.

MILKS

Cashew and oat milks are my favourite dairy-free items. They have the same creaminess as regular milk, but don't have that strong nutty taste you get with some nut milks, like almond milk, for example. It's really easy to make your own, too.

Coconut is a great dairy-free substitute for creamy sauces, but if you are using light versions, you may need to add a little starch to thicken.

CHEESES

There are lots of dairy-free cheeses on the market now. It's not an area I've experimented with much, but some definitely taste better than others, so it's worth doing some exploring.

SOY SAUCE

Coconut aminos is a great substitute for soy sauce if you have a soy allergy, and it's much more popular now than it was years ago, which means it's easier to source. It has a slightly sweeter taste, but works really well. You can also get some coconut aminos-based stir-fry sauces.

FLOURS

There are many types of gluten-free flours and starches available that you can use in recipes, however they are not all created equally so many do not work if doing a straight swap for a gluten version. Many gluten-free flours can be quite fibrous and so may need a completely different ratio of liquids and other ingredients.

Vegetarian Swaps

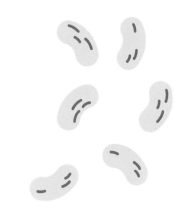

I have included some vegetarian meals in this book, as well as notes on what to use to make some of the non-vegetarian dishes veggie. Below are some other great ingredients to use to make a meal vegetarian.

BEANS, LENTILS, PULSES, ETC.
Great for bulking out a meal in place of meat, and a good source of protein. Try edamame beans, black beans, kidney beans, white beans, lentils, pinto beans, etc.

QUINOA
A great pseudo-grain that is a fantastic source of protein and fibre, it has a lovely nutty flavour.

MEAT SUBSTITUTES
Tofu, seitan, tempeh and soy mince are all great meat substitutes, and are versatile enough to use in a variety of recipes.

CHEESE
Paneer and halloumi makes particularly good meat substitutes, as they generally hold their shape when grilled or pan-fried.

EGGS
Eggs are a great quick source of protein and can be cooked in various ways – boiled, fried, poached, scrambled – or cooked into frittatas or omelettes.

AUBERGINE (EGGPLANT)
When roasted or sautéed with seasoning, spices or sauces, aubergine has a great texture and flavour.

VEGETABLES
Your favourite vegetables, roasted, sautéed, raw and grilled, are all great substitutes for meat. Enjoy them in tacos, stir-fries, curries, pasta dishes and more.

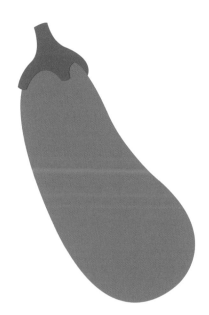

NUTS
Nuts add flavour, texture and protein, but they can be quite high in calories, so use in moderation.

HIGH-PROTEIN PASTAS
Pasta made from chickpeas, lentils or similar pulses can be a great way of getting additional protein into a meal.

Healthy Eating Tips

There are often things that happen in life that sabotage our healthy-eating journeys, such as stress, illness, anxiety or depression, and I know all too well through my own experiences how these can really affect our focus and motivation.

This is why I always stress to my readers that healthy eating should not mean depriving yourself of everything you love. Moderation is key. If you start depriving yourself, then it won't be sustainable. The changes made need to be a lifestyle change.

Healthy eating doesn't need to mean teeny portions that leave you feeling hungry. And don't fall into the trap of using all those foods advertised as diet, low-fat, sugar-free, etc. All too often, these options are not nearly as healthy as they claim to be.

Don't be scared to use real ingredients in your recipes. Food should still taste good and be enjoyable. Just because you are eating more healthily, or perhaps reducing calories if your goal is weight loss, it should not mean you have to consume boring or uninspiring food.

There is no reason to cut out good fats or natural sugars like maple syrup or honey; limit them to reduce calories, yes, but don't cut them out completely. They're ideal for when you want a healthy treat. As I've said already, a tablespoon of olive oil in a recipe that serves four people is hardly anything, and if a little drizzle of real maple syrup over some healthy pancakes is much more satisfying to you than a sugar-free artificial version, then have the maple syrup. If you don't enjoy your food, you will not be able to maintain these changes.

If your goal is weight loss, I understand the desire to lose the weight quickly, but sometimes extreme restricting will just cause you to binge once you get to your target weight. You might find you quickly revert back to your old eating habits – and we all know what happens then.

If you just make a few changes here and there to balance your meals, then, fine, it might take a little bit longer to reach your goal, but it won't feel quite so hard to stick to – and so when you do have those days where you struggle, it will be a little easier to manage, because you have not been depriving yourself of all the things you enjoy.

Take your journey one day at a time, and it will be much easier.

Here are some of my tips for staying motivated on your healthy-eating journey.

KEEP A FOOD DIARY

Don't just write down what you are eating. It's a good idea to also include your mood and how satiated you felt. A food diary is a really useful tool, as you can look back on your meals if you find yourself struggling and identify what foods make you feel better and more satisfied.

PLAN YOUR MEALS

Meal planning is important, if you can do it. I know it's not for everyone, as sometimes you plan a meal, but when the day comes, you don't fancy that particular food anymore. However, planning your meals really helps stop those moments in the kitchen when you are hungry and can't decide what to make. Those are the times when you are likely to grab something unhealthy instead.

MAKE SOME HOMEMADE READY MEALS AND GRAB-AND-GO SNACKS

Try not to have too many unhealthy convenience foods in the house. If they're not there, you can't grab them in moments of weakness.

It's OK to have the odd treat, and you don't need to deprive yourself completely. If you buy snacks, I recommend choosing items that are individually wrapped, as you are less likely to open up another one, whereas if there is an opened sharing bag of crisps, biscuits or sweets, they are easy to grab when you shouldn't.

If you can, spend a bit of time prepping some quick grab-and-go snacks and meals each week. Things like chopped fruit, portioned up in tubs, hard-boiled eggs, crustless quiche, soups, hummus and veggies crudites, will all mean you have something healthy at hand if you feel the need. Sometimes, a leftover portion from the day before is a great option for a quick lunch the next day (as long as it fits into your calorie goal).

MAKE USE OF ONLINE COMMUNITIES AND SOCIAL MEDIA

Slimming Eats started through me sharing my own personal journey on my blog. Sharing online can be great for keeping yourself accountable or motivated, because you will encounter others on a similar journey to you. Join a Facebook group or create an Instagram account and use it as a place to document your journey, get ideas and stay motivated.

FIND A NON-FOOD HOBBY

Find a hobby or activity you enjoy that takes the focus off food, especially at times of the day when you might normally struggle. I love drawing, painting and genealogy, as well as supporting members of my online Facebook group and interacting with people through my Slimming Eats social accounts.

EXERCISE

Exercise is another great way to keep you on plan and motivated. It doesn't have to be a strenuous workout; it can be whatever feels comfortable for you. Exercise creates endorphins that make you feel good, so getting moving is always a good thing. You could pair up with a friend and maybe try to go for a walk every other day to try and reach a goal of walking 10,000 steps a day. Start with a smaller number first if you think 10,000 is too much.

Another great option is a wearable fitness band. There are many out there to choose from, including cheaper options as well as the more expensive versions, like the Fitbit. Fitness bands are great because they set you daily step goals, and this can really encourage you to get moving to reach them, especially if you have the option of adding friends and seeing how many steps you all manage each day. I've been known to walk laps of the house at the end of the day to reach my step goals!

If you find that you hate working out at home, a good alternative is to find a fitness class you enjoy. For some, that group environment is much more appealing. Zumba is a fun and enjoyable workout, and the time flies by. There are many other similar classes too.

Lastly, there is also the option to join a gym or even go swimming. What works for one won't work for another. When it comes to fitness, it really has to be something you can maintain and enjoy, as otherwise, you won't keep it up.

Let's Get Started

That's all from me for now – it's time for the recipes. My belief is that if you can make cooking fun and enjoyable, then it will be much easier to stay motivated in the long run. It's one of the reasons I strongly believe that eating healthily should not mean having to cook separate meals or using strange 'diet' ingredients. In this book, you will find real ingredients, but in sensible amounts, so that what you cook can be enjoyed by the whole family.

Without further ado, I really hope you enjoy this cookbook – and thank you so much for making it possible for me to create it in the first place. I love seeing your tags, comments and mentions on my social media, so please do continue to tag me in your #slimmingeats creations.

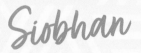

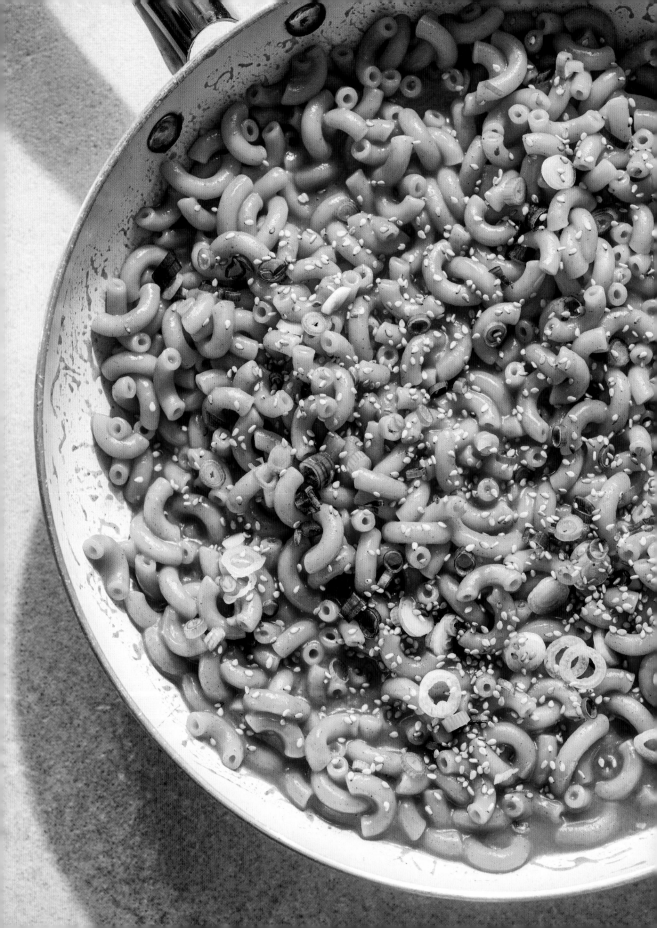

Simple
Stovetop

374 kcals
per serving

V

KCALS
374

FAT
4.8g

SAT FAT
0.6g

CARBS
58.5g

SUGARS
14.3g

FIBRE
13.4g

PROTEIN
17.3g

SALT
0.89g

Lentil Quinoa Shawarma Pittas

PREP TIME: **10 MINUTES**   COOK TIME: **25 MINUTES**   SERVES: **4**

olive oil spray
1 onion, halved and
    thinly sliced
2 garlic cloves, crushed
150g (5½oz) canned brown
    lentils, drained (you can
    also use green lentils)
1½ teaspoons ground cumin
1½ teaspoons ground
    coriander
1 teaspoon smoked paprika
½ teaspoon ground turmeric
pinch of red chilli flakes
1 tablespoon lemon juice
70g (2½oz) uncooked
    quinoa, rinsed
300ml (10fl oz) vegetable
    stock
1 tablespoon chopped
    fresh coriander (cilantro)
    (optional)
4 wholemeal pitta breads,
    warmed
salt and freshly ground
    black pepper

For the garlic mayo
2 tablespoons light
    mayonnaise
3 tablespoons fat-free
    Greek yogurt
1 garlic clove, crushed
1 teaspoon dried parsley
2 teaspoons lemon juice

To serve
250g (9oz) lettuce, chopped
1 cucumber, halved
    and sliced
4 medium ripe tomatoes,
    sliced
1 red onion, sliced

Here, brown lentils and nutty quinoa are flavoured with shawarma-inspired spices to create a delicious vegetarian shawarma pitta. Load up your pittas with the yummy filling, along with some garlic mayo and your favourite salad items, and you'll have a simple meat-free meal for the whole family.

1. To make the garlic mayo, mix all the ingredients together in a small bowl. Season with salt and pepper and set aside.

2. Heat a frying pan over a medium–high heat and spray with olive oil spray. Add the onion and fry for a couple of minutes until softened and golden, then add the garlic and fry for a further minute.

3. Add the lentils, along with the cumin, coriander, paprika, turmeric, red chilli flakes and lemon juice. Season with a pinch of salt and pepper and fry for a couple of minutes, stirring until everything is coated.

4. Add the quinoa and stock and give it a stir. Bring to the boil, then reduce the heat to low. Cover and simmer for about 10 minutes until the stock is just absorbed.

5. Turn off the heat and leave the mixture to rest with the lid on for 10–12 minutes – the quinoa will continue to cook in the trapped steam.

6. Once it's ready, remove the lid and stir, mashing the lentils slightly with the back of a wooden spoon. Add the coriander and stir to combine.

7. To serve, warm the pitta breads, then spread each one with garlic mayo. Add lettuce, cucumber, tomato and red onion to each, then spoon a quarter of the lentil and quinoa mix into each pitta. Enjoy straight away.

Optional add-ins:
These are also great with
some hummus, feta or
Cheddar added with the
other fillings.

Nutritional analysis:
Includes to serve options
as well.

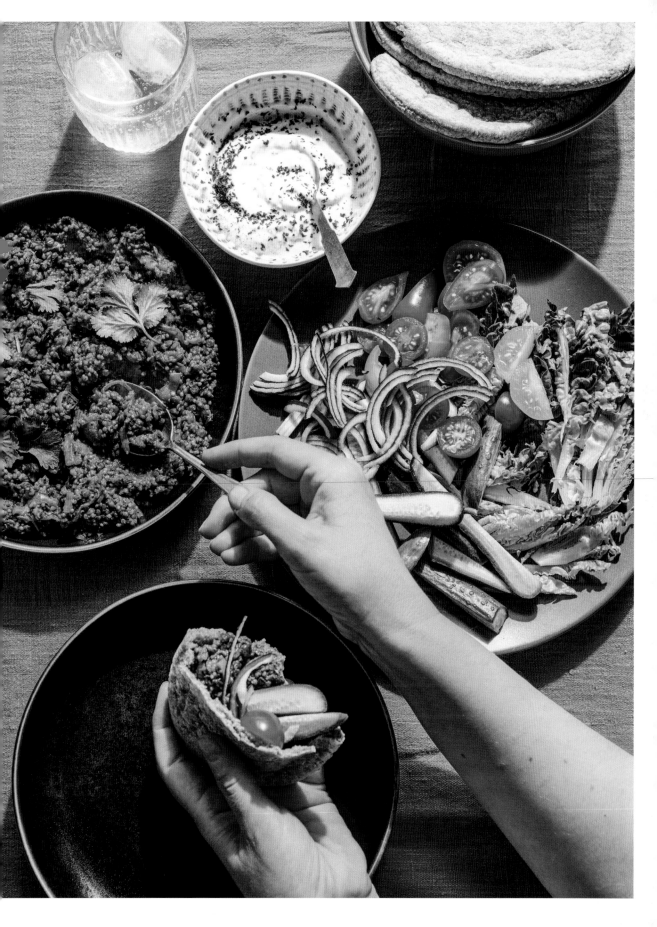

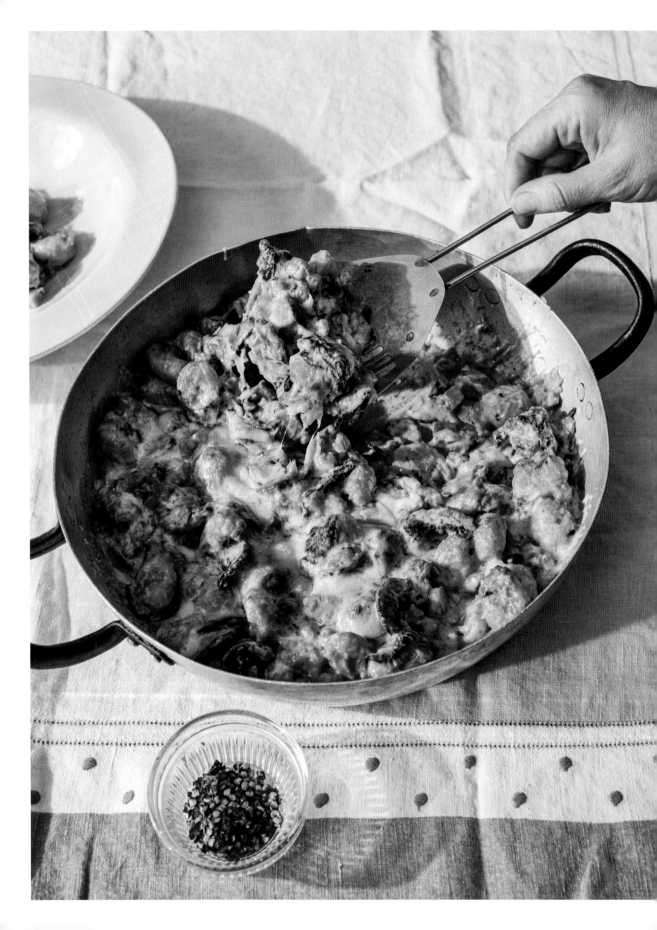

Creamy Sun-dried Tomato Gnocchi with Spinach, Mushrooms and Sweet Potato

PREP TIME: 15 MINUTES   **COOK TIME: 20 MINUTES**   **SERVES: 4**

olive oil spray
1 onion, finely diced
200g (7oz) mushrooms, thinly sliced
150g (5½oz) sweet potatoes, peeled and diced small
3 garlic cloves, crushed
50g (1¾oz) sun-dried tomatoes, chopped
500g (1lb 2oz) gnocchi
240ml (8½fl oz) vegetable stock
240ml (8½fl oz) semi-skimmed milk
80g (2¾oz) light cream cheese
1 tablespoon tomato purée (paste)
3 big handfuls of spinach
80g (2¾oz) Cheddar, grated
20g (¾oz) vegetarian Italian-style hard cheese or Parmesan, grated
salt and freshly ground black pepper

Optional add-ins:
For some additional protein, add some cooked chicken or a veggie protein of your choice.

Add a pinch of red chilli flakes with the sun-dried tomatoes for a slight spicy kick

Variation:
This is just as delicious without the cheese topping, so you can skip that step if you prefer.

As a family, we love gnocchi: it's so quick and easy, and goes well with a variety of sauces. This simple recipe combines mushrooms, sun-dried tomatoes, tender little cubes of sweet potato and spinach in a delicious creamy sauce. You can enjoy it just as it is from the pan or take it one step further with the golden melted cheese topping.

1. Heat an ovenproof frying pan over a medium–high heat and spray with olive oil spray.

2. Add the onion, mushrooms and sweet potato and fry for about 8 minutes until lightly golden.

3. Add the garlic and sun-dried tomatoes and fry for a further minute, then transfer the contents of the pan to a bowl and set aside.

4. Return the empty pan to the heat. Add the gnocchi and fry for a couple of minutes until lightly golden, then return the mushroom and sweet potato mixture to the pan.

5. Stir in the stock, milk, cream cheese and tomato purée and simmer for a few minutes until the mixture is creamy and well combined.

6. Stir in the spinach until wilted.

7. Taste the sauce and season with salt and pepper to taste.

8. Top the mixture with the Cheddar and Italian-style hard cheese or Parmesan and cover with the lid. Turn off the heat and leave for about 5 minutes until the cheese has all melted – or, for a golden topping, you can place the pan under the grill for a few minutes until melted and golden (my preferred method), then serve.

Gluten-free:
Use gluten-free gnocchi.

KCALS 448

FAT 11.7g

SAT FAT 6.9g

CARBS 61.7g

SUGARS 14.1g

FIBRE 6.9g

PROTEIN 20.4g

SALT 2.93g

448 kcals per serving

275 kcals per serving

DF

KCALS	**275**
FAT	**8.4g**
SAT FAT	**1.9g**
CARBS	**22.7g**
SUGARS	**12.6g**
FIBRE	**4.6g**
PROTEIN	**25g**
SALT	**1.93g**

Pork and Pineapple Stir-fry

PREP TIME: **15 MINUTES**   COOK TIME: **20 MINUTES**   SERVES: **4**

400g (14oz) pork loin chops, patted dry, trimmed of visible fat and thinly sliced (or use stir-fry pork)
2 tablespoons cornflour (cornstarch)
1 tablespoon vegetable oil
olive oil spray
1 onion, diced
1 red (bell) pepper, chopped
½ small green (bell) pepper, chopped
1 thumb-sized piece of fresh ginger, thinly sliced
2 garlic cloves, thinly sliced
1 red chilli, sliced, or a pinch of red chilli flakes (optional)
250g (9oz) beansprouts, rinsed and patted dry
2 tablespoons oyster sauce
1½ tablespoons light soy sauce
½ tablespoon dark soy sauce
1 tablespoon Shaoxing wine
225g (8oz) fresh pineapple chunks
3 spring onions (scallions), thinly sliced
salt and freshly ground black pepper

This simple stir-fry combines tender pieces of pork with crunchy vegetables and juicy pineapple, while the fresh red chilli adds a slightly spicy kick. It's delicious just as it is in a bowl, or served with your favourite sides – see my suggestions below.

1. In a large bowl, combine the pork with the cornflour and a pinch of salt and freshly ground black pepper. Toss to coat.

2. Heat half the vegetable oil in a large non-stick frying pan over a medium–high heat.

3. Add half of the pork and fry for a few minutes, making sure it gets really golden on the exterior. Don't move it around too much in the pan; let it get nice and brown underneath, then flip to repeat on the other side. Remove from the pan and set aside on a plate, then add the remaining vegetable oil and repeat with the other half of pork.

4. Once all the pork is browned and set aside, return the empty pan to the heat. Spray with some spray oil, then add the onion, peppers, ginger, garlic and red chilli, and fry for a few minutes just until tender.

5. Add the beansprouts and continue to fry for a further couple of minutes, then add the oyster sauce, soy sauces and Shaoxing wine. Toss everything to coat, then return the pork to the pan, along with the pineapple, spring onions and a pinch of black pepper. Toss once more to coat everything in the sauce, ensuring the pork is cooked through.

6. Serve and enjoy!!!

Side suggestions:
This is perfect just as it is for a lighter meal, but it's also great with cooked jasmine rice or egg noodles.

Low-carb side suggestion:
To get some additional veggies in and also bulk out your meal for bigger appetites, serve with some cauliflower rice.

Swaps:
Try swapping the pork for thinly sliced chicken (boneless, skinless thighs are best for flavour).

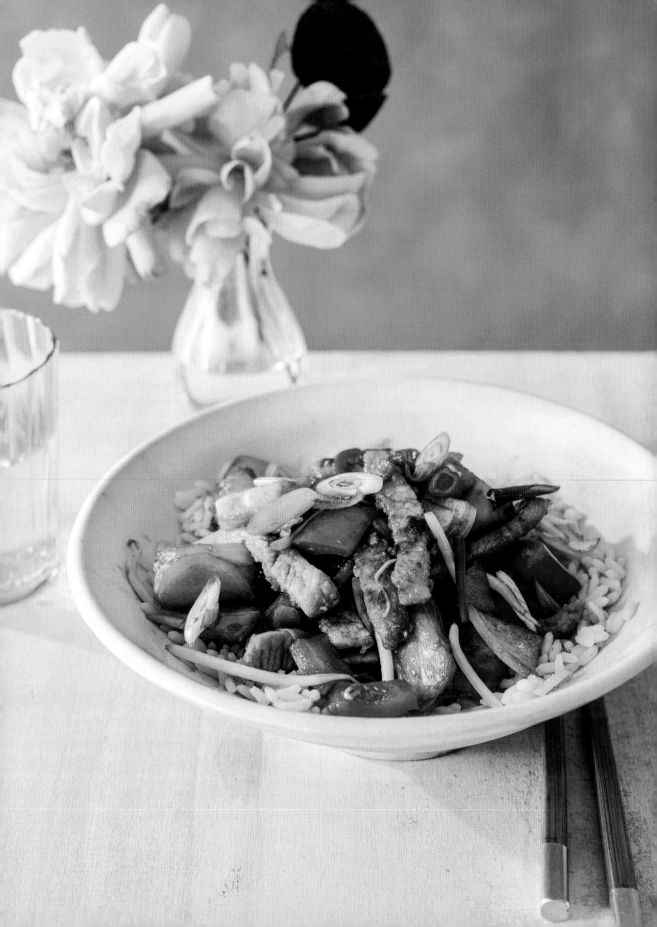

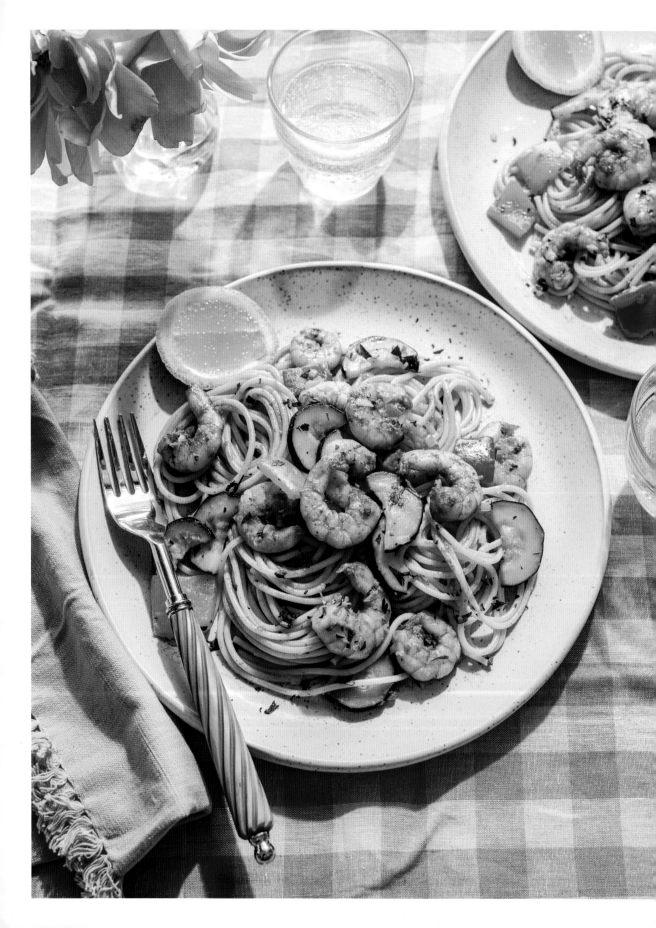

Garlic Butter Prawns and Vegetables

PREP TIME: **5 MINUTES**   COOK TIME: **15 MINUTES**   SERVES: **4**

400g (14oz) large frozen peeled prawns (shrimp), thawed

2 teaspoons sweet paprika

¼ teaspoon cayenne (or more if you prefer it spicy)

olive oil spray

1 small onion, finely diced

240ml (8½fl oz) chicken stock

6 garlic cloves, crushed

300g (10½oz) courgettes (zucchini), halved lengthways, then sliced

1 red (bell) pepper, diced

1 yellow or orange (bell) pepper, diced

juice of ½ lemon

2 tablespoons salted butter

1 tablespoon freshly chopped parsley (optional)

salt and freshly ground black pepper

fresh lemon wedges, to serve

Side suggestions:
This is delicious on its own, but you can also enjoy it with rice, pasta, roasted potato cubes or mashed potatoes.

Low-carb side suggestions:
Try it with cauliflower rice or cauliflower mash.

Deliciously seasoned sautéed prawns with tender vegetables cooked in a flavourful garlic butter sauce, this is a simple, quick one-pan meal that you can have on the table in less than 30 minutes.

1. In a bowl, combine the prawns with the paprika, cayenne and a pinch of salt and freshly ground black pepper and toss to coat.

2. Heat a frying pan over a medium–high heat and spray with olive oil spray. Add the spiced shrimp and cook, stirring occasionally, for a few minutes until it turns pink. Remove from the pan and set aside on a plate.

3. Return the empty pan to the heat and spray with some more spray oil, then add the onion and fry for a couple of minutes to soften. Gradually add half the stock, a little bit at a time, and allow it to reduce down around the onions until they are a lovely golden brown.

4. Add the garlic, courgettes, peppers and lemon juice, then add the remaining stock in the same way, adding it a little at a time and allowing it to reduce down between each addition. As you're adding the last of the stock, add the butter too, and stir until melted.

5. Return the prawns to the pan, along with the parsley and stir until everything is coated in the buttery sauce.

6. Serve with fresh lemon wedges for squeezing, and enjoy!

164 kcals per serving

KCALS
164

FAT
7.4g

SAT FAT
4.2g

CARBS
7.1g

SUGARS
5.8g

FIBRE
4.0g

PROTEIN
15.2g

SALT
1.56g

One-pot Spicy and Cheesy Korean Macaroni

PREP TIME: 5 MINUTES   **COOK TIME: 20 MINUTES**   **SERVES: 4**

KCALS
487

FAT
15.7g

SAT FAT
8.7g

CARBS
65.6g

SUGARS
8.6g

FIBRE
5.5g

PROTEIN
18.2g

SALT
1.68g

1 tablespoon salted butter
2 garlic cloves, finely chopped
960ml (32½fl oz) vegetable stock
3 tablespoons gochujang paste (you can use more or less depending on how spicy you like it)
1 tablespoon maple syrup or honey
300g (10½oz) dried macaroni pasta
120g (4¼oz) mature Cheddar or Red Leicester
1 spring onion (scallion), finely chopped
pinch of sesame seeds

Side suggestions:
To bulk out this meal, I recommend serving with some stir-fried veggies, like shredded cabbage, carrots, peppers and mushrooms. You can add the vegetables into the pasta if you prefer, but you may need slighty more stock if doing so.

Optional add-ins:
If you're not vegetarian, add some cooked chicken, or you can add a veggie protein of your choice.

As a family, one of our favourite Korean dishes is tteokbokki. Tteokbokki are Korean rice cakes – they're kind of like pasta, and have a similar shape to penne, but without the hole in the centre. Traditionally, they are served in a spicy sauce made from gochujang and gochugaru, and the flavours are just amazing. When I don't have tteokbokki on hand, I make this really easy macaroni pasta dish with Cheddar. It's the ideal comfort food.

1. In a saucepan over a high heat, combine the butter, garlic, stock, gochujang and maple syrup with the macaroni. Bring to the boil, then reduce the heat to medium–high and continue to bubble for 12–15 minutes until the pasta is cooked and the liquid is almost absorbed (you still want a little sauce to coat the pasta).

2. Add the cheese and stir until melted and cheesy.

3. Sprinkle with chopped spring onions and a pinch of sesame seeds.

4. Enjoy!

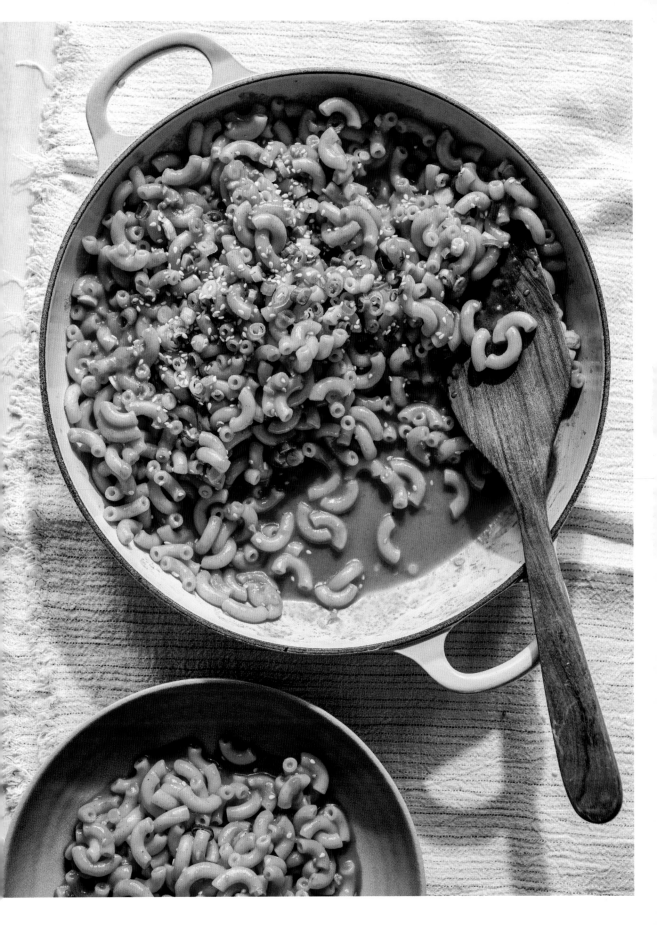

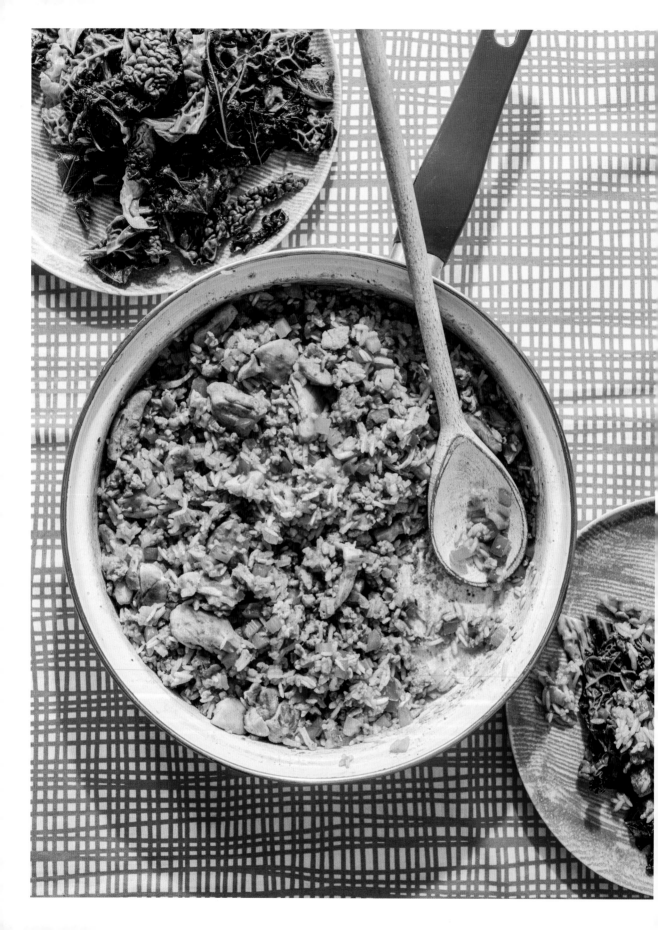

One-pot New Orleans Dirty Rice

PREP TIME: 10 MINUTES   **COOK TIME: 35 MINUTES**   **SERVES: 4**

olive oil spray

1 onion, diced

250g (9oz) 5% fat pork mince (ground pork)

3 slices of lean smoked bacon

1½ tablespoons Cajun Seasoning (page 281)

120ml (4fl oz) beer (I used an IPA)

250g (9oz) boneless, skinless chicken thighs, sliced into bite-sized pieces

2 celery stalks, chopped

2 garlic cloves, minced

1 green (bell) pepper, chopped

1 red (bell) pepper, chopped

175g (6oz) long-grain rice, uncooked

480ml (16¼fl oz) chicken stock

salt and freshly ground black pepper

Side suggestions:
For a more filling meal, pair this with some sautéed garlic collard greens or kale.

Swaps:
Swap the pork mince for chicken, turkey or beef mince.

Don't let the name put you off: dirty rice is a classic dish, traditionally featuring a delicious blend of Cajun spices along with chicken livers (or gizzards) and minced (ground) meat. In my version, I create a spicy mixture with minced pork, bacon and beer, and add some tender chicken thighs for even more flavour. It's one of my children's favourite rice dishes, and so simple to make too.

1. Heat a deep frying pan over a medium–high heat and spray with olive oil spray.

2. Add the onion and cook for a couple of minutes until golden and softened.

3. Add the minced pork, bacon and 1 tablespoon of the Cajun seasoning. Fry for a few minutes until lightly browned, then gradually add the beer, adding a little at a time and letting it reduce between additions until it's all absorbed.

4. Add the chicken and fry for a few minutes until golden, then add the celery, garlic and peppers and fry for another 5 minutes until softened.

5. Stir in the remaining Cajun seasoning, then add the rice and stir for about a minute until the rice is translucent.

6. Add the stock and bring to the boil, then reduce the heat to low and simmer for 10–15 minutes until the stock is just absorbed.

7. Turn off the heat and cover the pan with a lid. Leave for about 12 minutes until the rice is perfectly cooked (do not stir or remove the lid for this part; the rice will finish cooking in the residual heat).

8. Taste and season with salt and pepper as needed, then serve.

433 kcals per serving

DF

KCALS
433

FAT
11.5g

SAT FAT
3.8g

CARBS
42.7g

SUGARS
5.7g

FIBRE
4.3g

PROTEIN
36.2g

SALT
2.37g

421 kcals
per serving

KCALS
421

FAT
27.8g

SAT FAT
16.8g

CARBS
13.7g

SUGARS
11.1g

FIBRE
3.9g

PROTEIN
27g

SALT
0.3g

Paneer in Spicy Tomato Sauce

PREP TIME: **10 MINUTES**   COOK TIME: **30 MINUTES**   SERVES: **4**

1 tablespoon ghee or
    vegetable oil
350g (12oz) paneer, cubed
1 large onion, diced
3 garlic cloves, crushed
2 teaspoons freshly grated
    ginger
2 teaspoons ground cumin
2 teaspoons ground
    coriander
1 teaspoon ground turmeric
¾ teaspoon hot chilli powder
low-calorie cooking oil spray
1½ tablespoons tomato
    purée (paste)
400g (14oz) can chopped
    tomatoes
1 courgette (zucchini), diced
240ml (8½fl oz) vegetable
    stock
4 green cardamom pods
4 whole cloves
1 bay leaf
1 teaspoon granulated sugar
    or granulated sweetener
120ml (4fl oz) light coconut
    milk
3 handfuls of spinach
salt and freshly ground
    black pepper

Side suggestions:
This pairs well with rice, or
for a low-carb side, serve with
cauliflower rice or roasted
cauliflower florets.

In this tasty dish, golden cubes of paneer cheese are mixed with vegetables in a rich tomato sauce. The beautiful blend of spices gives it the ultimate flavour, while the coconut milk adds a silky, creamy finish.

1. Heat half the ghee or oil in a large, flat-bottomed frying pan over a medium–high heat. Once hot, add the paneer and fry until golden. Remove from the pan and set aside on a plate.

2. Add the remaining ghee to the empty pan. Once hot, add the onion and fry for a few minutes until golden and softened, then add the garlic and ginger and fry for another couple of minutes just to infuse the ghee with flavour.

3. Add the ground cumin, coriander, turmeric and hot chilli powder, along with a little spray of oil, and cook for a couple of minutes, taking care not to burn the spices.

4. Add the tomato purée and 2 tablespoons water. Stir well, then add the chopped tomatoes, courgette, stock, cardamom pods, cloves, bay leaf and sugar. Bring to the boil, then reduce the heat to low and simmer for 10 minutes.

5. Next, stir in the coconut milk, then return the paneer to the pan. Stir, then leave to simmer for 5 minutes. Season to taste. If you wish, you can discard the bay leaf, cardamom and cloves at this point, but I usually just leave them in.

6. Add the spinach and stir until wilted, then serve.

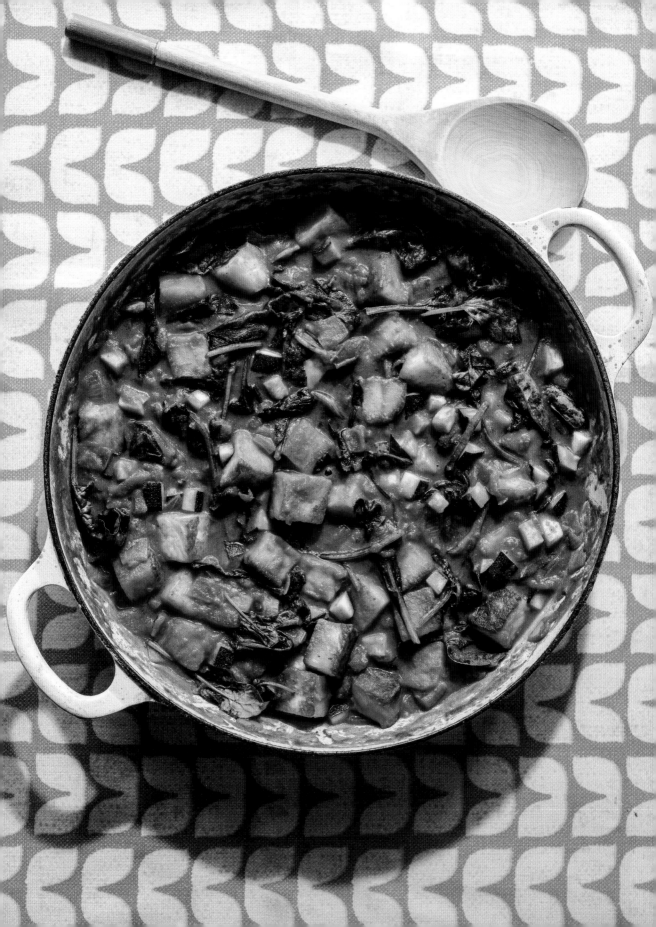

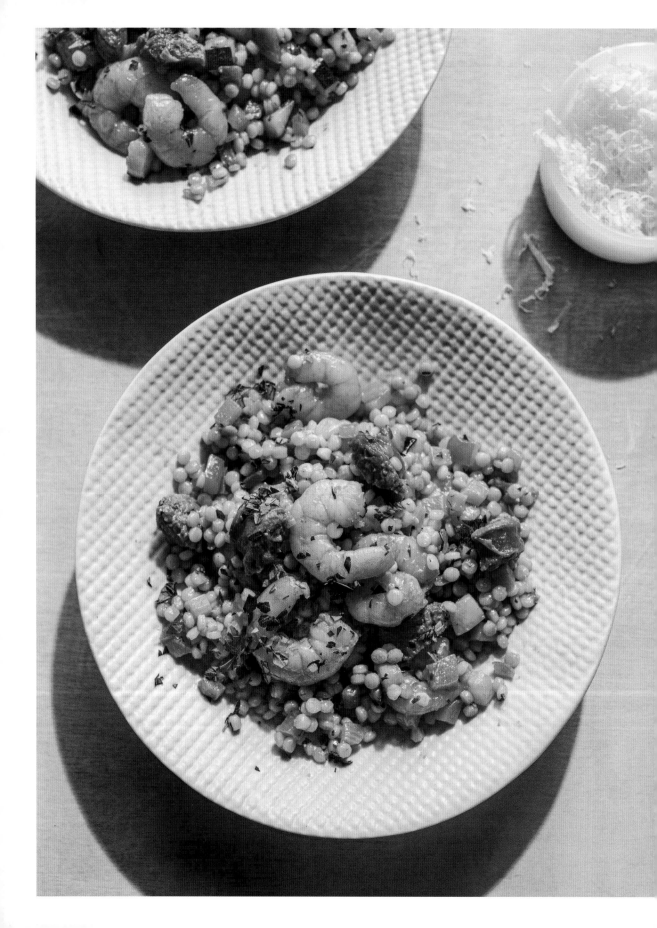

One-pot Chorizo and Prawn Israeli Couscous

PREP TIME: **10 MINUTES**   COOK TIME: **25 MINUTES**   SERVES: **4**

333 kcals per serving

DF

olive oil spray
400g (14oz) frozen peeled
    prawns (shrimp), thawed
½ teaspoon paprika
80g (2¾oz) chorizo,
    chopped
1 onion, diced
100g (3½oz) carrot,
    finely diced
1 small red (bell) pepper,
    finely diced
1 green (bell) pepper,
    finely diced
3 garlic cloves, crushed
100g (3½oz) courgette
    (zucchini), finely diced
½ teaspoon red chilli flakes
150g (5½oz) Israeli couscous
400ml (14fl oz) chicken
    stock
salt and freshly ground
    black pepper
1 tablespoon freshly chopped
    parsley (optional)

Swaps:
The prawns can be swapped
for chicken if you prefer
(thighs are best).

Optional add-ons:
Serve topped with a little
grated Parmesan.

Side suggestions:
Delicious with long-stem
broccoli, green beans,
spinach, kale or a mixed
salad.

Israeli or pearl couscous is a great ingredient to use in one-pot recipes. It has a similar texture to pasta and pairs well with a variety of flavours and ingredients. This one-pot recipe with tender prawns and vegetables includes chorizo and chilli flakes for a delicious, smoky, spicy flavour.

1. Heat a frying pan over a medium–high heat and spray with olive oil spray.

2. Add the prawns, paprika and a pinch of salt and pepper, and fry for a few minutes, turning occasionally until the prawns turn pink. Remove from the pan and set aside on a plate.

3. Spray the empty pan with more spray oil, then add the chorizo and onion and fry for a couple of minutes until the onion takes on the colour of the chorizo and softens.

4. Add the carrot, peppers and garlic and fry for a couple of minutes, then add the courgettes, chilli flakes and Israeli couscous, along with a little bit of stock. Stir to combine, scraping any bits from the bottom of the pan, then add the rest of the stock.

5. Bring to then boil, then cover and reduce the heat to low. Simmer for 10–12 minutes until the stock is just absorbed, then return the prawns to the pan. Cover with the lid once more, then turn off the heat and leave to rest for a few minutes, just to ensure the couscous is fully cooked.

6. Season to taste with salt and pepper, then sprinkle with fresh parsley and serve.

KCALS	**333**
FAT	**8.4g**
SAT FAT	**2.8g**
CARBS	**36.8g**
SUGARS	**8.0g**
FIBRE	**6.0g**
PROTEIN	**24.6g**
SALT	**2.37g**

One-pot French Onion Beef Pasta

PREP TIME: 10 MINUTES   **COOK TIME: 40 MINUTES**   **SERVES: 4**

400g (14oz) 5% fat beef
  mince (ground beef)
olive oil spray
400g (14oz) onions, halved
  and thinly sliced
1 teaspoon granulated sugar
½ teaspoon dried thyme
960ml (32½fl oz) beef stock
2 garlic cloves, crushed
2 tablespoons good-quality
  balsamic vinegar
200g (7oz) dried fusilli pasta
80g (2¾oz) Swiss cheese,
  such as Gruyère, or
  mozzarella, thinly sliced
salt and freshly ground
  black pepper
freshly chopped parsley
  or thyme, to serve

Side suggestions:
Serve with long-stem
broccoli, green beans,
cauliflower, roasted or
sautéed Brussels sprouts
or a simple salad.

Freezing:
Only the beef mixture is
freezable. To reheat after
freezing, defrost in the fridge,
then follow steps 4–5.

If there is one soup my family loves above all others, it's French onion soup, so it seemed like the perfect idea to turn it into a one-pot recipe with the addition of pasta and minced beef – and, boy, was this heavenly! Sweet caramelized onions, rich beef mince and fusilli pasta, all finished off with delicious melted cheese for a quick, easy dinner for the whole family.

1. Heat a deep frying pan over a medium–high heat. Add the beef mince and season with a pinch of salt and pepper. Fry for a few minutes until browned, then remove from the pan and set aside in a bowl.

2. Spray the empty pan with olive oil spray and add the onions, sugar, dried thyme and a pinch of salt. Fry for about 15 minutes until the onions have really softened and caramelized. During this time, add about 120ml (4fl oz) of the beef stock, adding it a little at a time and allowing it to evaporate off between additions. This will prevent the onions from sticking or burning.

3. Once the onions are really softened and golden, add the garlic and balsamic vinegar and cook for a couple of minutes until the liquid evaporates.

4. Return the beef mince to the pan, along with the pasta, and stir to combine. Pour in the remaining stock and increase the heat to high. Bring to the boil, then reduce the heat to medium–high and let it bubble for 15 minutes until the pasta is cooked and the stock is absorbed: the sauce should just loosely coat the pasta.

5. Scatter the cheese over the top, then cover with the lid and turn off the heat. Leave for 6–7 minutes until the cheese has all melted, then top with a pinch of black pepper and some freshly chopped parsley or thyme before serving.

474 kcals
per serving

KCALS
474

FAT
13.7g

SAT FAT
6.7g

CARBS
47.0g

SUGARS
9.7g

FIBRE
6.0g

PROTEIN
37.6g

SALT
1.04g

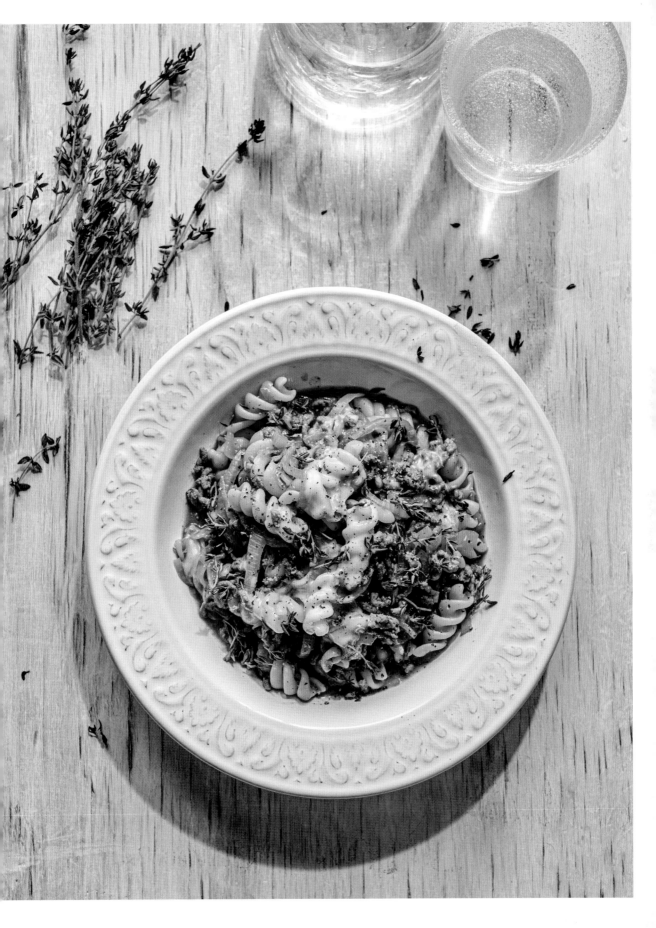

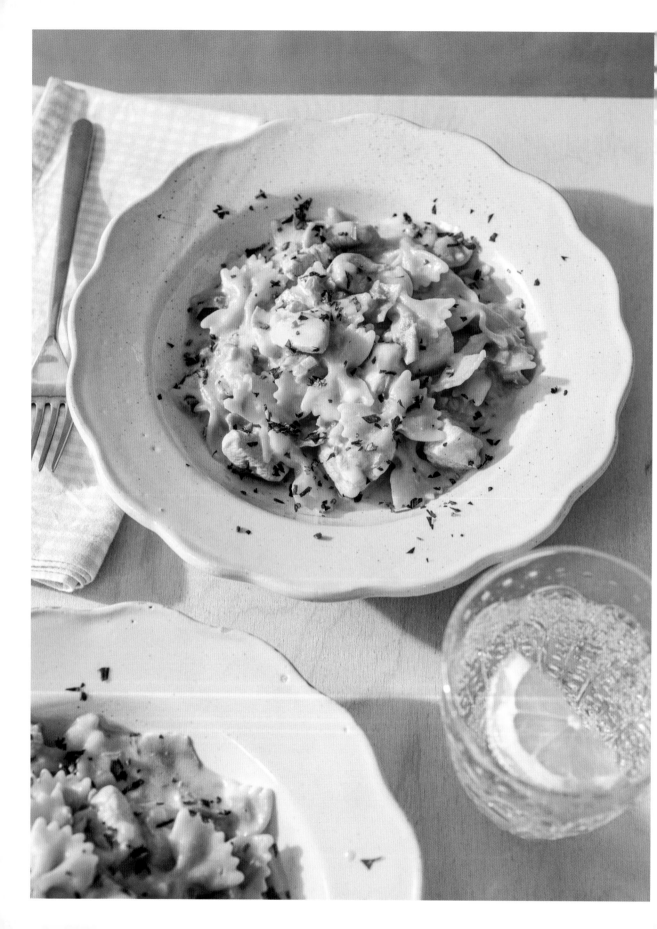

One-pot Chicken Cordon Bleu Pasta

PREP TIME: 10 MINUTES   **COOK TIME: 25 MINUTES**   **SERVES: 4**

350g (12oz) boneless, skinless chicken breast, diced into bite-sized pieces

½ teaspoon garlic powder

olive oil spray

1 small onion, finely chopped

100g (3½oz) lean ham, chopped

250g (9oz) dried farfalle pasta

840ml (28½fl oz) chicken stock

1½ tablespoons Dijon mustard (not wholegrain)

1 tablespoon freshly chopped parsley

50g (1¾oz) light cream cheese

100ml (3½fl oz) semi-skimmed milk

15g (½oz) Parmesan, grated

80g (2¾oz) Swiss cheese, sliced

salt and freshly ground black pepper

Side suggestions:

Pair with some greens, like asparagus, green beans or broccoli.

Swaps:

If you prefer, you can use mozzarella instead of Swiss cheese.

A super-simple way to enjoy the delicious flavours of Cordon Bleu in an easy one-pot recipe for the whole family: tender pieces of chicken breast with diced ham and pasta bows in a creamy Dijon sauce with melted Swiss cheese.

1. Season the chicken with the garlic powder and some salt and freshly ground black pepper, then set aside.

2. Heat a frying pan over a medium–high heat and spray with olive oil spray. Add the onion and fry for a couple of minutes until golden and softened, then add the chicken and fry for a further few minutes until lightly browned. Stir in the diced ham and fry for 1 minute more.

3. Now add the pasta, along with 720ml (24¾fl oz) of the stock, as well as the Dijon mustard and parsley. Stir to combine. Bring to the boil, then reduce the heat to medium and let it bubble for 12–15 minutes, stirring occasionally, until the pasta is cooked and the stock is almost absorbed. If needed, add the remaining 120ml (4fl oz) stock to ensure the pasta is cooked.

4. Stir in the cream cheese, milk and Parmesan until melted and creamy (ensure the cream cheese is fully melted). Place the Swiss cheese slices on top, then cover with a lid and turn off the heat. Leave for a couple of minutes until the Swiss cheese has melted.

5. Enjoy!

KCALS	518
FAT	13.9g
SAT FAT	6.5g
CARBS	50.5g
SUGARS	5.2g
FIBRE	4.2g
PROTEIN	45.6g
SALT	2.58g

388 kcals
per serving

KCALS
388

FAT
9.2g

SAT FAT
3.7g

CARBS
44.1g

SUGARS
7.6g

FIBRE
6.1g

PROTEIN
29.3g

SALT
1.47g

One-pot Moroccan-style Lamb Pilaf

PREP TIME: **10 MINUTES**   COOK TIME: **30 MINUTES**   SERVES: **4**

olive oil spray
400g (14oz) lean lamb steak,
    thinly sliced
1½ tablespoons Moroccan
    Seasoning (page 280)
4 garlic cloves, minced
1 onion, finely diced
1 small carrot, finely diced
200g (7oz) aubergine
    (eggplant) chopped
½ red (bell) pepper,
    thinly sliced
500ml (18fl oz) chicken
    stock
100g (3½oz) courgette
    (zucchini), chopped
6 cherry tomatoes, chopped
1 tablespoon tomato purée
    (paste)
175g (6oz) basmati rice,
    uncooked
1 tablespoon freshly chopped
    parsley
1 tablespoon freshly chopped
    coriander (cilantro)
salt and freshly ground
    black pepper

Freezing:
The rice is not freezer-
friendly so only freeze
the mixture up to the end
of step 3. To reheat after
freezing, defrost in the fridge,
then follow steps 4–6.

In this delicious recipe, tender pieces of lamb are pan-fried with vegetables, basmati rice and a homemade blend of Moroccan spices, all cooked together in one pan for a simple yet yummy family meal.

1. Heat a large, deep frying pan over a medium–high heat and spray with olive oil spray.

2. Add the lamb and fry for a couple of minutes until browned. Add the Moroccan seasoning and garlic and continue to fry for another couple of minutes, stirring until the lamb is coated in the seasoning. Remove from the pan and set aside on a plate.

3. Add the onion and carrot to the empty pan and fry for a couple minutes until golden, then add the aubergine and pepper and fry for another couple of minutes until softened. As you cook them, add a couple of tablespoons of the stock and let it reduce around the vegetables: this will help them to soften.

4. Return the lamb to the pan, along with the courgette, cherry tomatoes, tomato purée and rice. Stir to combine, then pour in the stock. Bring to the boil, then cover and reduce the heat to low. Simmer for 10–15 minutes until the stock is almost all absorbed.

5. Turn off the heat and leave, untouched, with the lid still on, for 10 minutes.

6. Now fluff up the rice with a spoon and season to taste with salt and pepper. Finally, stir in the fresh parsley and coriander and serve.

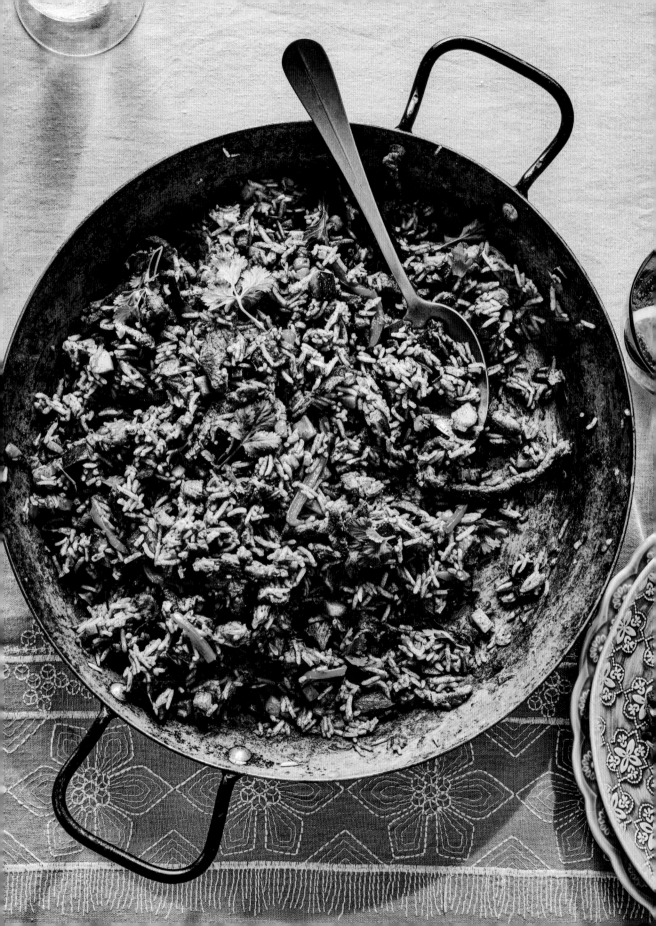

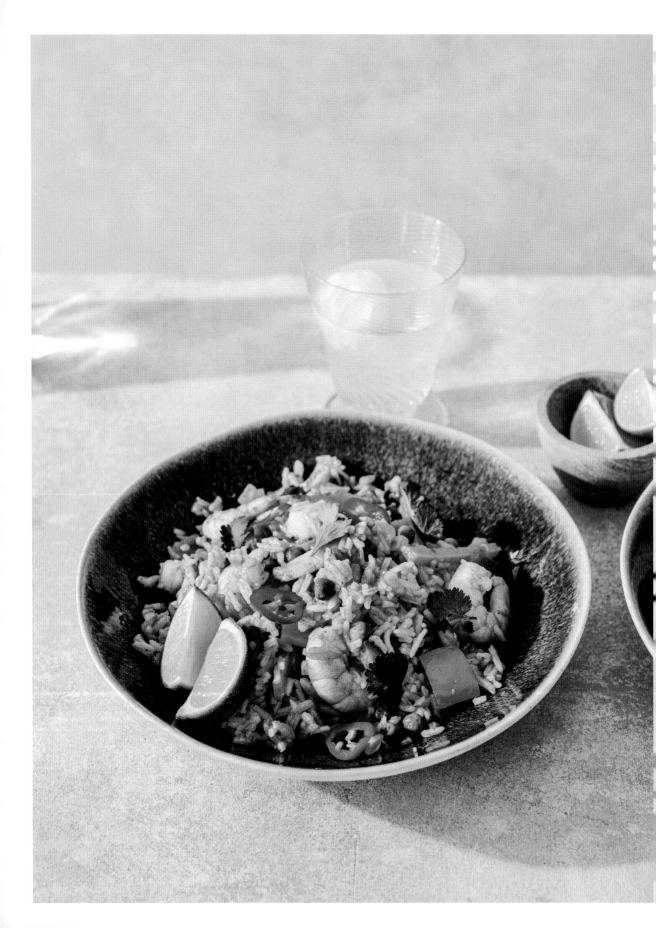

One-pot Thai Red Prawn and Vegetable Rice

PREP TIME: 10 MINUTES   **COOK TIME: 25 MINUTES**   **SERVES: 4**

GF
DF

olive oil spray
1 small onion, finely diced
2 garlic cloves, finely chopped
2 teaspoons grated fresh ginger
2–3 tablespoons red Thai curry paste (depending on your preferred spice level)
175g (6oz) long-grain rice, rinsed
½ red (bell) pepper, diced
½ green (bell) pepper, diced
½ yellow (bell) pepper, diced
1 small carrot, sliced into thin batons
240ml (8½fl oz) chicken stock
1 tablespoon fish sauce
½ tablespoon light brown sugar, or granulated sweetener if you prefer
240ml (8½fl oz) light coconut milk
400g (14oz) frozen peeled prawns (shrimp), thawed
80g (2¾oz)) frozen peas
handful of fresh coriander (cilantro)
1 fresh red Thai chilli, sliced
1 lime, sliced into wedges

If you love Thai-inspired dishes, this one-pot recipe is the perfect dish for you. It has the delicious flavours of a Thai red curry, with tender prawns, tasty vegetables, creamy coconut milk and rice, all cooked in one pan. It's a nourishing yet simple meal that can be on the table in less than half an hour, and you can vary it by using different proteins to suit your tastes.

1. Heat a large, deep non-stick frying pan over a medium–high heat and spray with olive oil spray. Add the onion, garlic and ginger and fry for a couple of minutes until lightly golden and softened. Add the red Thai curry paste and a couple of tablespoons of water, and stir until the paste is well combined with the onions.

2. Add the rice and stir to coat, then add the peppers, carrot, stock, fish sauce, brown sugar and coconut milk. Give it all a good stir to make sure nothing is stuck to the bottom of the pan. Bring to the boil, then reduce the heat to low and simmer, covered, for about 10 minutes until the liquid is almost absorbed.

3. Add the prawns and peas, and give it a little stir to combine, but don't overmix. Cover once more, then turn off heat and leave for 10–12 minutes until the prawns are pink and cooked and the rice is fluffy.

4. Once ready, garnish with the coriander and chilli and serve with lime wedges for squeezing.

KCALS	348
FAT	7.6g
SAT FAT	4.1g
CARBS	48.9g
SUGARS	9.6g
FIBRE	5.3g
PROTEIN	18.5g
SALT	2.73g

Side suggestions:
Don't like prawns? Swap them for some chicken. If you do this, I recommend browning the chicken with the onion and keeping it in the pan for the entire cooking time.

Variation:
This can also be made with Thai green curry paste.

KCALS
392

FAT
3.6g

SAT FAT
1.0g

CARBS
53.9g

SUGARS
14.5g

FIBRE
7.6g

PROTEIN
32.3g

SALT
3.58g

Chicken Vegetable Yaki Udon

PREP TIME: 8 MINUTES   **COOK TIME: 12 MINUTES**   **SERVES: 4**

low-calorie cooking oil spray

350g (12oz) boneless, skinless chicken thighs

1 tablespoon dark soy sauce

2 garlic cloves, minced

125g (4½oz) shiitake mushrooms

200g (7oz) shredded green cabbage

1 carrot, cut into long, thin batons

100g (3½oz) sugar snap peas or mangetout (snow peas)

600g (1lb 5oz) straight-to-wok udon noodles

5 spring onions (scallions), sliced

For the sauce

3 tablespoons dark soy sauce

1½ tablespoons oyster sauce

2 tablespoons mirin

1 tablespoon rice vinegar

1 tablespoon maple syrup

Swaps:
You can use dried udon noodles if you prefer: just cook them according to the packet instructions and then weigh once cooked to get the quantity required.

Vegetarian:
Swap out the chicken for more veggies or a meat-free protein to make this vegetarian.

This is probably one of quickest and easiest noodle dishes you will ever make, yet it doesn't compromise on flavour. Tender chicken and vegetables with thick udon noodles (my family's favourite type of noodle) all coated in a delicious sauce. It will become a regular feature on your menu.

1. To make the sauce, mix together all the ingredients in a bowl, then set aside.

2. Heat a large, deep frying pan or wok over a medium–high heat and spray with low-calorie cooking spray. Add the chicken, along with the soy sauce and garlic, and fry for a few minutes until the chicken is a deep golden brown. Remove from the pan and set aside on a plate.

3. Spray the empty pan with low-calorie cooking spray once more, then add the shiitake mushrooms and fry for a couple of minutes. Add the cabbage and carrots, and fry for a further few minutes until tender. Now return the chicken to the pan, along with the sugar snap peas, and continue to stir-fry for a few minutes until the chicken is cooked through.

4. Meanwhile, put the udon noodles into a large bowl and cover with boiling water. Leave to soak for 2 minutes, then carefully separate, and drain.

5. Add the drained noodles to the frying pan, along with the spring onions, then pour in the sauce.

6. Continue to fry for a few minutes, tossing the noodles until everything is well coated in the sauce. Serve and enjoy!

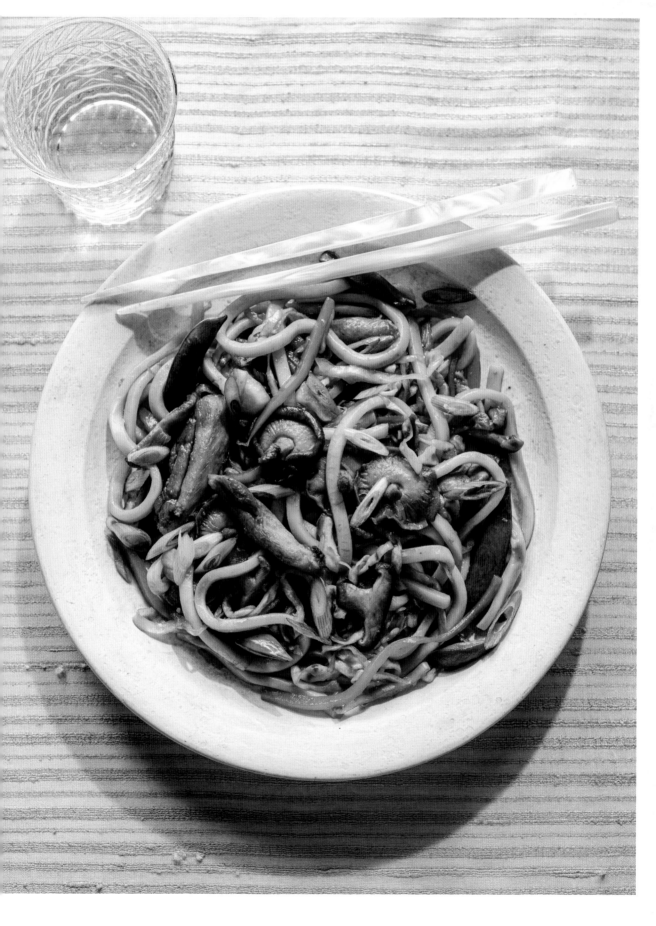

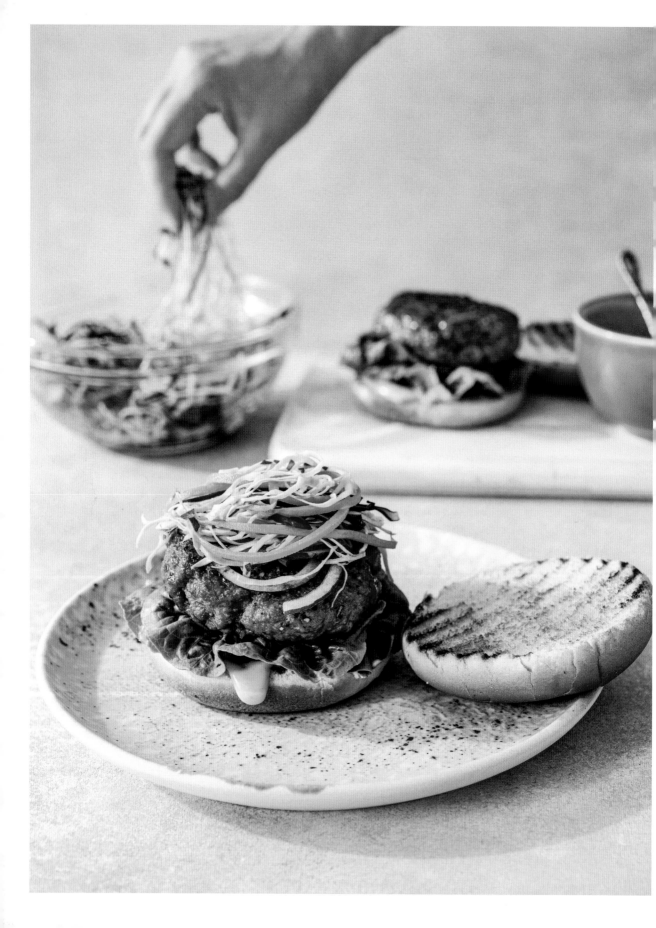

Teriyaki Turkey Burgers with Slaw and Sriracha Mayo

PREP TIME: 10 MINUTES   **COOK TIME: 5 MINUTES**   **SERVES: 4**

4 tablespoons light
  mayonnaise
2 teaspoons sriracha (or
  more if you like it spicy)
olive oil spray
450g (1lb) 5% fat turkey
  mince (ground turkey)
2 garlic cloves, minced
1 teaspoon grated fresh
  ginger
1 small shallot, finely
  chopped
olive oil spray
4 low-calorie burger buns
  of your choice
a few lettuce leaves
salt and freshly ground
  black pepper

For the teriyaki sauce
2 tablespoons soy sauce
2 tablespoons mirin
2 tablespoons rice vinegar
1 tablespoon honey
½ teaspoon garlic powder
½ teaspoon onion powder
½ teaspoon sesame oil

For the slaw
100g (3½oz) green cabbage,
  shredded
100g (3½oz) red cabbage,
  shredded
1 carrot, grated or julienned
½ small red onion, thinly
  sliced
1 tablespoon freshly chopped
  coriander (cilantro)
2 tablespoons rice vinegar
1 teaspoon granulated sugar
  or granulated sweetener

The easiest burgers you will ever make. These delicious, tender turkey burgers are seared in a pan and then coated in a homemade teriyaki sauce that's reduced around the burgers to give them the ultimate flavour. Paired with some Asian slaw and sriracha mayo and served in bun, they are a real crowd-pleaser.

1. Combine all the ingredients for the teriyaki sauce in a bowl. Whisk to combine, then set aside.

2. To make the slaw, combine all the ingredients in a bowl, season with salt and pepper and set aside.

3. To prepare the burgers, mix together the mayonnaise and sriracha, then set aside.

4. In a large bowl, mix together the turkey mince, garlic, ginger and shallot. Once combined, form into four patties and season the outsides with salt and pepper.

5. Heat a large frying pan over a medium–high heat and spray with olive oil spray. Add the burgers to the pan and fry for a couple of minutes on each side until browned.

6. Pour the teriyaki sauce into the pan and keep cooking for a few minutes, turning the burgers in the sauce until they are well coated and the sauce reduces down around the burgers (be careful not to burn the sauce).

7. Lightly toast the buns, then spread the sriracha mayo on the bottom halves of the buns. Top with lettuce, then add the burgers and some slaw. Top with the other bun halves and enjoy!

Swaps:
You can swap the turkey mince for the mince of your choice.

Variations:
These can also be served without the buns: just serve the burgers with slaw, mayo and extra salad. They're also delicious with rice, if you prefer.

Freezing:
Only the burger patties are freezer-friendly. Freeze after step 4. To reheat after freezing, defrost in the fridge, then follow steps 5–7. These can also be frozen after cooking.

433 kcals per serving

KCALS	**433**
FAT	**12.6g**
SAT FAT	**2.1g**
CARBS	**49.8g**
SUGARS	**16.9g**
FIBRE	**4.9g**
PROTEIN	**27.6g**
SALT	**2.72g**

One-pot Chicken Riesling Pasta

PREP TIME: 15 MINUTES   **COOK TIME: 30 MINUTES**   **SERVES: 4**

400g (14oz) boneless, skinless chicken breast, sliced
olive oil spray
2 slices of lean back bacon, fat removed
1 shallot, finely chopped
250g (9oz) mushrooms, sliced
5 garlic cloves, crushed
120ml (4fl oz) Riesling wine
250g (9oz) dried spaghetti
720–840ml (24¾–28½fl oz) chicken stock
120ml (4fl oz) semi-skimmed milk
80g (2¾oz) low-fat cream cheese
20g (¾oz) Parmesan, freshly grated
salt and freshly ground black pepper
freshly chopped parsley, to serve

Side suggestions:
Pair with a side salad or some steamed greens, like asparagus or green beans.

This is a quick and simple dinner to make any night of the week feel special. Tender chicken breast, mushrooms and garlic are cooked in one pan with spaghetti in a light, creamy, white wine sauce. It's all finished off with golden bacon and Parmesan for a delicious combination of flavours.

1. Season the chicken well all over with salt and freshly ground black pepper.

2. Heat a frying pan over a medium–high heat and spray with olive oil spray. Add the bacon and fry for a couple of minutes until really golden (you need to be patient to get a nice colour on the bacon). Remove from the pan and set aside on a plate.

3. Spray the empty pan with olive oil spray once more, then add the chicken and fry for a few minutes on each side until golden. Remove from the pan and set aside on a plate.

4. Add the shallot to the empty pan and fry for a couple of minutes until softened and golden, then add the mushrooms and garlic and fry for a further few minutes until the mushrooms are lightly golden. Add a little more olive oil spray if needed.

5. Pour in the wine and deglaze the pan, scraping up any bits stuck to the bottom.

6. Return the chicken to the pan and stir, then add the spaghetti. Pour in 720ml (24¾fl oz) of the stock and bring to the boil, then reduce the heat to medium and let it bubble for 10–12 minutes, stirring occasionally, until the pasta is cooked and the stock is almost absorbed. If needed, add the remaining 120ml (4fl oz) stock to ensure the pasta is cooked.

7. Add the milk, cream cheese and Parmesan and stir until the cheeses are melted and everything is coated in a light, creamy sauce.

8. Season to taste with salt and freshly ground black pepper, then sprinkle with the parsley and the cooked bacon and enjoy!

KCALS	**483**
FAT	**7.6g**
SAT FAT	**4.3g**
CARBS	**51.4g**
SUGARS	**5.4g**
FIBRE	**4.1g**
PROTEIN	**45.4g**
SALT	**1.79g**

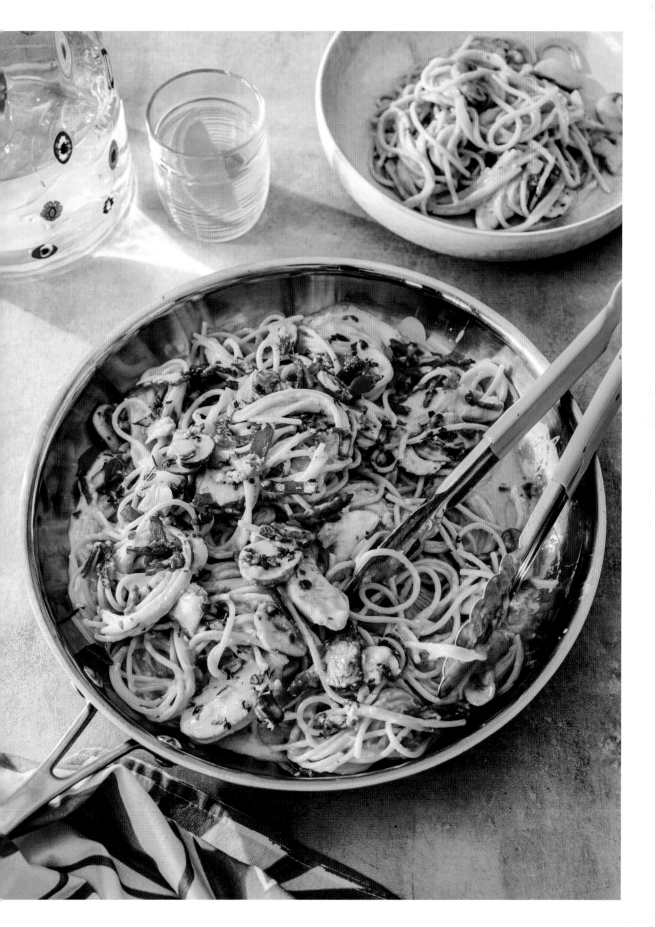

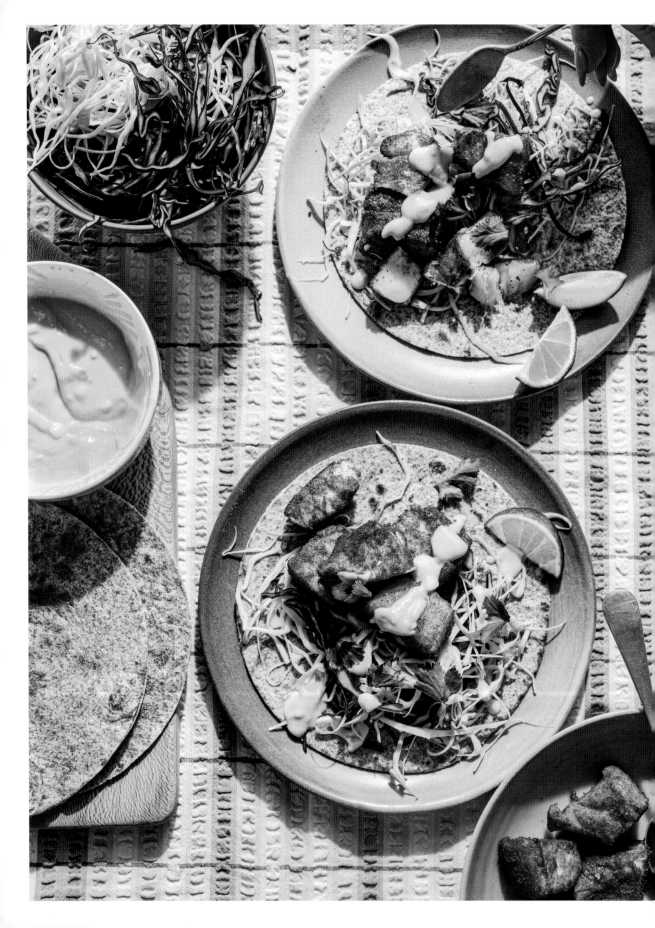

Fish Tacos with Avocado Sauce

PREP TIME: 8 MINUTES   **COOK TIME: 8 MINUTES**   **SERVES: 4**

500g (1lb 2oz) firm white fish (such as tilapia or haddock), cut into large, bite-sized chunks

1½ tablespoons All-purpose Seasoning (page 280)

¼ teaspoon cayenne pepper (optional)

olive oil spray

4 low-calorie tortillas

80g (2¾oz) red cabbage, shredded

80g (2¾oz) green cabbage, shredded

salt and freshly ground black pepper

freshly chopped coriander (cilantro), to serve

lime wedges, to serve

For the avocado sauce

60g (2oz) avocado flesh

2 tablespoons low-fat Greek yogurt

½ tablespoon lime juice

½ teaspoon garlic powder

½ teaspoon onion powder

small handful of coriander (cilantro)

Swaps:

Don't like fish? Swap the fish for chicken – or, for a vegetarian option, roast some cauliflower, then fry it in the pan with the seasoning.

Optional add-ons:

Try this with Pineapple Salsa (page 261), feta, Cheddar, sweetcorn or diced red onion.

Side suggestions:

For a more filling meal, you can serve these with rice, potato wedges, homemade oven fries or a side salad.

Creamy avocado sauce:

This is really versatile and can be used in other recipes or as a salad dressing.

A real family favourite, this fish taco recipe is so quick and easy to make. I've used my homemade All-purpose Seasoning to flavour the fish, which is then pan-fried until golden and served on tortillas with shredded cabbage and coriander. It's all drizzled with a creamy avocado sauce for a delicious combination of textures and flavours.

1. In a bowl, toss the fish in the all-purpose seasoning mix, adding a pinch of cayenne if you like it spicy. Set aside.

2. To make the avocado sauce, place the avocado in a mini food-processor along with the yogurt, lime juice, garlic powder, onion powder and a pinch of salt. Add 2 tablespoons water and blend, adding a little more water as needed (4–6 tablespoons in total) until your sauce is creamy but of a drizzling consistency. Set aside.

3. Heat a frying pan over a medium–high heat and spray with olive oil spray. Once hot, add the fish and season with a pinch of salt and pepper. Cook for about 3 minutes, then flip and cook for another 3 minutes on the other side. It should have a lovely deep golden colour all over. Remove from the pan and set aside on a warmed plate.

4. Wipe the empty pan with paper towels, then spray with a little more olive oil spray and heat the tortillas briefly on each side until warm and browned in spots.

5. When you are ready to enjoy your tacos, you can quickly return the fish back to the pan for a minute just to warm up if you wish.

6. To serve, add some red and green cabbage to each tortilla, then top with the fish. Drizzle over the avocado sauce and some fresh coriander, then serve with lime wedges for squeezing. Enjoy!

KCALS	**289**
FAT	**7.5g**
SAT FAT	**2.0g**
CARBS	**24.0g**
SUGARS	**3.2g**
FIBRE	**4.2g**
PROTEIN	**29.2g**
SALT	**1.87g**

419 kcals per serving

DF

KCALS
419

FAT
5.9g

SAT FAT
1.8g

CARBS
61.4g

SUGARS
13.0g

FIBRE
10.9g

PROTEIN
24.8g

SALT
2.13g

One-pot Smoky Paprika Sausage Penne

PREP TIME: **10 MINUTES**   COOK TIME: **20 MINUTES**   SERVES: **4**

olive oil spray
1 onion, diced
6 low-calorie sausages (approx. 350g/12oz in weight), skin removed
1 red (bell) pepper
1 green (bell) pepper
3 garlic cloves, minced
1½ teaspoons smoked paprika
1½ teaspoons sweet paprika
½ tablespoon Worcestershire sauce
1 teaspoon dried parsley
300g (10½oz) fresh ripe tomatoes, peeled and chopped
2 tablespoons tomato purée (paste)
240g (8½oz) dried penne pasta
720–960ml (24¾–32½fl oz) chicken stock
85g (3oz) frozen peas
1 tablespoon freshly chopped parsley
a few torn basil leaves
salt and freshly ground black pepper

I love using fresh tomatoes in pasta dishes. Canned tomatoes are always great to have on hand, but fresh tomatoes have a beautiful, natural sweetness and create such a lovely sauce. I use my trusty serrated peeler, which effortlessly peels the skin of any soft fruit or vegetable without the need to score or blanch first.

This is a favourite recipe with my kids. They love the sausages with the smoky paprika flavours and pasta. A simple one-pot meal for any night of the week.

1. Heat a large frying pan over a medium–high heat and spray with olive oil spray.

2. Add the onion and sausages and fry for a couple of minutes until golden brown, breaking up the sausages with the back of a wooden spoon as they cook.

3. Add the peppers, garlic, paprika, Worcestershire sauce and dried parsley and stir to combine, then add the fresh tomatoes and cook for a few minutes until they start to soften and break down.

4. Add the tomato purée, pasta and 720ml (24¾fl oz) of the stock. Bring to the boil, then reduce the heat to medium and allow to bubble for 12–14 minutes until the pasta is cooked, adding more stock if needed to cook the pasta). Add the frozen peas halfway through the cooking time.

5. Taste and season with salt and freshly ground black pepper, then stir in the fresh parsley and torn basil. Serve and enjoy!

Swaps:
The sausage can be swapped for the protein of your choice: chicken, pork and prawns will all work great, although if you opt for prawns, I recommend adding them towards the end, as they won't take long to cook.

Optional add-ins:
Once the pasta is cooked, stir in some grated Cheddar until creamy and silky in appearance (I add about 15g/½oz per person).

Side suggestions:
Pair with a mixed salad or some steamed greens of your choice.

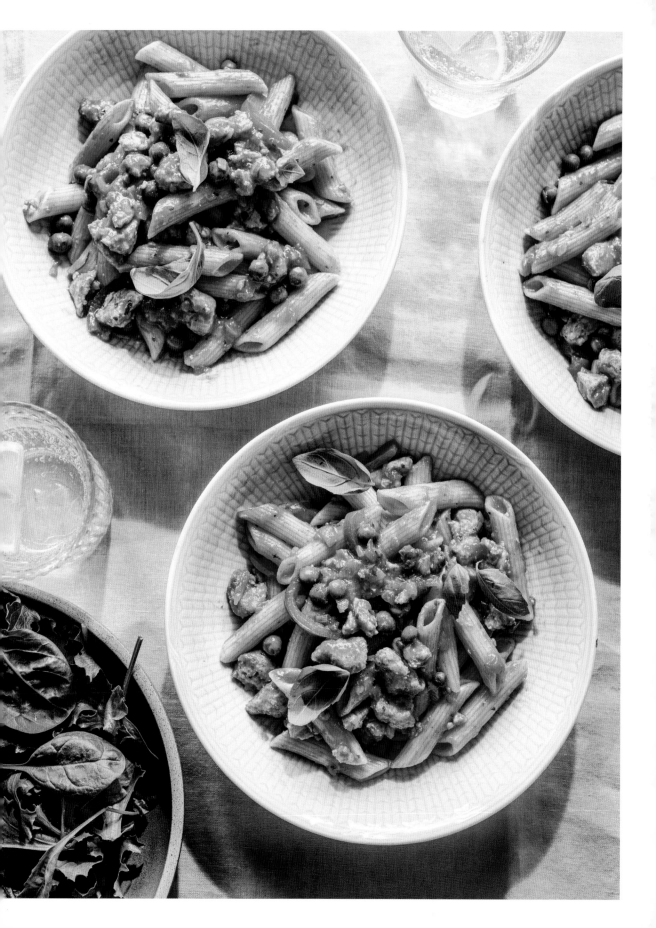

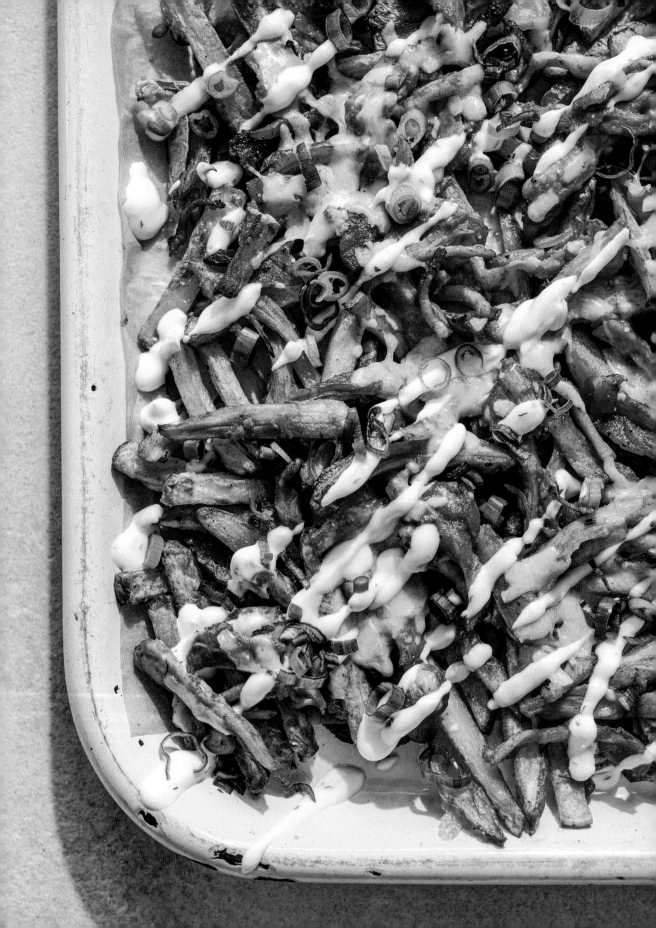

Sheet-pan Meals Made Simple

Hoisin Pork Tenderloin with Special Fried Rice

PREP TIME: **10 MINUTES**   COOK TIME: **30 MINUTES**   SERVES: **4**

olive oil spray
500g (1lb 2oz) pork
   tenderloin (fillet),
   visible fat removed
1 onion, diced
1 carrot, diced
450g (15½oz) cooked
   rice (uncooked weight
   160g/5¾oz) – see Note
1 tablespoon light soy sauce
½ tablespoon dark soy sauce
1 teaspoon sesame oil
85g (3oz) frozen peas
2 medium eggs, whisked
2 spring onions (scallions),
   chopped
freshly ground black pepper

For the sauce
4 tablespoons hoisin sauce
2 tablespoons dark soy sauce
1 tablespoon honey
80g (2¾oz) passata
2 garlic cloves, crushed
½ teaspoon onion powder

Cooking pork tenderloin:
Pork should have an internal
temperature of 63°C (145°F)
when cooked through. It's
important to let it rest for at
least 8 minutes before slicing.

Note:
Cooked rice should be
refrigerated.

Optional add-ins:
If you like Chinese five spice,
add ½–1 teaspoon to the hoisin
sauce mix for extra flavour.

The ultimate all-in-one dinner. Create the perfect fake-away at home with this easy baking-tray meal of tender pork fillet in a delicious hoisin sauce, served with perfectly cooked special fried rice.

1. Preheat the oven to 220°C/200°C fan/425°F/gas 7. Line a large baking tray with baking paper and spray with olive oil spray.

2. To make the sauce, combine all the ingredients in a bowl and set aside.

3. Use foil to make a 'boat' about a third of the size of the baking tray. Place the pork tenderloin in the boat, then pour all the sauce over the top, turning the pork in the sauce to ensure it's covered.

4. Spread out the chopped onion and carrot across the rest of the tray and spray with olive oil spray. Place in the oven and bake for 15 minutes.

5. Remove from the oven and add the rice, soy sauces, sesame oil and frozen peas on top of the carrots and onion. Mix to combine, breaking up any clumps of rice, then spread out across the tray and spray with olive oil spray once more. Baste the pork tenderloin with the sauce, then return to the oven for another 10 minutes.

6. Remove from the oven and carefully lift out the foil boat containing the pork. Set aside to rest for 8 minutes.

7. Meanwhile, make 2 hollows in the rice mixture. Spray them with spray oil, then pour in the beaten eggs. Return the tray to the oven for 4 minutes; the eggs should now be cooked.

8. Toss all the rice mixture together, breaking up the eggs to combine. Season with a little black pepper and sprinkle the spring onions over the top.

9. Slice the rested pork and serve with the fried rice. Enjoy!

Side suggestions:
This is great served just as it is, or with some additional vegetables of your choice.

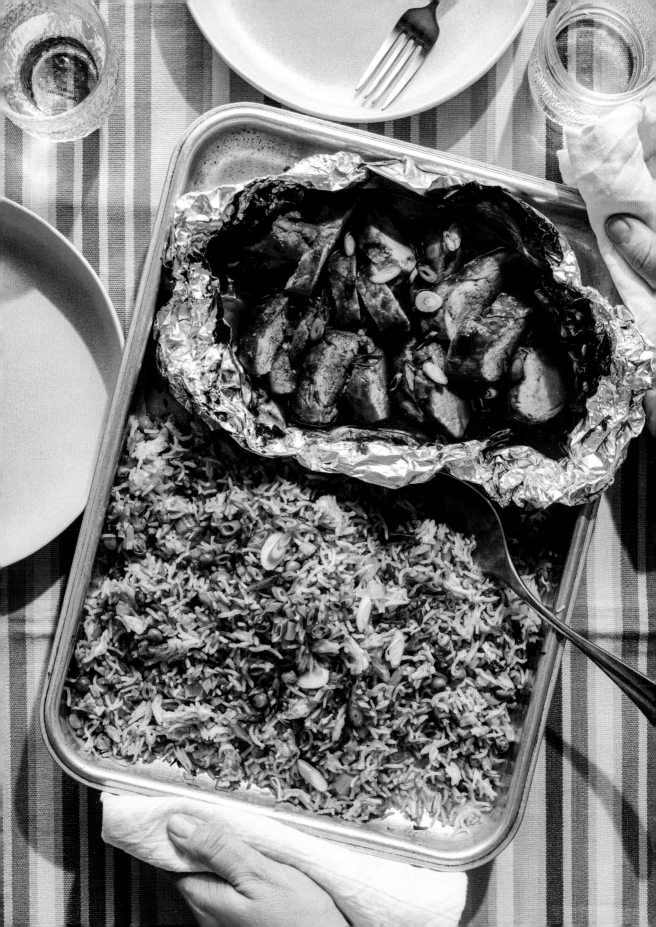

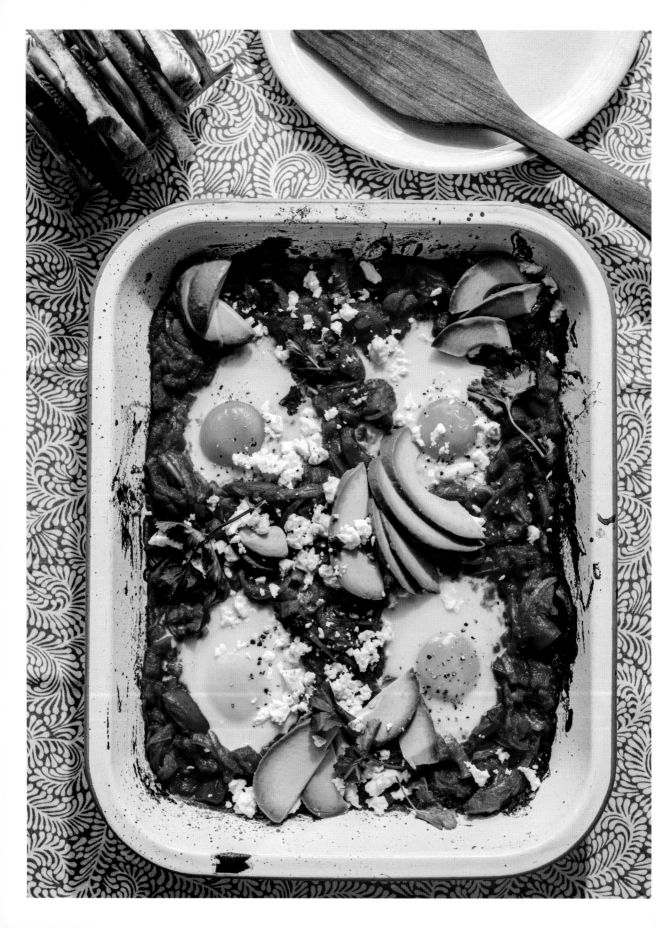

Easy Shakshuka with Crispy Oven-baked Toast

PREP TIME: 5 MINUTES   **COOK TIME: 35 MINUTES**   **SERVES: 4**

1 small onion, quartered and thinly sliced
3 garlic cloves, minced
300g (10½oz) fresh ripe tomatoes, roughly chopped
1 red (bell) pepper, finely diced
300g (10½oz) passata
2 tablespoons tomato purée (paste)
1 tablespoon paprika
½ teaspoon smoked hot paprika
1 teaspoon ground cumin
pinch of red chilli flakes
2 teaspoons extra virgin olive oil
4 large eggs
4 slices of low-calorie bread, halved diagonally
olive oil spray
50g (1¾oz) feta, crumbled
small handful of fresh coriander (cilantro) or parsley
90g (3oz) avocado, sliced

Gluten-free:
Use a gluten-free bread of your choice.

Breakfast is one of my family's favourite meals of the day, so when everyone is home in the mornings, it's a great time to all sit down and enjoy a filling breakfast together. However, as an often tired and busy mum, I generally like breakfasts that are simple and easy, so that I can enjoy my morning coffee. This easy shakshuka is a great throw-it-in-the-oven breakfast – even the toast's made in the oven!

1. Preheat the oven to 220°C/200°C fan/425°F/gas 7.

2. Place the onion, garlic, tomatoes, red pepper, passata and tomato purée in a large baking tray. Scatter over the spices and drizzle with the olive oil, then toss to combine.

3. Bake for 20 minutes, then remove from the oven. Make 4 holes in the tomato mixture and crack an egg into each one. Place the bread slices on a second tray and spray with olive oil spray.

4. Reduce the oven temperature to 200°C/180°C fan/400°F/gas 6 and place both trays in the oven. Bake for 12–15 minutes until the eggs are cooked to your liking and the toast is golden and crispy.

5. Sprinkle the shakshuka with feta and coriander, and serve with the avocado and toast.

KCALS	**291**
FAT	**15.5g**
SAT FAT	**4.7g**
CARBS	**18.3g**
SUGARS	**9.9g**
FIBRE	**7.1g**
PROTEIN	**15.8g**
SALT	**0.81g**

GF
DF

KCALS
408

FAT
17.3g

SAT FAT
4.4g

CARBS
22.3g

SUGARS
18.0g

FIBRE
5.6g

PROTEIN
38.0g

SALT
0.38g

Maple Turmeric Chicken Traybake

PREP TIME: 10 MINUTES   **COOK TIME: 40 MINUTES**   **SERVES: 4**

8 boneless, skinless chicken thighs, trimmed of visible fat (approx. 720g/1lb 9oz)
1½ teaspoons ground turmeric
½ teaspoon paprika
2½ tablespoons maple syrup or honey
3 garlic cloves, crushed
1 cauliflower, broken into florets
1 small carrot, finely diced
1 onion, halved and sliced
2 teaspoons extra virgin olive oil
1 large courgette (zucchini), halved lengthways and sliced
1 red (bell) pepper, finely diced
½ teaspoon garlic powder
½ teaspoon onion powder
olive oil spray
salt and freshly ground black pepper
freshly chopped coriander (cilantro), to serve
lime wedges, to serve (optional)

Side suggestions:
This is perfect just as it is, or you can serve it with rice or potatoes.

A simple but elegant traybake with beautiful colours and gorgeous flavours from the maple syrup, turmeric and garlic. It's a great dish for including plenty of healthy vegetables into your meal, and can be enjoyed just as it is or with a side of your choice.

1. Preheat the oven to 220°C/200°C fan/425°F/gas 7 and line a baking tray with baking paper.

2. Place the chicken in a large bowl with the turmeric, paprika, maple syrup and garlic. Toss until well coated and set aside to marinate while you prepare the other ingredients.

3. Place the cauliflower, carrot and onion in the prepared baking tray. Drizzle over the olive oil and toss to coat, then season with salt and pepper. Roast for 10 minutes.

4. Remove the tray from the oven and add the courgette and red pepper. Sprinkle over the garlic and onion powder and toss to coat, then spread out in an even layer. Make 8 spaces in the mixture and place a piece of chicken in each one. Season with salt and pepper, then spray everything with olive oil spray.

5. Bake for 20 minutes, then remove the tray from the oven and toss everything together so that all the veg gets coated in the chicken juices. This will give it all a beautiful colour and flavour. Spread everything back out and return to the oven for another 10 minutes.

6. Sprinkle with fresh coriander and serve with lime wedges (if liked) for squeezing.

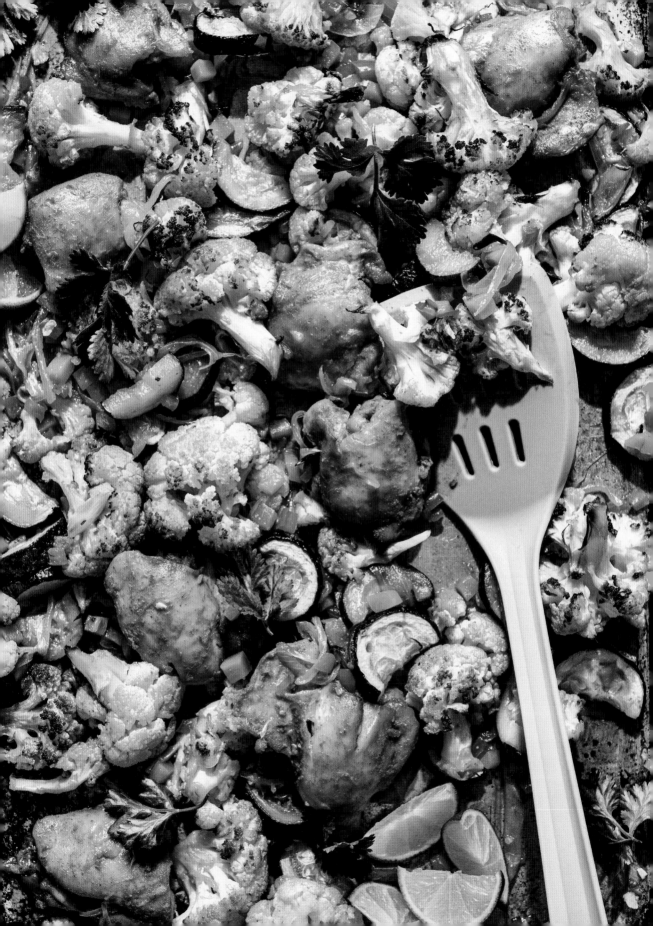

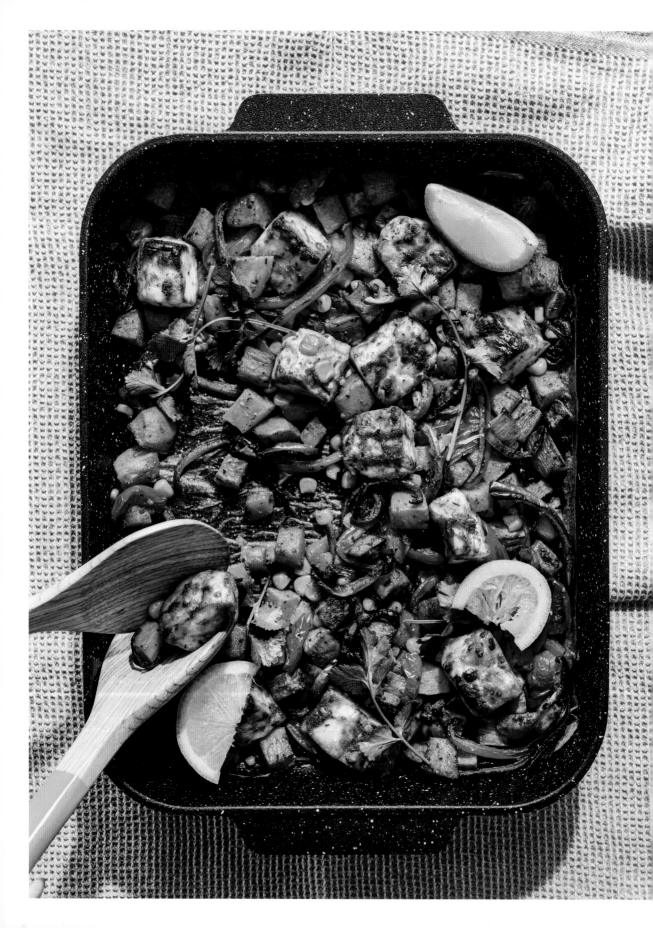

Piri Piri Halloumi Traybake

PREP TIME: 10 MINUTES   **COOK TIME: 45 MINUTES**   **SERVES: 4**

800g (24oz) sweet potatoes, peel and cubed

1 large red onion, halved and sliced

1½ tablespoons homemade Piri Piri Seasoning (page 281)

2 teaspoons extra virgin olive oil

1 red (bell) pepper, sliced

1 green (bell) pepper sliced

12 grape tomatoes (baby plum tomatoes) or cherry tomatoes, halved

1 tablespoon maple syrup or honey

1 tablespoon tomato purée (paste)

1 tablespoon lemon juice

250g (9oz) halloumi cheese, sliced

100g (3½oz) canned sweetcorn, drained

olive oil spray

salt and freshly ground black pepper

handful of freshly chopped coriander (cilantro), to serve

1 lemon, sliced into wedges, to serve

Even non-vegetarians will love this delicious vegetarian traybake. It's made with tasty roasted vegetables in a homemade piri piri spice mix, all finished off with some seasoned grilled halloumi for a simple one-tray dinner for the whole family.

1. Preheat the oven to 220°C/200°C fan/425°F/gas 7 and line a baking tray with baking paper.

2. Place the sweet potato chunks and red onion in the prepared tray. Scatter over 1 tablespoon of the piri piri seasoning and drizzle over the olive oil, then toss to coat. Bake for 20 minutes.

3. Remove from the oven and add the peppers and tomatoes. Toss to coat once more, then return to the oven for another 20 minutes.

4. Meanwhile, in a bowl, mix the remaining piri piri seasoning with the maple syrup, tomato purée and lemon juice. Add the halloumi and toss to coat.

5. Remove the tray from the oven and add the sweetcorn. Toss to combine, then place the halloumi slices on top of the vegetables. Spray with olive oil spray, then heat the grill to medium and place under the grill for 5–7 minutes until the halloumi is golden brown around the edges.

6. Season as needed with salt and freshly ground black pepper, then sprinkle with fresh coriander and serve with lemon wedges for squeezing.

Side suggestions:
This is delicious just as it is, but it can also be paired with some rice or homemade oven chips for a more filling meal.

Low-carb side suggestions:
Serve with some cauliflower rice or additional vegetables of your choice.

Swaps:
Don't like halloumi? Swap it for the protein of your choice, coating it in the same seasoning used in step 4 and adjust the cooking method to suit. You can also swap the sweet potato for butternut squash.

999 kcals
per serving

V

GF

KCALS
499

FAT
18.0g

SAT FAT
11.1g

CARBS
58.3g

SUGARS
35.5g

FIBRE
11.9g

PROTEIN
20.0g

SALT
2.67g

Breakfast Quesadillas

PREP TIME: 10 MINUTES   **COOK TIME: 35 MINUTES**   **SERVES: 4**

4 low-calorie tortillas
olive oil spray
2 low-calorie sausages,
   skin removed, or vegetarian
   sausages
1 small onion, finely diced
½ red (bell) pepper, finely
   diced
½ green red (bell) pepper,
   finely diced
2 spring onions (scallions),
   sliced
4 grape (baby plum
   tomatoes) or cherry
   tomatoes, diced
4 large eggs, whisked
60g (2oz) Cheddar, grated
salt and freshly ground
   black pepper

Side suggestions:
These are perfect just as they
are, or with a small serving
of avocado (30g/1oz per
person) and a couple of
tablespoons of your favourite
salsa.

Swaps:
Swap the sausage for bacon
or ham. You can also try
using different veg, such
as spinach: just be careful
that any veg you add is not
too wet, or it will make the
quesadillas soggy.

Gluten-free:
Use gluten-free wraps
and sausages.

My kids love breakfast quesadillas, but sometimes when you are making them for the whole family, it can be a bit time-consuming doing them one at a time on the stove. These yummy quesadillas are all baked together in the oven once the filling is done, so that you can all sit down for breakfast and enjoy them at the same time.

1. Preheat the oven to 200°C/180°C fan/400°F/gas 6.

2. Line a baking sheet with baking paper and spray with cooking oil spray. Arrange the tortillas on the tray and set aside.

3. Heat a frying pan over a medium–high heat and spray with olive oil spray. Add the sausages, onion and peppers and cook for a few minutes until browned and golden, breaking up the sausages into small pieces as you cook.

4. Season with salt and pepper, then add the spring onions and tomatoes and stir to combine.

5. Pour the eggs into the pan, gently mixing them into a scramble. Take care not to overcook them: you want the scramble to be slightly undercooked.

6. Divide the scramble mixture between the tortillas, placing it on one half of each. Divide the Cheddar over the top, then fold each tortilla so you have 4 semicircles. Spray with olive oil spray.

7. Place another baking sheet (base down) over the top of the tortillas, then bake for 20 minutes. Remove the top tray and bake for an additional 4–5 minutes until the quesadillas are crisp and golden.

8. Slice each one in in half and enjoy!

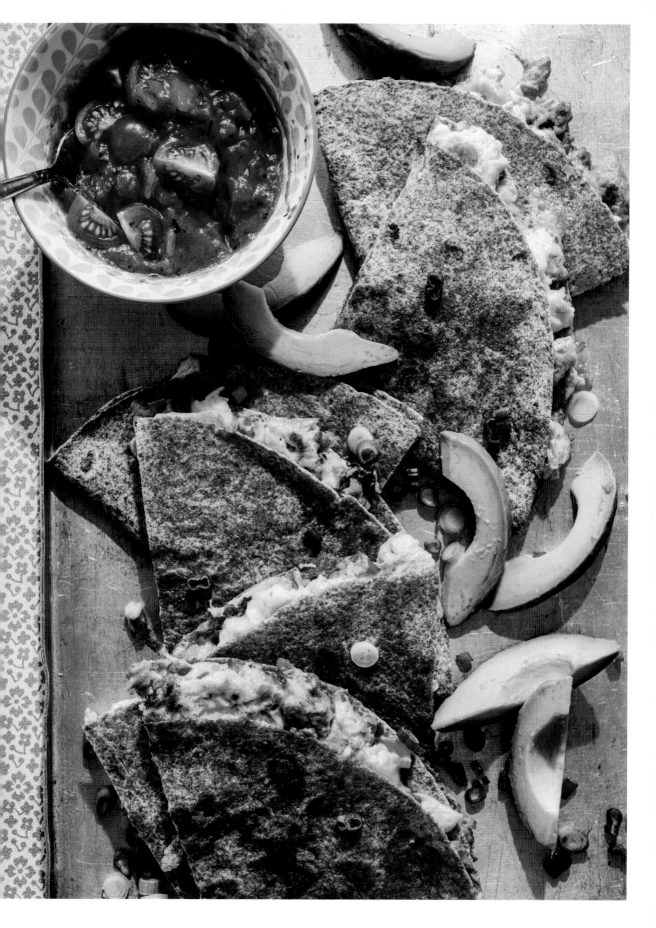

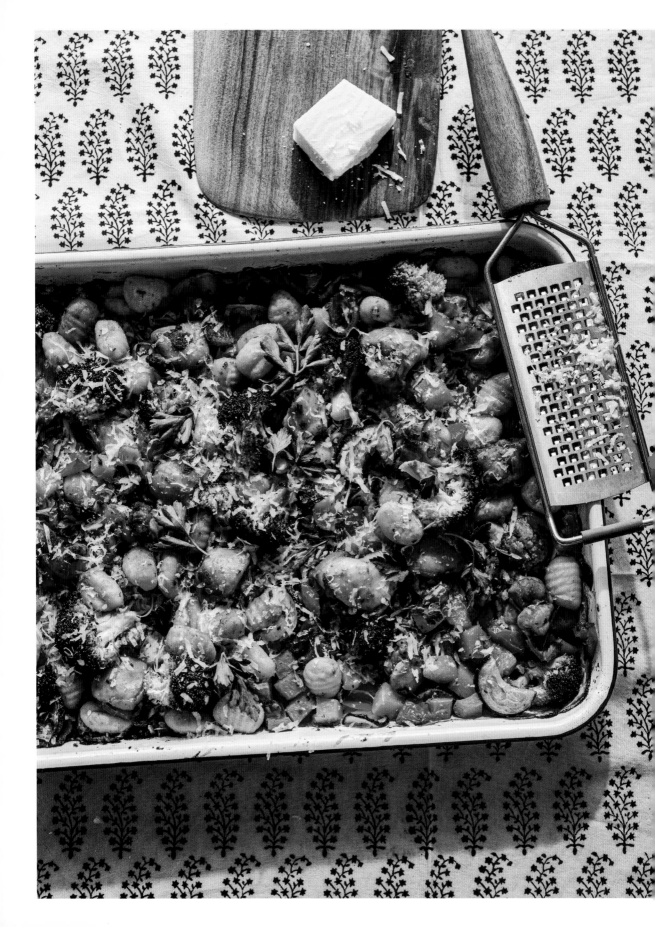

Chicken, Vegetable and Gnocchi Traybake

PREP TIME: 15 MINUTES   **COOK TIME: 35 MINUTES**   **SERVES: 4**

olive oil spray

600g (1lb 5oz) boneless, skinless chicken thighs, halved

1 tablespoon tomato purée (paste)

1 teaspoon smoked paprika

1½ tablespoons Garlic and Herb Seasoning (page 280)

160g (5¾oz) broccoli florets

160g (5¾oz) carrots, halved and thinly sliced

160g (5¾oz) butternut squash, cubed

1 red (bell) pepper, cubed

1 green (bell) pepper, cubed

1 red onion, chopped

1 small courgette (zucchini), halved lengthways and sliced

10 cherry tomatoes, halved

2 teaspoons extra virgin olive oil

400g (14oz) fresh gnocchi

salt and freshly ground black pepper

60g (2oz) Parmesan or Cheddar, grated, to serve

freshly chopped parsley, to serve

Gluten-free:
Use gluten-free gnocchi.

If you have only ever tried gnocchi boiled in a pan, you are missing out. Oven-baked gnocchi is amazing: golden, crispy and delicious. Here, it's paired with smoky, seasoned pieces of chicken and tasty roasted veg.

1. Preheat the oven to 200°C/180°C fan/400°F/gas 6. Line a baking sheet with baking paper and spray with olive oil spray.

2. In a bowl, combine the chicken with the tomato purée, smoked paprika and half of the garlic and herb seasoning. Toss to combine and set aside to marinate while you prepare the vegetables.

3. Place all the veg in the prepared tray. Scatter over the remaining garlic and herb seasoning, and drizzle with the olive oil. Toss to combine, then spread out evenly across the tray. Place in the oven and bake for 10 minutes.

4. Remove the tray from the oven and add the gnocchi. Toss everything together, then make spaces among the veg and gnocchi for the chicken pieces and add them to the tray. Spray with olive oil spray, then season everything with salt and pepper.

5. Bake for another 25–30 minutes, until the chicken is cooked through, the veggies are tender and the gnocchi is golden on the edges.

6. Sprinkle over the Parmesan or Cheddar, along with some parsley, and serve.

KCALS	498
FAT	15.6g
SAT FAT	4.1g
CARBS	48.4g
SUGARS	12.7g
FIBRE	10.2g
PROTEIN	35.8g
SALT	2.74g

Honey Cajun Salmon with Succotash

PREP TIME: 10 MINUTES   **COOK TIME: 35 MINUTES**   **SERVES: 4**

GF

DF

KCALS	**421**
FAT	**20.4g**
SAT FAT	**3.8g**
CARBS	**20.6g**
SUGARS	**17.7g**
FIBRE	**5.1g**
PROTEIN	**36.2g**
SALT	**1.16g**

600g (1lb 5oz) salmon fillet
5 teaspoons Cajun Seasoning (page 281)
2½ tablespoons honey
1 tablespoon lime juice
1 small onion, diced
1 garlic clove, finely chopped
1 small courgette (zucchini), finely chopped
1 red (bell) pepper, finely chopped
1 green (bell) pepper, finely chopped
5 cherry tomatoes, quartered
olive oil spray
85g (3oz) frozen edamame, defrosted
85g (3oz) canned sweetcorn
salt and freshly ground black pepper
a few fresh basil leaves, to serve
lime wedges, to serve

Side suggestions:
This is delicious just as it is, or paired with potaotes or some rice like the seasoned rice on page 278. For a low-carb side you could serve it with some additional vegetables (see the low-carb sides on page 18).

Salmon is one of my favourite types of fish: it cooks super quickly and can easily be varied with different seasonings and sauces. In this recipe, the salmon is seasoned with a simple homemade Cajun mix and drizzled with honey for a delicious golden glaze. I've paired it with an oven-baked succotash. A perfect combination!

1. Preheat the oven to 200°C/180°C fan/400°F/gas 6 and line a baking sheet with baking paper.

2. Pat the salmon fillet dry with some paper towels, then rub it with 4 teaspoons of the Cajun seasoning. In a small bowl, mix the honey with the lime juice, just to loosen it a little, and brush this over the top of the salmon. Set aside.

3. Place the onion, garlic, courgette, peppers and tomatoes on one half of the prepared baking sheet. Sprinkle with the remaining 1 teaspoon of Cajun seasoning and a pinch of salt and pepper, then spray with olive oil spray and toss to coat. Place in the oven and bake for 20 minutes.

4. Remove from the oven and add the edamame and sweetcorn to the veg mixture and toss again. Place the salmon on the other half of the tray and season with salt and pepper, then spray with olive oil spray.

5. Return the tray to the oven for another 12–15 minutes until the salmon is cooked through. (If you prefer, you can finish this off under the grill for the last couple of minutes, just to make the top of the salmon a little more golden, but incorporate this into the 12–15 minutes' cooking time, otherwise the fish will be overcooked.)

6. Scatter the succotash with the fresh basil leaves, then serve the salmon, with lime wedges on the side for squeezing.

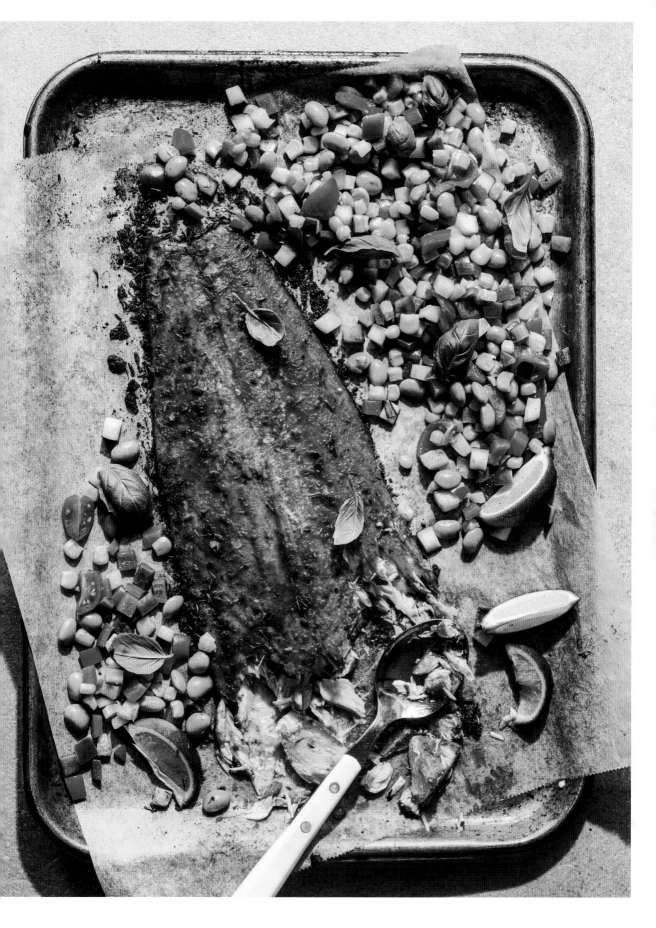

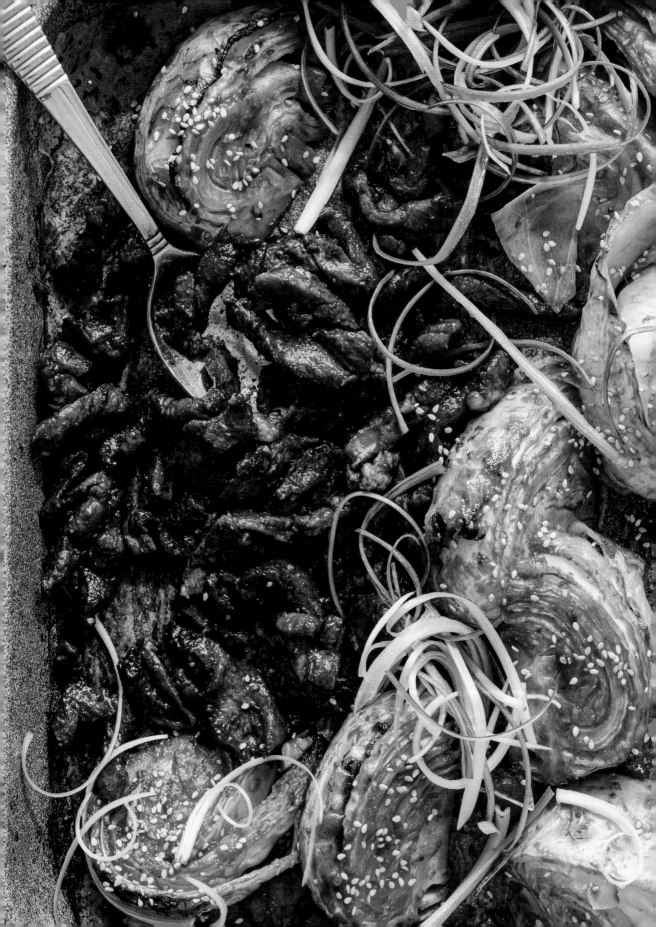

Korean Barbecue Pork with Spicy Gochujang Cabbage Wedges

272 kcals per serving

PREP TIME: **10 MINUTES + MARINATING**   COOK TIME: **35 MINUTES**   SERVES: **4**

500g (1lb 2oz) pork shoulder steaks (trimmed of visible fat), very thinly sliced
1 small green cabbage, sliced into 8 wedges
olive oil spray
2 spring onions (scallions), sliced, to serve
pinch of toasted sesame seeds, to serve

For the barbecue marinade
80g (2¾oz) fresh ripe pear, chopped
1 tablespoon light brown sugar
2 tablespoons light soy sauce
2 tablespoons dark soy sauce
3 garlic cloves
1 teaspoon grated fresh ginger
1 teaspoon sesame oil
2 spring onions (scallions)

For the spicy gochujang marinade
2 tablespoons gochujang
1 teaspoon sesame oil
½ tablespoon maple syrup
1 garlic clove, crushed

Side suggestions:
Delicious served with rice.

Low-carb side suggestions:
Pair with cauliflower rice, or serve with stir-fried vegetables, like carrots, beansprouts and mushrooms.

Over the past couple of years, I've really been enjoying cooking Korean food. I love the amazing combinations of flavours you get in Korean dishes, and it's great experimenting with different ingredients to make my own recipes. Here is my take on Korean barbecue in a simple traybake, where I've paired the pork with some spicy cabbage wedges. It's perfect just as it is, or with some additional sides of your choice. The pork needs at least 4 hours to marinate, so bear that in mind when you're planning your meals.

1. Combine all the barbecue marinade ingredients in a mini food-processor and pulse until smooth.

2. Transfer to a bowl and add the pork, tossing to coat. Leave to marinate in the fridge overnight or for at least 4 hours.

3. When you're ready to cook, preheat the oven to 220°C/200°C fan/425°F/gas 7 and line a baking tray with baking paper.

4. In a bowl, mix together all the ingredients for the gochujang marinade, along with 1 tablespoon water.

5. Arrange the cabbage wedges on one half of the prepared baking tray and brush with the marinade. Spray with olive oil spray and bake for 15 minutes.

6. Remove the tray from the oven and add the pork and its marinade to the other side of the tray. Spread it out in a thin, even layer and spray with olive oil spray. Return to the oven and bake for 20 minutes until the pork is cooked and slightly golden around the edges. (If you like, you can place it under the grill for a couple of minutes at the end, just to slightly char the edges of the meat.)

7. Sprinkle the spring onions over the pork and scatter the sesame seeds over the cabbage, then serve and enjoy!

KCALS
272

FAT
9.1g

SAT FAT
2.7g

CARBS
18.0g

SUGARS
14.6g

FIBRE
3.6g

PROTEIN
27.7g

SALT
2.54g

Southwestern Beef Potato Traybake

PREP TIME: 10 MINUTES   **COOK TIME: 40–45 MINUTES**   **SERVES: 4**

GF

KCALS	**458**
FAT	**13.8g**
SAT FAT	**7.0g**
CARBS	**43.1g**
SUGARS	**11.6g**
FIBRE	**11.4g**
PROTEIN	**34.6g**
SALT	**1.91g**

600g (1lb 5oz) russet potatoes, skin on
olive oil spray
1 teaspoon paprika
½ teaspoon onion powder
½ teaspoon salt
1 onion, sliced
1 red (bell) pepper, sliced
1 green (bell) pepper, sliced
400g (14oz) 5% fat beef mince (ground beef)
2 tablespoons Taco Seasoning (page 281)
100ml (3½fl oz) passata
1 tablespoon tomato purée (paste)
1 ripe tomato, diced
150g (5½oz) canned black beans
150g (5½oz) frozen or canned sweetcorn
50g (1¾oz) Red Leicester, grated
50g (1¾oz) mozzarella, grated

To serve
2 spring onions (scallions), sliced
handful of fresh coriander (cilantro)
6 tablespoons reduced-fat soured cream

Note:
If you don't have a microwave, you can parboil the potatoes instead. Simply place in a pan of water and bring to the boil, then turn off heat and leave in the water for 5 minutes. Drain fully and then follow the recipe as above.

Optional add-ins:
Try adding some extra toppings, like chopped avocado or fresh tomatoes.

Get ready for the ultimate southwestern-style traybake: taco-seasoned beef, delicious golden potato cubes, peppers, onion, black beans and corn, all finished off with some melted cheese. I like to serve it with some soured cream. It makes a perfect sharing meal for the whole family.

1. Preheat the oven to 220°C/200°C fan/425°F/gas 7.

2. Microwave the potatoes on high for 5 minutes, then, once cool enough to handle, dice into cubes. Transfer to a bowl and spray with olive oil spray, then toss with the paprika, onion powder and salt.

3. Transfer the potato cubes to a baking tray. Add the onion and peppers and spray with olive oil spray, then bake for 20 minutes.

4. Meanwhile, in a bowl, mix together the mince and the taco seasoning, ensuring it's fully combined.

5. Remove the tray from the oven and push the potato-and-pepper mixture over to one half of the tray. Place a piece of foil on the empty half of the tray and crumble the mince on to the foil in a single layer, trying to spread it out evenly.

6. Return the tray to the oven for 8 minutes, or until the beef is cooked through and golden.

7. Add the passata and tomato paste to the beef and mix to combine, breaking up any big clumps of mince. Don't drain the juices: this is all flavour and stops the beef from becoming dry. Carefully lift up the foil holding the beef and remove it from the tray. Spread out the potatoes and peppers across the whole tray once more, then scatter with the browned seasoned beef, followed by the diced tomato, black beans, corn and cheese. Return to the oven for 8–10 minutes until the cheese is melted.

8. Scatter with the spring onions and coriander, and serve with the soured cream.

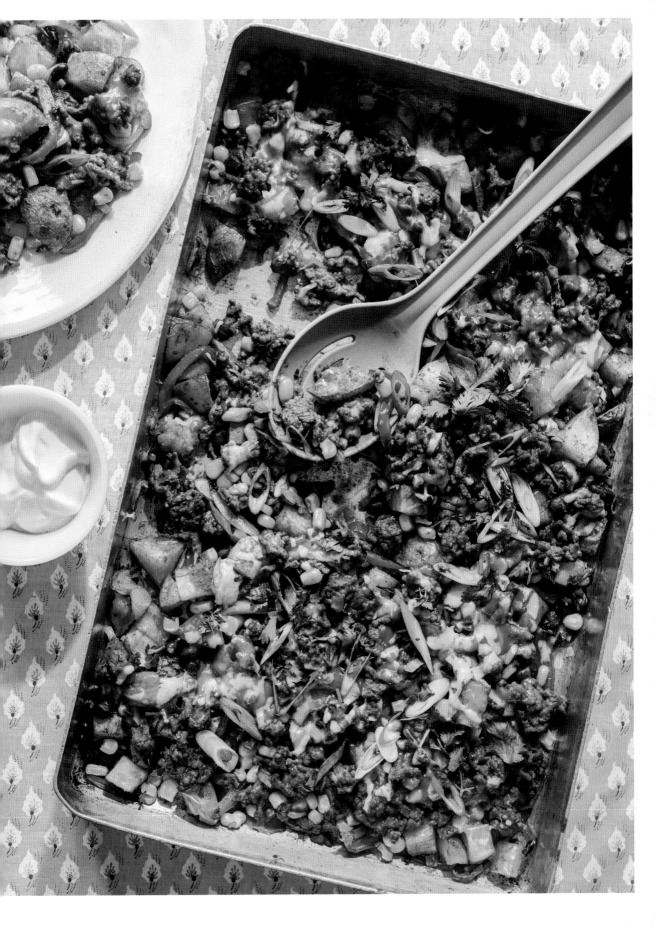

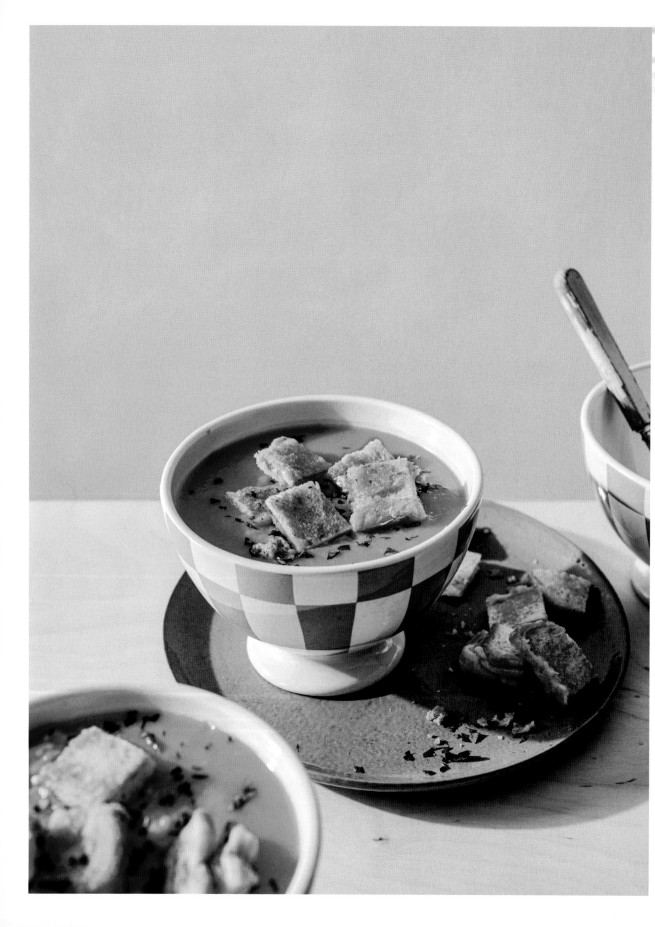

Roasted Vegetable Soup with Grilled Cheese Bites

PREP TIME: 15 MINUTES   **COOK TIME: 30 MINUTES**   SERVES: **4**

400g (14oz) sweet potatoes, peeled and cubed
250g (9oz) carrots, chopped
1 large onion, chopped
3 garlic cloves, peeled
1 large sweet apple, cored and chopped (no need to peel)
½ tablespoon extra virgin olive oil
720ml (24¾fl oz) vegetable stock
freshly chopped parsley, to serve
salt and freshly ground black pepper

For the grilled cheese bites
3 slices of low-calorie bread
60g (2oz) Cheddar, grated or sliced
olive oil spray

Variations:
There are so many variations you can do; it's a great way to use up any leftover veg lurking in your fridge. Just dump them all on a baking tray with some seasoning and roast until softened, then blend up with some hot stock and it's done.

Freezing:
Only the soup is freezer-friendly. To reheat after freezing, simply defrost in the fridge, warm through over a medium heat, and finish making the grilled cheese bites.

As a family, we absolutely love soup, but sometimes a plain old bowl of soup can be a little bit boring, and it doesn't always feel like a filling meal. So I always serve my soups with a delicious topping or little add-ons to keep things interesting, and this simple roasted vegetable soup with grilled cheese bites ticks all the boxes. The kids absolutely love it, too, and it's a great way to sneak some healthy vegetables into even the fussiest of eaters.

1. Preheat the oven to 220°C/200°C fan/425°F /gas 7 and line one large and one small baking tray with baking paper.

2. Place the sweet potatoes, carrots, onion, garlic and apple on the prepared large baking tray. Drizzle over the olive oil and season with salt and pepper, then toss to coat. Spread out into an even layer and roast for 30 minutes until the vegetables and apple are softened and caramelized at the edges.

3. Meanwhile, prepare the grilled cheese bites. Slice each slice of bread in half widthways, then and roll flat with a rolling pin. Divide the cheddar between three of the halves, then top with the other halves, so you have three half-sandwiches.

4. Spray the small lined baking tray with olive oil spray, then add the half-sandwiches and spray over the top.

5. Add the small tray to the oven for the last 16 minutes of the roasted vegetables' cooking time. Flip the sandwiches over after 8 minutes so they get golden on both sides.

6. Once the veggies are roasted, add them to a blender with 500ml (18fl oz) of the hot stock (always be careful when blending hot liquids!). Blend until smooth. Add more stock, a little at a time, until it reaches your desired consistency. Ladle the soup into four bowls.

7. Using a sharp knife, slice the grilled cheese sandwiches into smaller bites and divide these between the bowls of soup, floating them on top. Scatter over a little fresh parsley and season with salt and pepper to taste.

8. Enjoy!

KCALS	**294**
FAT	**8.2g**
SAT FAT	**3.8g**
CARBS	**41.6g**
SUGARS	**24.2g**
FIBRE	**9.7g**
PROTEIN	**8.6g**
SALT	**1.02g**

294 kcals per serving

Barbecue Chicken, Bacon and Ranch Loaded Fries

PREP TIME: **15 MINUTES**   COOK TIME: **55 MINUTES**   SERVES: **4**

KCALS
497

FAT
14.9g

SAT FAT
87.6g

CARBS
49.8g

SUGARS
14.1g

FIBRE
5.6g

PROTEIN
38.2g

SALT
2.10g

1kg (2.25lb) floury potatoes, sliced into chips
1 teaspoon paprika
olive oil spray
250g (9oz) cooked chicken, shredded (see Note)
3 cooked lean bacon medallions, chopped
100g (3½oz) Cheddar, grated
2 spring onions (scallions), chopped
1 batch Ranch Dressing (see Ranch Seasoning, page 280)
salt

For the barbecue sauce
120g (4¼oz) passata
1½ tablespoons maple syrup
1 tablespoon balsamic vinegar
½ tablespoon Worcestershire sauce
1 teaspoon dark soy sauce
1 teaspoon smoked paprika
1 teaspoon yellow American mustard
½ teaspoon garlic powder
½ teaspoon onion powder

As a family, we love building different variations on loaded fries, and this has to be our favourite. It's so easy to make and a great way to use up any leftover chicken you may have. Homemade oven-baked chips, tender cooked chicken tossed in easy homemade barbecue sauce, topped with melted cheesy goodness and a homemade ranch yogurt dressing. What's not to like? Simple but delicious! We love it paired with a mixed crisp salad.

1. Preheat the oven to 220°C/200°C fan/425°F/gas 7 and line a large baking tray with baking paper.

2. Place the chips in a large saucepan of boiling water. Bring to the boil, then turn off the heat and leave to sit in the water for 3 minutes.

3. Drain the chips and blot dry with a clean towel, then transfer them to the prepared baking tray. Scatter over the paprika and season with salt, then spray with olive oil spray and toss to coat. Spread out in an even layer to ensure even cooking, and bake for about 45 minutes until golden, flipping over halfway through and giving them another spray of olive oil.

4. Meanwhile, make the barbecue sauce. Place all the ingredients in a small saucepan over a high heat and just bring to the boil, then simmer for 10 minutes. Remove from the heat, add the cooked chicken and stir to ensure it is all coated.

5. Once the chips are cooked, remove from the oven and scatter the barbecue chicken over the top. Sprinkle over the cooked bacon, followed by the grated Cheddar. Return the tray to the oven for 8–10 minutes until the cheese is melted.

6. Sprinkle with the chopped spring onions and drizzle with the ranch dressing, then serve and enjoy.

Variation:
If you prefer, you can use your favourite shop-bought low-calorie barbecue sauce.

Side suggestions:
I serve these with a big mixed salad. You can choose some of your favourite salad items – we like crisp romaine, cucumber, red onion, tomatoes and shredded carrot.

Note:
If you don't have any leftover cooked chicken, just add some boneless, skinless chicken breasts to a pan of stock and boil until cooked through, then roughly shred.

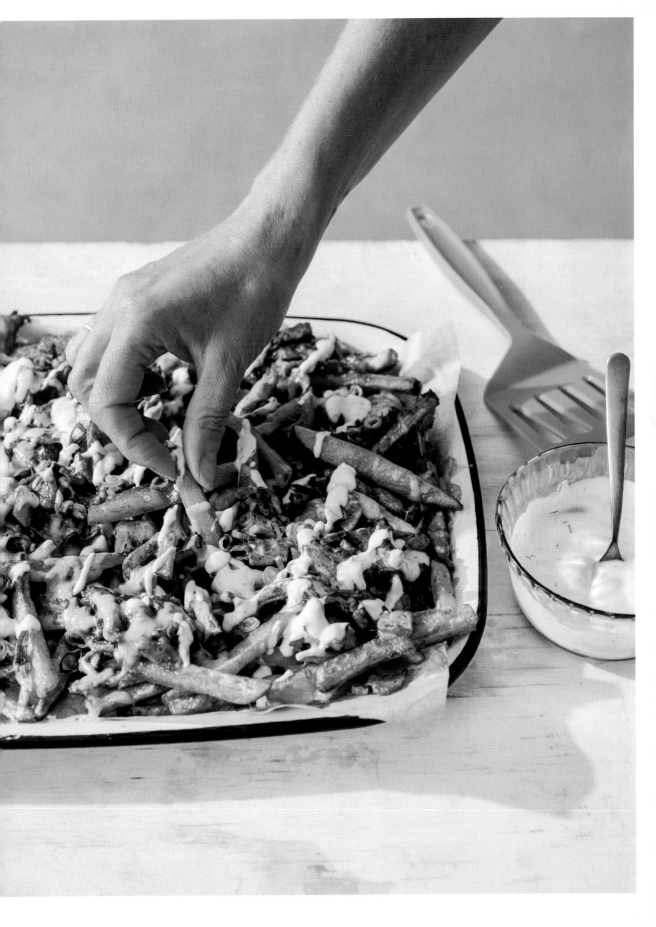

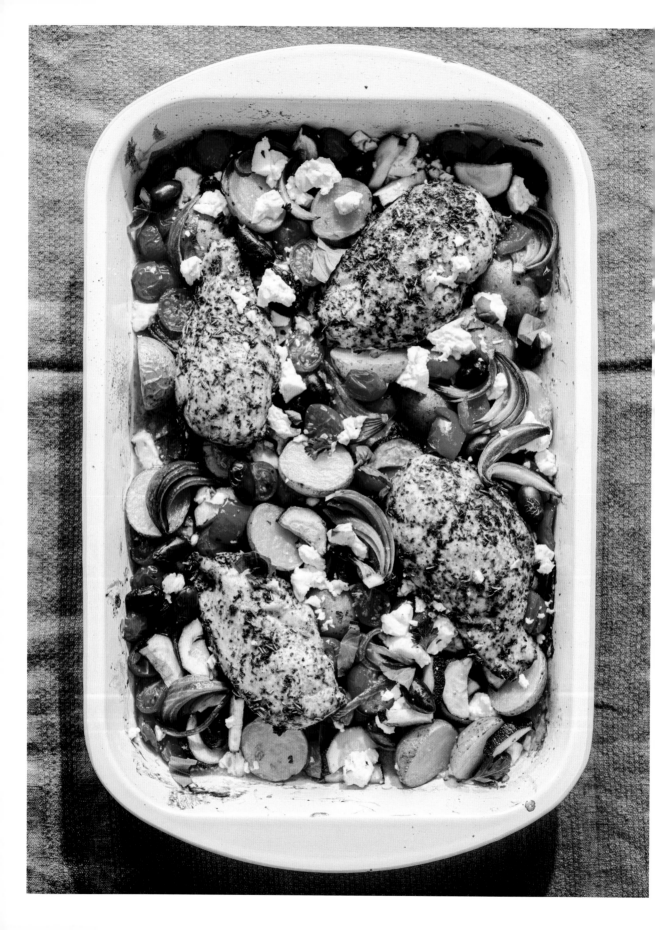

Greek Chicken Tray Bake

PREP TIME: **10 MINUTES**   COOK TIME: **45 MINUTES**   SERVES: **4**

GF

4 boneless, skinless chicken breasts (approx. 175g/6oz)
400g (14oz) baby potatoes, halved
1 red onion, chopped
½ teaspoon garlic powder
½ teaspoon onion powder
olive oil spray
1 red (bell) pepper, chopped
300g (10½oz) cherry tomatoes, halved
300g (10½oz) courgettes (zucchini), halved lengthways, then sliced
100ml (3½fl oz) chicken stock
24 pitted kalamata olives (black olives)
100g (3½oz) feta, crumbled
salt and freshly ground black pepper
fresh basil and parsley, to serve
lemon wedges, to serve

For the marinade
1 tablespoon extra virgin olive oil
1 garlic clove, crushed
1 teaspoon dried oregano
1 teaspoon dried rosemary
1 teaspoon dried parsley
½ teaspoon dried thyme
½ teaspoon sweet paprika
¾ teaspoon salt
½ teaspoon black pepper

Enjoy all your favourite Greek flavours with this delicious and easy traybake: tender seasoned chicken breast, baby potatoes, peppers, onion and tomatoes, all finished off with some salty, creamy feta and kalamata olives. It can transport you to the Greek islands any night of the week. If you have time, marinate the chicken the day before, so it can take on all the flavours of the herbs.

1. Place the chicken breasts in a bowl or dish with all the marinade ingredients and mix to ensure it's well coated. Leave to marinate in the fridge overnight if you can; if not, just let it marinate while you're preparing the other ingredients.

2. When you're ready to cook, preheat the oven to 200°C/180°C fan/400°F/gas 6 and line a large baking tray with baking paper.

3. Spread out the potatoes and onion on the prepared baking tray, then sprinkle with the onion and garlic powders. Spray with olive oil spray and toss to coat, then spread out once more and bake for 20 minutes.

4. Remove the tray from the oven and add the pepper, tomatoes and courgette. Pour over the chicken stock and toss to coat, then season with salt and pepper and spread out in an even layer once more. Make 4 spaces among the vegetables and place a chicken breast in each one. Return the tray to the oven and bake for 20 minutes.

5. Remove from the oven and add the olives and feta, then bake for an additional 5 minutes. The chicken should be cooked through.

6. Sprinkle the traybake with fresh parsley and basil and serve with fresh lemon wedges for squeezing. Enjoy!

KCALS
493

FAT
21.0g

SAT FAT
6.8g

CARBS
26.0g

SUGARS
9.4g

FIBRE
6.7g

PROTEIN
46.7g

SALT
2.45g

Panko-Parmesan Pork Loin Chops with Lemon and Garlic Shredded Brussels

PREP TIME: **20 MINUTES**   COOK TIME: **25 MINUTES**   SERVES: **4**

KCALS	**351**
FAT	**14.7g**
SAT FAT	**5.2g**
CARBS	**12.6g**
SUGARS	**3.7g**
FIBRE	**6.4g**
PROTEIN	**38.9g**
SALT	**0.70g**

olive oil spray
1 medium egg
1½ teaspoons Dijon mustard
4 pork loin chops, trimmed of visible fat (approx. 125g/4½oz each)
40g (1½oz) panko breadcrumbs
¾ teaspoon paprika
30g (1oz) Parmesan, grated
½ teaspoon onion powder
½ teaspoon garlic powder
salt and freshly ground black pepper

For the lemon and garlic Brussels
400g (14oz) Brussels sprouts
½ tablespoon olive oil
zest and juice of ½ lemon
3 garlic cloves, crushed
½ teaspoon onion powder

Side suggestions:
This is great as it is, but if you fancy a side, try it with mashed potatoes, roast potatoes or rice.

Low-carb side suggestions:
Cauliflower mash or any other vegetables of choice.

The amazing panko-Parmesan coating on these pork loin chops means the meat stays lovely and tender when baked in the oven. I've paired them with some truly delicious lemon and garlic shredded Brussels sprouts: it's a flavour sensation!

1. Preheat the oven to 200°C/180°C fan/400°F/gas 6.

2. Line a large baking tray with baking paper and spray with olive oil spray.

3. In a shallow dish, whisk together the egg and mustard. Add the pork chops and ensure they are well coated in the mixture.

4. On a large plate, combine the panko breadcrumbs with the paprika, Parmesan, onion and garlic powders, along with a pinch of salt and pepper.

5. Add the egg-and-mustard-coated pork loins to the panko mixture and turn to ensure they are fully covered.

6. Transfer to one half of the prepared baking tray. Sprinkle any excess breadcrumbs left on the plate on the top of the pork chops and pat down to secure.

7. To prepare the sprouts, remove their hard stems and slice each one in half, then use a sharp knife to finely shred them.

8. Add the shredded sprouts to a bowl with the olive oil, lemon zest and juice, garlic and onion powder. Season with salt and pepper, then toss to coat.

9. Spread out the Brussels sprouts on the other half of the tray, then spray the pork and Brussels with olive oil spray.

10. Place in the oven and bake for 20–25 minutes until the pork is golden and cooked through.

11. Serve and enjoy!

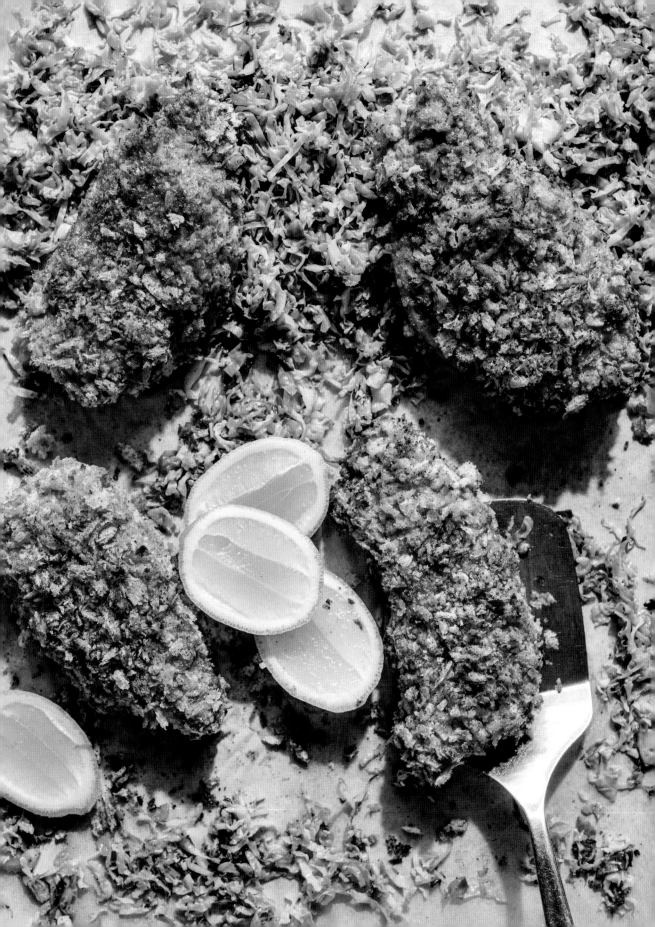

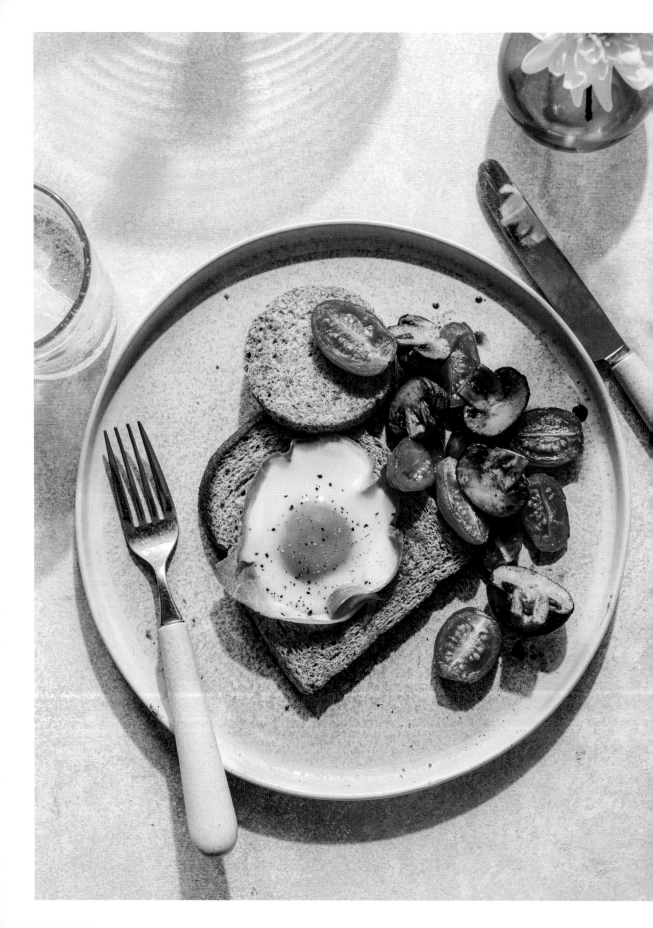

Egg-in-a-Hole with Balsamic Mushrooms and Tomatoes

PREP TIME: **5 MINUTES**   COOK TIME: **22 MINUTES**   SERVES: **4**

olive oil spray

4 slices of low-calorie bread (I used wholemeal)

250g (9oz) button mushrooms, halved

250g (9oz) cherry tomatoes, halved

½ teaspoon garlic powder

4 slices of lean ham

4 large eggs

1 tablespoon balsamic vinegar

salt and freshly ground black pepper

Optional add-ins:

These are great with a little grated Cheddar sprinkled on top of the eggs, and my kids also love these with some baked beans.

Vegetarian:

Omit the ham.

This is a fun yet effortless breakfast that the whole family can enjoy: a perfectly cooked egg made in the oven with crispy toast, tasty ham and delicious balsamic mushrooms and tomatoes. It's perfect for enjoying at the weekend; I love to have it with a freshly brewed pot of coffee.

1. Preheat the oven to 200°C/180°C fan/400°F/gas 6.

2. Line a large baking tray with baking paper and spray with olive oil spray.

3. Using a 7.5cm (3in) cookie cutter, cut a hole in each slice of bread. Place the bread and the cut-out circles on one half of the prepared baking tray.

4. Place the mushrooms and tomatoes on the other half of the tray. Sprinkle with the garlic powder and season salt and pepper. Spray with olive oil spray, toss to combine, then spread out in an even layer. Spray the bread with olive oil spray too, then place the tray in the oven and bake for 10 minutes.

5. Remove from the oven and flip the bread slices over (including the cut out bread circles). Place a slice of ham in each hole in the bread, then crack an egg into each one, so that the ham acts as a kind of bowl for the egg.

6. Drizzle the mushrooms and tomatoes with the balsamic vinegar, then return the tray to the oven for about 12 minutes until the eggs are cooked. (This should give you a soft yolk; if you prefer a firm yolk, cook for a further couple of minutes.)

7. Serve and enjoy!

187 kcals per serving

DF

KCALS
187

FAT
7.5g

SAT FAT
2.1g

CARBS
11.5g

SUGARS
3.6g

FIBRE
2.8g

PROTEIN
16.9g

SALT
0.92g

Bourbon Chicken with Vegetables

PREP TIME: 10 MINUTES   **COOK TIME: 30 MINUTES**   **SERVES: 4**

KCALS	**370**
FAT	**10.7g**
SAT FAT	**2.9g**
CARBS	**26.5g**
SUGARS	**21.3g**
FIBRE	**5.9g**
PROTEIN	**34.3g**
SALT	**1.72g**

olive oil spray
400g (14oz) broccoli, broken into small florets
125g (4½oz) carrots, sliced into thin sticks
600g (1lb 5oz) boneless, skinless chicken thighs, chopped into small pieces
1 tablespoon cornflour (cornstarch)
2 spring onions (scallions)
salt and freshly ground black pepper

For the Bourbon sauce
2 tablespoons Bourbon whiskey
60ml (4 tablespoons) apple juice
1 garlic clove, minced
1 teaspoon grated fresh ginger
2 tablespoons tomato purée (paste)
1 tablespoon apple cider vinegar
1½ tablespoons dark soy sauce
1½ tablespoons light soy sauce
3 tablespoons honey
½ teaspoon red chilli flakes (add more if you like additional heat)

Bourbon chicken is a delicious dish of tender pieces of chicken in a rich, Bourbon-infused marinade. It's popular in New Orleans and Louisiana, and can be found in the food court of any mall in America. My traybake version is probably one of the easiest recipes you could make, and it's a real crowd-pleaser. Just make the sauce, add the ingredients to a tray, and 30 minutes later, it's done.

1. Preheat the oven to 220°C/200°C fan/425°F/gas 7.

2. Line a large baking tray with baking paper and spray with olive oil spray.

3. Place the broccoli and carrots on one half of the prepared baking tray. Season with salt and pepper, then spray with olive oil spray. Toss to coat, then spread out in an even layer.

4. On the other side of the baking tray, use foil to make a 'boat'. Spray the foil with olive oil spray, then add the chicken and cornflour and toss to coat. Sprinkle with the chopped spring onions.

5. In a bowl, whisk together all the sauce ingredients with some freshly ground black pepper and 4 tablespoons water until well combined. Pour the sauce over the chicken, ensuring the sides of the 'boat' are high enough so the water doesn't leak out.

6. Bake for 30 minutes until the chicken is cooked, the sauce thickened and the broccoli and carrots tender.

7. Serve and enjoy!

Note:
If you prefer your broccoli softer, you can blanch in hot water prior to cooking.

Side suggestions:
Bourbon chicken is often served with white rice and any vegetables you like, so feel free to switch out the broccoli and carrot for something else if you prefer.

Low-carb side suggestions:
This would be perfect with some cauliflower rice.

Variation:
There isn't really a good substitute for that Bourbon flavour, but if you prefer not to use it, this is still equally tasty without.

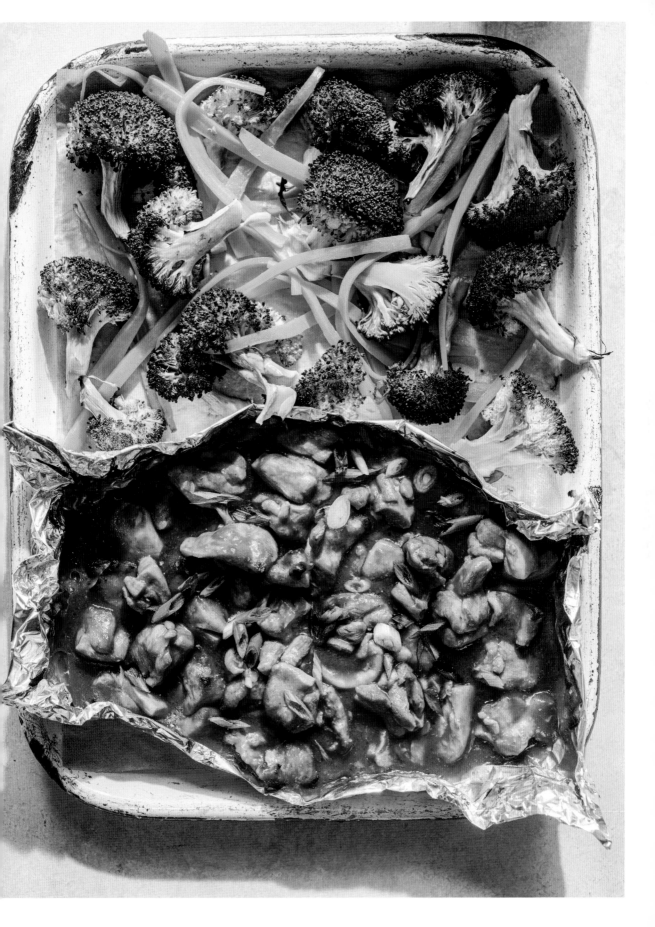

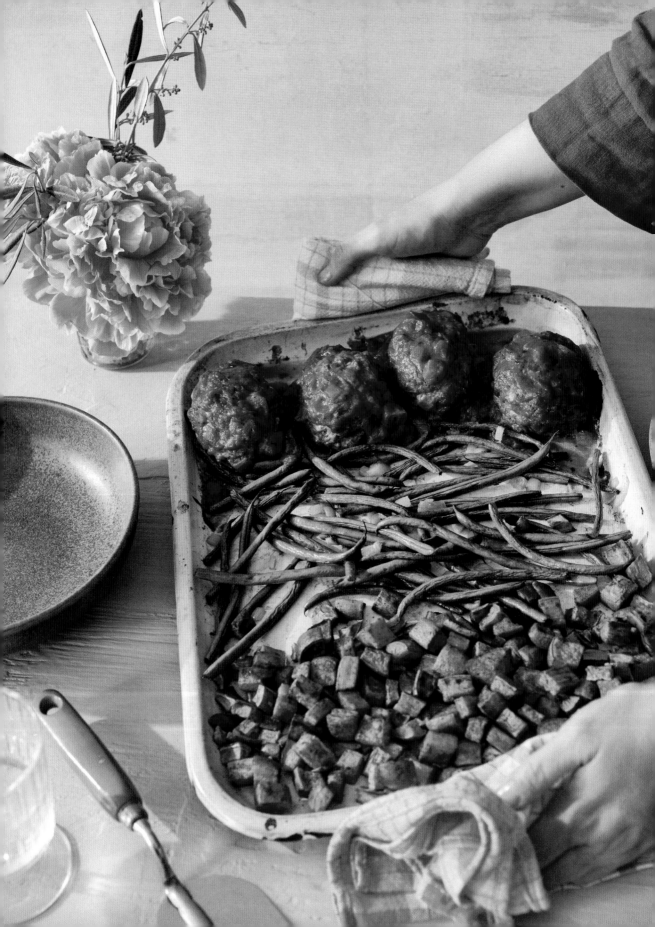

Salsa Meatloaves with Green Beans and Sweet Potato

PREP TIME: 15 MINUTES   **COOK TIME: 35 MINUTES**   **SERVES: 4**

500g (1lb 2oz) sweet potato, diced
olive oil spray
1 teaspoon paprika
350g (12oz) green beans, trimmed
½ small onion, finely diced
½ teaspoon garlic powder
salt and freshly ground black pepper

For the mini meatloaves
455g (1lb) 5% fat beef mince (ground beef)
30g (1oz) breadcrumbs
1 egg
70g (2½oz) Cheddar, grated
1 teaspoon paprika
½ teaspoon garlic powder
½ teaspoon onion powder
pinch of cayenne pepper (optional)
½ teaspoon salt
200g (7oz) shop-bought chunky salsa (mild or medium heat)
1 tablespoon tomato purée (paste)
1 tablespoon maple syrup

Swaps:
Swap the sweet potato for cubes of butternut squash for a lower-carb option.

Gluten-free:
Use gluten-free breadcrumbs.

Freezing:
Only the meatloaves are freezer-friendly. Defrost fully before reheating.

In this fun take on a traditional meatloaf, everyone gets their own miniature one. The mini meatloaves are made with beef mince, Cheddar and seasonings, all topped with chunky, tangy salsa to really bring the flavours to life. It's all baked in the same tray with seasoned cubes of sweet potato and roasted green beans to create a delicious family dinner in just one tray.

1. Preheat the oven to 220°C/200°C fan/425°F/gas 7 and line a baking tray with baking paper.

2. Place the sweet potato in the prepared baking tray. Spray with olive oil spray, then sprinkle with the paprika and a pinch of salt. Toss to coat, then spread out on the tray and bake for 10 minutes.

3. Meanwhile, in a large bowl, mix together the mince, breadcrumbs, egg, Cheddar, paprika, garlic powder, onion powder, cayenne (if using) and salt until well combined.

4. Remove the baking tray from the oven and push the sweet potato cubes to one side so they're taking up a third of the tray. Spray them with olive oil spray once more.

5. Add the green beans and onion to the middle of the tray, and sprinkle with garlic powder and a pinch of salt and pepper. Spray with the oil spray and toss to coat.

6. Divide the meatloaf mixture into four equal-sized balls and form each ball into a mini meatloaf shape. Spray the final third of the baking tray with olive oil spray, then place the meatloaves on it.

7. In a bowl, mix the salsa with the tomato purée and maple syrup, then spoon this mixture over the meatloaves.

8. Return the tray to the oven and bake for 20–25 minutes until the meatloaves are cooked through and the vegetables tender.

9. Arrange on four plates and enjoy!

456 kcals
per serving

KCALS
456

FAT
15.1g

SAT FAT
7.0g

CARBS
41.5g

SUGARS
22.0g

FIBRE
8.6g

PROTEIN
34.3g

SALT
1.52g

Cornflake Halibut with Garlic Potatoes, Leeks, Courgette and Peas

PREP TIME: 20 MINUTES   **COOK TIME: 50 MINUTES**   **SERVES: 4**

KCALS
349

FAT
6.1g

SAT FAT
2.6g

CARBS
36.7g

SUGARS
4.3g

FIBRE
7.3g

PROTEIN
33.1g

SALT
0.63g

For the potatoes

600g (1lb 5oz) potatoes, peeled and diced
¾ teaspoon garlic powder
½ teaspoon onion powder
1 teaspoon dried mixed herbs
olive oil spray
salt and freshly ground black pepper

For the minty leeks, courgette and peas

2 small leeks, halved lengthways, then sliced
1 courgette (zucchini), halved lengthways, then sliced
1 garlic clove, crushed
100ml (3½fl oz) chicken stock
1 tablespoon white wine vinegar
300g (10½oz) can marrowfat peas
a few fresh mint leaves, chopped

For the fish

4 cod fillets (approx. 140g/5oz each), or a similar white fish
1 egg, beaten
50g (1¾oz) cornflakes, crushed
1 tablespoon salted butter melted
½ tablespoon freshly chopped parsley

To serve

lemon wedges (optional)

This all-in-one traybake is a decadent take on your typical fish and chips – and so easy to make, too. Garlicky herbed potatoes, delicious leeks, courgette and peas with mint, and beautifully golden cornflake-topped cod: what more could you want?

1. Preheat the oven to 220°C/200°C fan/425°F/gas 7 and line a baking tray with baking paper.

2. Place the potatoes on the prepared tray. Scatter over the garlic powder, onion powder, mixed herbs and a good pinch of salt and pepper, then spray with olive oil spray and toss to coat. Spread the potatoes out on the tray and bake for 20 minutes.

3. Meanwhile, use a piece of foil to make a 'boat' and fill it with the leeks, courgette, garlic, stock and white wine vinegar. Toss to coat, then season with salt pepper and spray with olive oil spray.

4. Remove the baking tray from the oven and push the potatoes over to take up a third of the tray. Place the foil boat in the middle of the tray, then return to the oven for 15 minutes.

5. Meanwhile, season the fish all over with salt and pepper, then place in a bowl with the beaten egg, making sure the fish is well coated.

6. In a bowl, mix the crushed cornflakes with the butter and fresh parsley.

7. Remove the baking tray from the oven. Add the peas to the leeks and courgette and stir to combine.

8. Place the fish pieces on the remaining space on the tray and top each one with some of the cornflake mix, pressing it down slightly. Spray with olive oil spray, then return the tray to the oven and bake for 12–15 minutes until the fish is cooked through and flakes easily (it may take slightly longer for thicker cuts of fish).

9. Just before serving, stir the mint into the leeks, peas and courgette, then season to taste with salt and pepper. Arrange the fish, chips and minty green veg on four plates and serve with lemon wedges (optional).

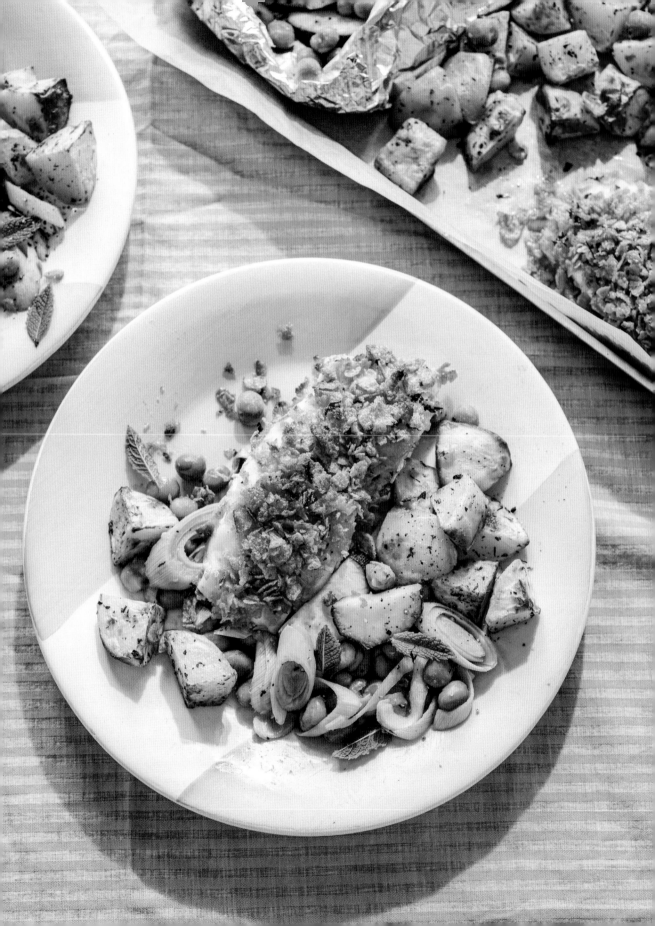

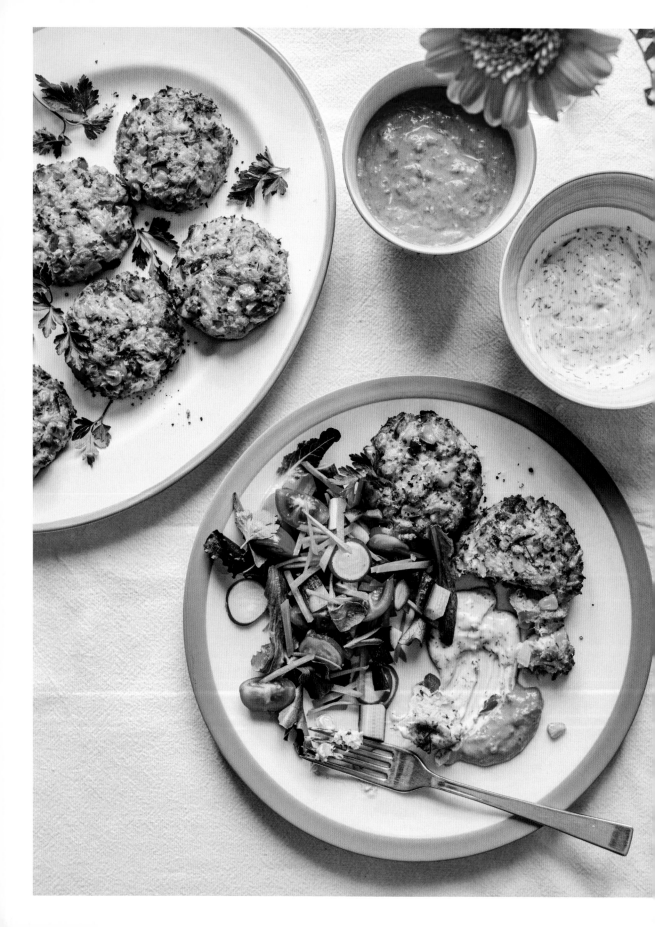

Salmon Patties with Two Dips

PREP TIME: 10 MINUTES   **COOK TIME: 25 MINUTES**   **SERVES: 4 (2 PATTIES PER PERSON)**

olive oil spray
1 small onion, finely chopped
⅓ red (bell) pepper,
   finely diced
⅓ green (bell) pepper,
   finely diced
1 tablespoon All-purpose
   Seasoning (page 280)
350g (12oz) cooked salmon,
   chilled
4 tablespoons fat-free
   Greek yogurt
1 tablespoon freshly chopped
   parsley
30g (1oz) panko breadcrumbs
4 tablespoons canned
   sweetcorn, drained
1 egg

For the lemon dill dip
3 tablespoons light
   mayonnaise
5 tablespoons fat-free
   Greek yogurt
1 tablespoon fresh lemon juice
1 teaspoon dried dill
1 garlic clove, crushed

For the spicy red pepper dip
125g (4½oz) roasted red
   peppers in brine, drained
1 garlic clove
6 tablespoons fat-free
   Greek yogurt
2 tablespoons light
   mayonnaise
pinch of cayenne pepper
½ tablespoon granulated
   sweetener

I love making patties like these with salmon. They're so quick and simple to make, and are perfect for lunch with a mixed salad. I like to use leftover cooked salmon for that fresher taste, but they can also be made with canned salmon if that's all you have on hand. The recipe makes eight mini patties, but if you prefer, you could make four bigger patties instead and serve them as burgers.

1. Preheat the oven to 200°C/180°C fan/400°F/gas 6. Line a baking tray with baking paper and spray with olive oil spray.

2. Heat the frying pan over a medium–high heat and spray with olive oil spray. Add the onion and peppers and fry for a couple of minutes until softened. Add the all-purpose seasoning and continue to fry for another minute.

3. Transfer the onion mixture to a large bowl. Flake in the salmon, then add the yogurt, parsley, breadcrumbs, sweetcorn and egg, and mix well to combine.

4. Grease your hands with olive oil spray and form the mixture into eight patties. Place the patties on the prepared baking tray and spray with olive oil spray. Bake for 20 minutes until golden, carefully flipping halfway through.

5. Meanwhile, make your chosen dip (or both!). For the lemon dill dip, just mix together all the ingredients in a bowl and season with salt and pepper.

6. For the roasted red pepper dip, squeeze the roasted red peppers to remove as much liquid as possible, then place in a blender with the garlic and half the yogurt. Blend until smooth, then stir in the remaining yogurt, along with the mayonnaise, cayenne pepper and sweetener.

7. Serve the fishcakes with your choice of dip.

Freezing:
Only the burger patties
are freezer-friendly.

Side suggestions:
Serve these patties with
a simple mixed salad.

Note:
The patties can be enjoyed
hot or cold and make a great
portable lunch.

365 kcals
per serving

**Salmon Patties
with Lemon
Dill Dip**

KCAL: **365**

FAT: **18.0g**

SAT FAT: **3.1g**

CARBS: **14.3g**

SUGARS: **7.1g**

FIBRE: **2.2g**

PROTEIN: **35.2g**

SALT: **1.07g**

379 kcals
per serving

**Salmon Patties
with Red
Pepper Dip**

KCAL: **379**

FAT: **17.1g**

SAT FAT: **3.0g**

CARBS: **18.6g**

SUGARS: **7.2g**

FIBRE: **2.1g**

PROTEIN: **36.7g**

SALT: **1.08g**

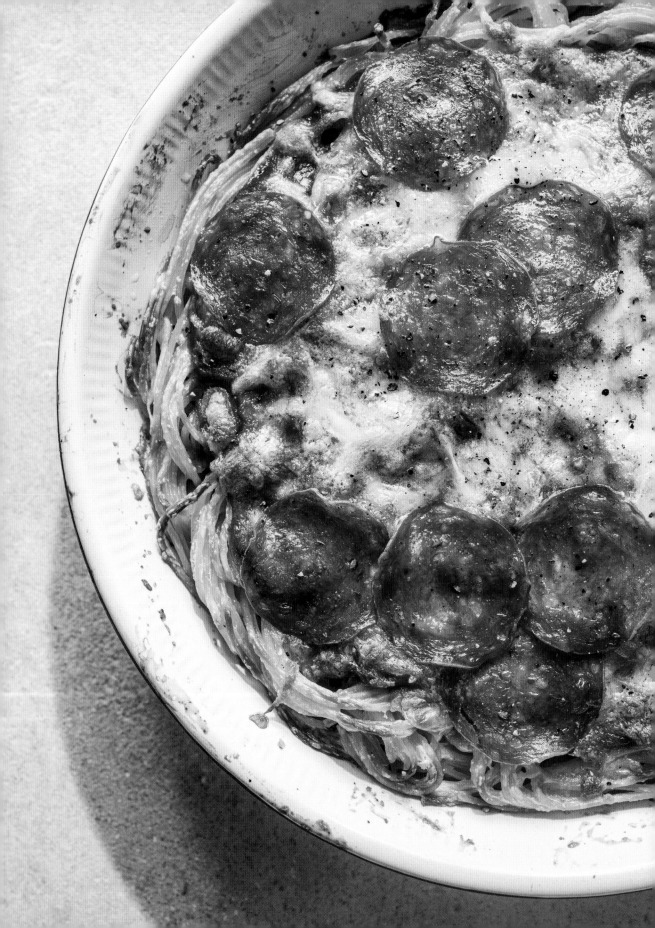

Made
Simple in
the Oven

Butternut Squash and Black Bean Enchilada Casserole

PREP TIME: **20 MINUTES**   COOK TIME: **35 MINUTES**   SERVES: **6**

KCALS	**383**
FAT	**13.6g**
SAT FAT	**5.3g**
CARBS	**44.7g**
SUGARS	**14.8g**
FIBRE	**11.1g**
PROTEIN	**14.8g**
SALT	**1.19g**

1 tablespoon olive oil
150g (5½oz) onions, finely diced
300g (10½oz) butternut squash, finely diced
1 tablespoon paprika
½ tablespoon ground cumin
1 teaspoon dried oregano
½ teaspoon onion powder
½ teaspoon garlic powder
½ teaspoon cayenne pepper
1 red (bell) pepper, diced
2 jalapeños, deseeded and diced
160g (5¾oz) canned sweetcorn
400g (14oz) can black beans, drained
6 low-calorie tortilla wraps
60g (2oz) Cheddar
50g (1¾oz) mozzarella

For the enchilada sauce
400g (14oz) passata
2 tablespoons tomato purée (paste)
120ml (4fl oz) vegetable stock
1½ tablespoons sweet paprika
2 teaspoons ground cumin
1½ teaspoons dried oregano
1 teaspoon onion powder
½ teaspoon garlic powder
½ teaspoon cayenne pepper
1 tablespoon cider vinegar
1 tablespoon maple syrup
salt and freshly ground black pepper

For the topping
1 spring onion (scallion), chopped,
1 ripe tomato, chopped,
handful of freshly chopped coriander (cilantro)
1 jalapeño, sliced
1 small avocado (70g/2½oz), chopped

This is a delicious vegetarian dish of seasoned butternut squash with black beans, sweetcorn and peppers, layered between tortilla wraps with an easy homemade enchilada sauce. It's all topped with cheese and baked in the oven until melted and invitingly golden.

1. Preheat the oven to 180°C/160°C fan/350°F/gas 4.

2. Heat the olive oil in a frying pan over a medium–high heat. Add the onions and fry for a couple of minutes until golden, then add the butternut squash and fry for a further few minutes until slightly caramelized.

3. Stir in the dried herbs and spices, then add the red pepper, jalapeño, sweetcorn and black beans. Continue to fry for a couple of minutes until well combined.

4. Meanwhile, place all the enchilada sauce ingredients in a saucepan over a medium heat. Season with salt and pepper and simmer for 15 minutes until thickened.

5. Spread a quarter of the sauce in a thin layer across the base of a 23 x 28cm (9 x 11in) casserole dish. Top with a third of the bean and butternut mixture, followed by two tortilla wraps, slightly overlapping them to fit. Top with another quarter of the enchilada sauce, then another third of the bean and butternut mixture, and two more tortilla wraps. Repeat once more, then finish with the remaining enchilada sauce. Top with the Cheddar and mozzarella, then cover with foil and bake for 20 minutes.

6. After 20 minutes, remove the foil and bake for a further 10–15 minutes until the cheese is melted and lightly golden.

7. Scatter over the toppings and serve.

Side suggestions:
This is delicious served with some reduced-fat soured cream and a mixed salad.

Variation:
If you're not vegetarian, some cooked shredded chicken added to the bean mix is delicious.

Freezing:
Freeze without the toppings.

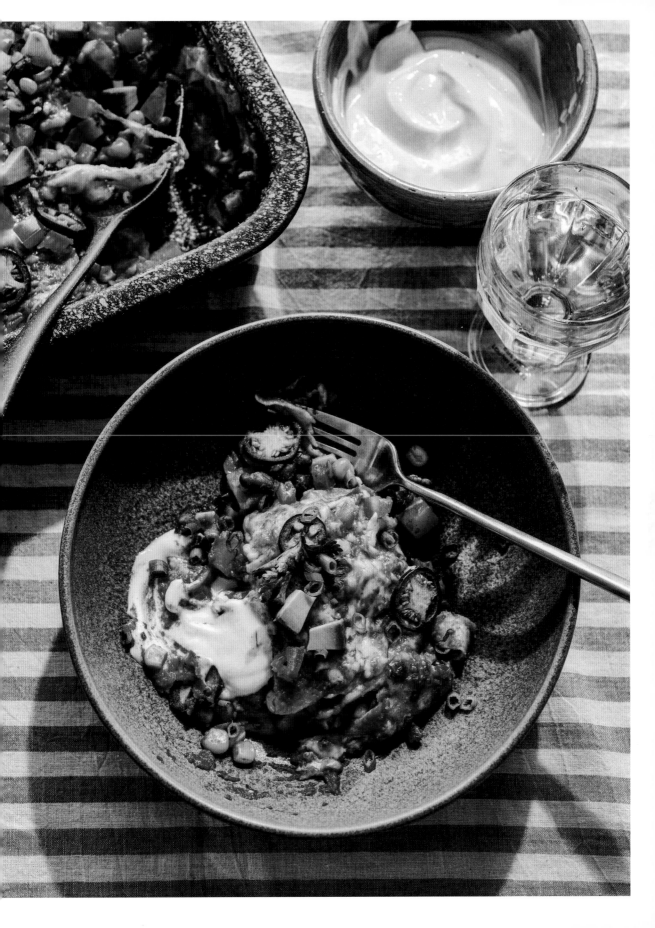

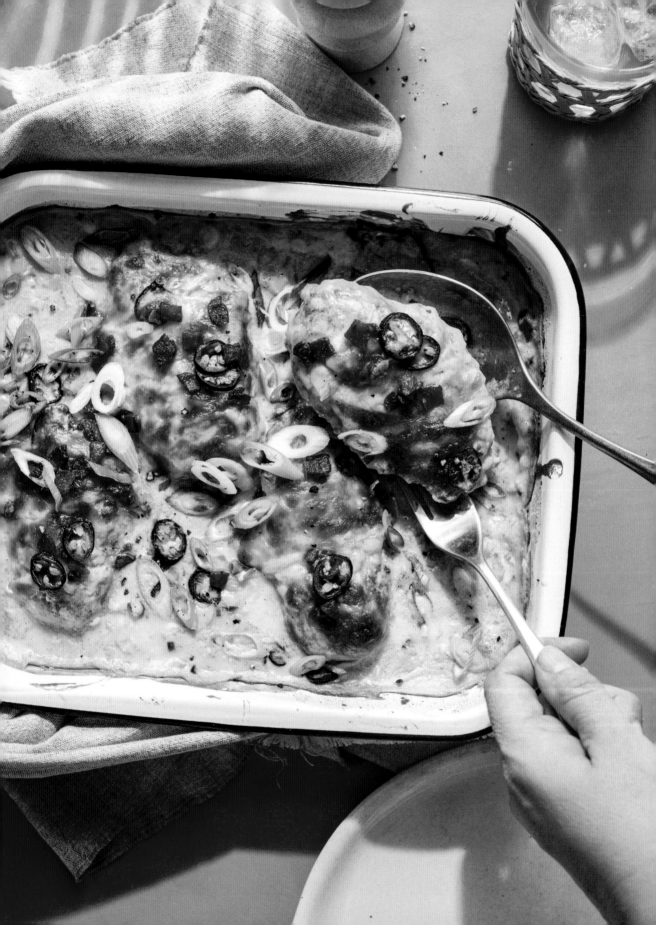

Cheesy Jalapeño Chicken Bake

PREP TIME: 15 MINUTES   **COOK TIME: 45 MINUTES**   **SERVES: 4**

437 kcals
per serving

4 boneless, skinless
  chicken breasts (approx.
  175g/6oz each)
¾ teaspoon coarse sea salt
½ teaspoon freshly ground
  black pepper
½ teaspoon paprika
½ teaspoon ground cumin
½ teaspoon garlic powder
½ teaspoon onion powder
olive oil spray
2 lean bacon medallions,
  diced
1 small onion, finely diced
2 jalapeños, 1 sliced,
  1 deseeded and finely diced
2 garlic cloves
125g (4½oz) canned
  sweetcorn
1 tablespoon freshly chopped
  chives
100g (3½oz) light cream
  cheese
250ml (9fl oz) chicken stock
1 tablespoon cornflour
  (cornstarch)
50g (1¾oz) Cheddar or
  Red Leicester, grated
50g (1¾oz) mozzarella,
  grated
1 spring onion (scallion), sliced

Side suggestions:
This is delicious with rice,
or potatoes cooked however
you like. For veggies, we like
steamed or roasted broccoli
or green beans.

This cheesy jalapeño chicken bake is one of my favourites to make, and it pairs well with so many different sides. Tender, seasoned chicken thighs in a creamy sauce, topped with Cheddar, mozzarella, golden bacon and jalapeños for that spicy kick. What's not to like?

1. Preheat the oven to 200°C/180°C fan/400°F/gas 6.

2. Place the chicken into a bowl and add the salt, pepper, paprika, cumin, garlic powder and onion powder. Toss to coat.

3. Heat a large, ovenproof frying pan over a medium–high heat and spray with olive oil spray. Add the bacon and fry for a few minutes until golden, then remove from the pan and set aside on a plate.

4. Add the chicken breasts to the empty pan and cook them for 2–3 minutes on each side until golden, then remove from the pan and set aside on a plate.

5. Add the onion and diced jalapeño to the pan and fry for 5 minutes until softened and the onion is lightly golden. Add the garlic and fry for a further minute, then add the sweetcorn, chives, cream cheese and stock.

6. In a small bowl or mug, mix the cornflour with a little water to make a slurry, then stir this into the pan until combined. Let it all bubble away for 5–6 minutes until the sauce thickens and the cream cheese is fully melted.

7. Once the sauce has fully thickened, return the chicken breasts to the pan, placing them on top of the sauce. Top the chicken with the Cheddar and mozzarella, followed by the jalapeño slices, then scatter over the bacon.

8. Transfer to the oven and bake for 20–25 minutes until the cheese is all melted and lightly golden and the chicken is cooked through. (If you prefer a more golden cheese topping, you can place it under the grill for a couple of minutes at the end.)

9. Remove from the oven and sprinkle with the chopped spring onion to serve.

KCALS
437

FAT
18.4g

SAT FAT
8.3g

CARBS
10.9g

SUGARS
5.0g

FIBRE
2.2g

PROTEIN
55.7g

SALT
2.73g

Harissa Meatballs with Whipped Feta

PREP TIME: **20 MINUTES**   COOK TIME: **30 MINUTES**   SERVES: **4**

KCALS	**442**
FAT	**17.2g**
SAT FAT	**7.9g**
CARBS	**25.4g**
SUGARS	**11.2g**
FIBRE	**6.4g**
PROTEIN	**43.2g**
SALT	**2.49g**

olive oil spray
1 onion, finely chopped
2 garlic cloves, finely chopped
120ml (4fl oz) chicken stock
400g (14oz) can chopped tomatoes
3 tablespoons tomato purée (paste)
½ teaspoonground cumin
1 teaspoon sweet paprika
2½ tablespoons harissa paste (adjust depending on how spicy you like it)
pinch of granulated sugar (optional)
200g (7oz) canned chickpeas

For the meatballs
500g (1lb 2oz) 5% fat beef mince (ground beef)
1 garlic clove, crushed
½ small onion, very finely diced
1 large egg
30g (1oz) breadcrumbs
1 teaspoon paprika
1 tablespoon freshly chopped parsley, plus extra to serve
1 tablespoon freshly chopped coriander (cilantro), plus extra to serve
¾ teaspoon salt
pinch of freshly ground black pepper
olive oil spray

For the whipped feta
120g (4¼oz) feta
80g (2¾oz) fat-free Greek yogurt
40g (1½oz) low-fat cream cheese
pinch of dried dill
pinch of dried oregano
1 garlic clove
juice of ½ lemon
½ teaspoon extra virgin olive oil
freshly chopped parsley, to garnish

This is an amazing flavour-packed dinner for the whole family that you can serve with a variety of different sides to keep things exciting. The spicy harissa tomato sauce goes brilliantly with the meatballs, but for the perfect finish, a dollop of salty, creamy whipped feta is a must!

1. Preheat the oven to 200°C/180°C fan/400°F/gas 6 and spray a baking dish with olive oil spray.

2. Begin by making the whipped feta. Place the feta, yogurt, cream cheese, dill, oregano, garlic and lemon juice into a mini food-processor and pulse until smooth and creamy. Transfer to a bowl and season with a little black pepper. Drizzle with the olive oil and garnish with the parsley.

3. In a large bowl, mix together all the meatball ingredients until well combined.

4. Spray your hands with olive oil spray and use them to form the meat mixture into 16 equal-sized meatballs. Place the meatballs in the prepared baking dish.

5. Scatter the finely chopped onion and garlic between the meatballs, then bake for 10 minutes.

6. Meanwhile, in a bowl, mix together the stock, tomatoes, tomato purée, cumin, paprika and harissa paste, along with the sugar (if using).

7. Remove the meatballs from the oven and pour the sauce over them. Mix well so all the meatballs are evenly covered, then add the chickpeas.

8. Bake for another 15–20 minutes until the sauce is thickened.

9. Sprinkle with fresh coriander or parsley and serve with the whipped feta.

Optional add-ins:
Sprinkle the meatballs with some pomegranate seeds for a sweet crunch.

Note:
The whipped feta also works well as a dip.

Freezing:
Only the meatballs are freezer-friendly.

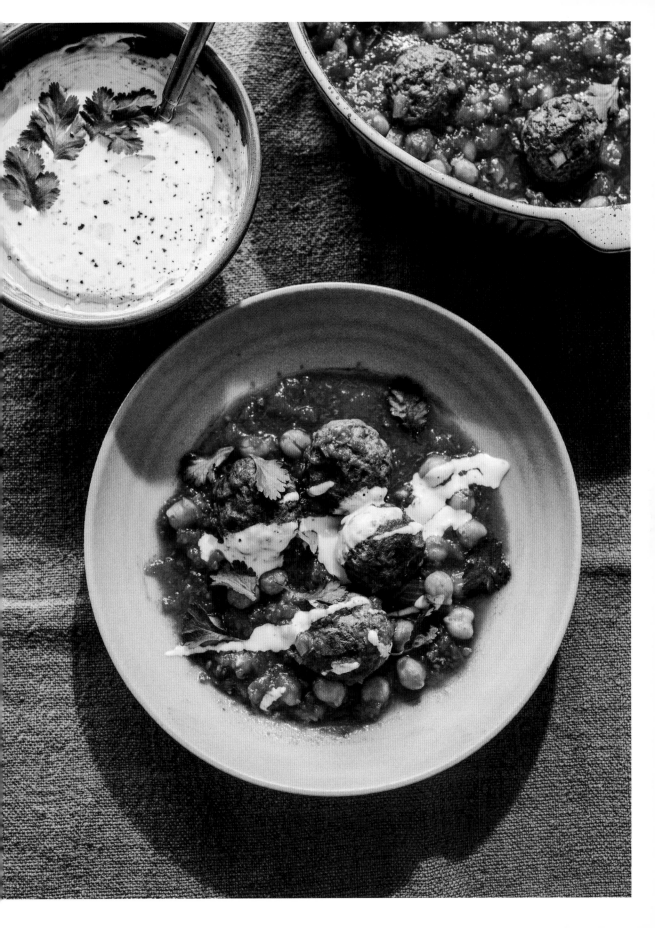

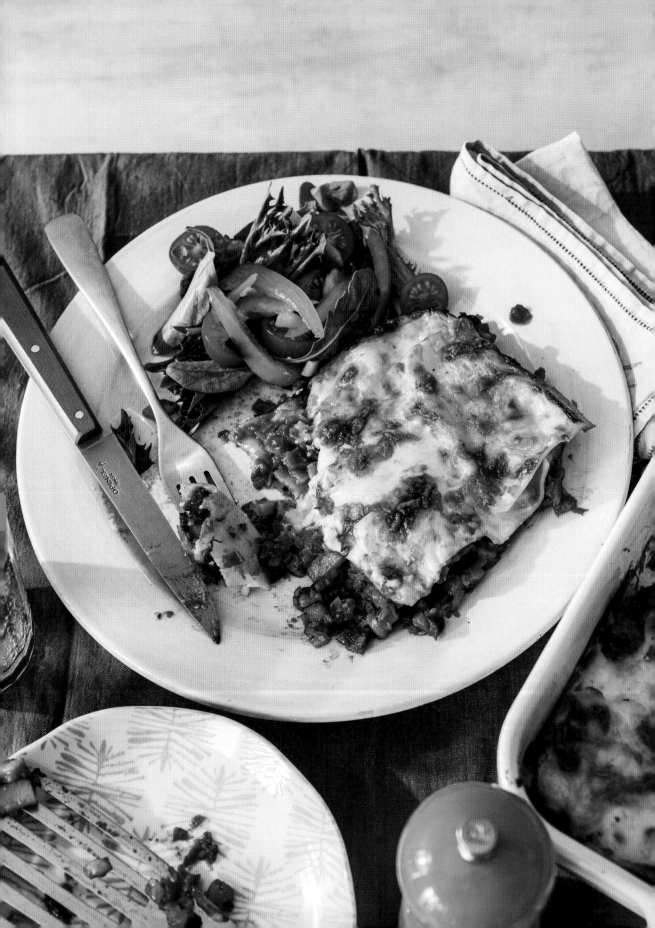

Ratatouille Lasagne

PREP TIME: **20 MINUTES**   COOK TIME: **55 MINUTES**   SERVES: **4**

438 kcals per serving

2 teaspoons extra virgin olive oil

1 large onion, finely diced

½ red (bell) pepper, diced

½ yellow or orange (bell) pepper, diced

200g (7oz) aubergine (eggplant), diced

200g (7oz) courgette (zucchini), diced

4 garlic cloves, crushed

400g (14oz) can chopped tomatoes

3 tablespoons tomato purée (paste)

5 basil leaves, chopped

1 tablespoon freshly chopped parsley

pinch of dried thyme

pinch of dried oregano

½ tablespoon maple syrup or granulated sweetener

6 dried lasagne sheets

50g (1¾oz) Cheddar, grated

50g (1¾oz) mozzarella, grated

salt and freshly ground black pepper

For the bechamel sauce

300ml (10fl oz) semi-skimmed milk

100ml (3½fl oz) vegetable stock

2 tablespoons cornflour (cornstarch)

½ teaspoon garlic powder

30g (1oz) Cheddar, grated

If you love ratatouille, just wait until you try this delicious meat-free lasagne. It's packed with healthy veggies, and has an amazing light bechamel sauce that is really easy to make and is my go-to topping when making a lasagne.

1. Preheat the oven to 180°C/160°C fan/350°F/gas 4.

2. Heat the olive oil in a large, deep frying pan over a medium–high heat. Once hot, add the onion, peppers, aubergine and a good pinch of salt and pepper and fry for about 7–10 minutes until really softened, stirring every now and then. Add the courgette and garlic and cook for another 2 minutes.

3. While the vegetables are cooking, you can make the bechamel sauce. Combine the milk, stock, cornflour and garlic powder in a saucepan over a medium heat and gently bubble until it thickens. Stir in the Cheddar until melted, then season with a pinch of black pepper and set aside.

4. Returning to the vegetables, add the chopped tomatoes, tomato purée, basil, parsley, thyme, oregano and maple syrup to the pan. Stir well and continue to simmer for about 5 minutes. Taste and season as needed with salt and pepper.

5. Pour half the ratatouille mixture into a 23cm (9in) square baking dish. Top with 3 lasagne sheets, then add the other half of the ratatouille mix. Top with the remaining lasagne sheets and pour over the bechamel sauce. Scatter over the Cheddar and mozzarella and bake for 30 minutes, then place under the grill for a couple of minutes to brown the top.

6. Remove from the oven and let the lasagne rest for about 10 minutes before slicing and serving.

Optional add-ins:

If you are not vegetarian, you can add some shredded cooked chicken to the ratatouille mix. Cooked sausage works well too.

KCALS **438**

FAT **13.7g**

SAT FAT **7.3g**

CARBS **55.4g**

SUGARS **18.3g**

FIBRE **7.2g**

PROTEIN **19.5g**

SALT **0.67g**

Oven-baked Poached Fish in Coconut Milk

PREP TIME: **8 MINUTES**   COOK TIME: **30 MINUTES**   SERVES: **4**

KCALS
237

FAT
8.9g

SAT FAT
6.6g

CARBS
10.2g

SUGARS
3.6g

FIBRE
2.1g

PROTEIN
27.9g

SALT
1.90g

1 small onion, finely chopped
3 garlic cloves, thinly sliced
1 red Thai chilli, thinly sliced
olive oil spray
1 lemongrass stalk, tough
    outer leaves removed,
    then halved and bashed
½ tablespoon grated
    fresh ginger
175g (6oz) baby pak choi,
    hard stems removed
    and leaves separated
400g (14oz) can light
    coconut milk
1 tablespoon cornflour
    (cornstarch)
1½ tablespoons fish sauce
4 white fish fillets, such as cod
    (approx. 140g/5oz each)
75g (2½oz) frozen peas
handful of freshly chopped
    coriander (cilantro)
salt and freshly ground
    black pepper
lime wedges, to serve

Swaps:
You can substitute the
lemongrass stalk for
1 teaspoon lemongrass
powder or 1 tablespoon
lemongrass paste.

I love recipes with coconut milk, and you will see it used frequently on Slimming Eats. It lends a beautiful creaminess to curries and is popular in Thai-style dishes. In this easy oven-baked recipe, white fish fillets are delicately poached with lemongrass, red chilli, pak choi and peas. The tender flaked fish in a beautiful coconut milk broth is perfect served over rice with lime wedges and coriander.

1. Preheat the oven to 200°C/180°C fan/400°F/gas 6.

2. Put the onion, garlic, and half of the Thai chilli into an ovenproof dish. Season with a pinch of salt and spray with olive oil spray, then bake for 10 minutes.

3. Remove from the oven and add the lemongrass, ginger and pak choi.

4. In a bowl, mix the coconut milk with the cornflour and fish sauce. Pour this mixture into the dish, ensuring the majority of the pak choi is submerged in the coconut milk.

5. Place the fish fillets into the sauce in the dish (they don't need to be fully submerged) and season with salt and pepper. Scatter in the peas, then loosely cover the dish with foil and bake for 20 minutes until the fish flakes easily.

6. Sprinkle with the remaining fresh chilli and some fresh coriander, and serve with lime wedges.

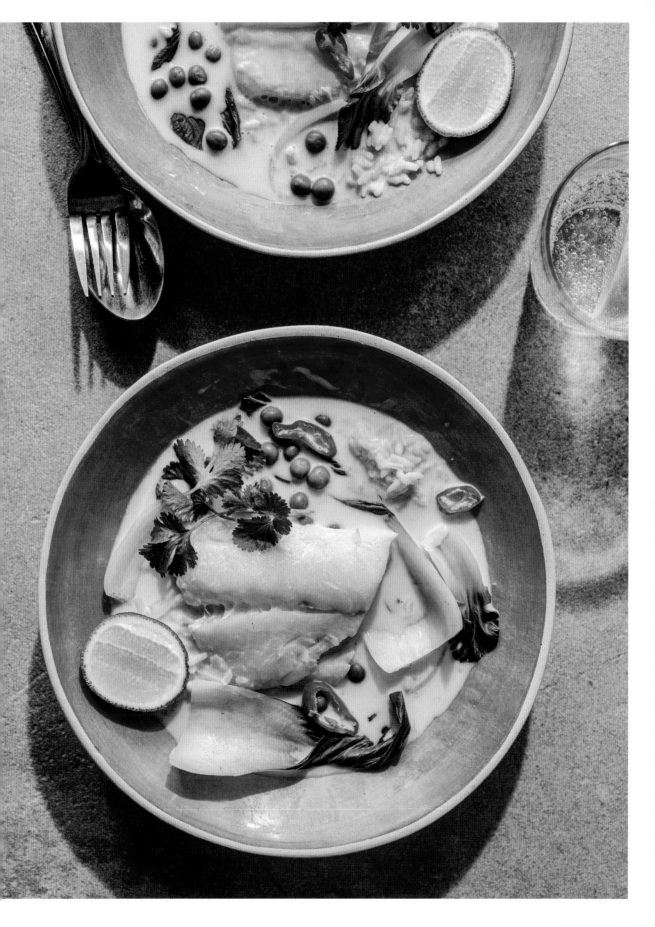

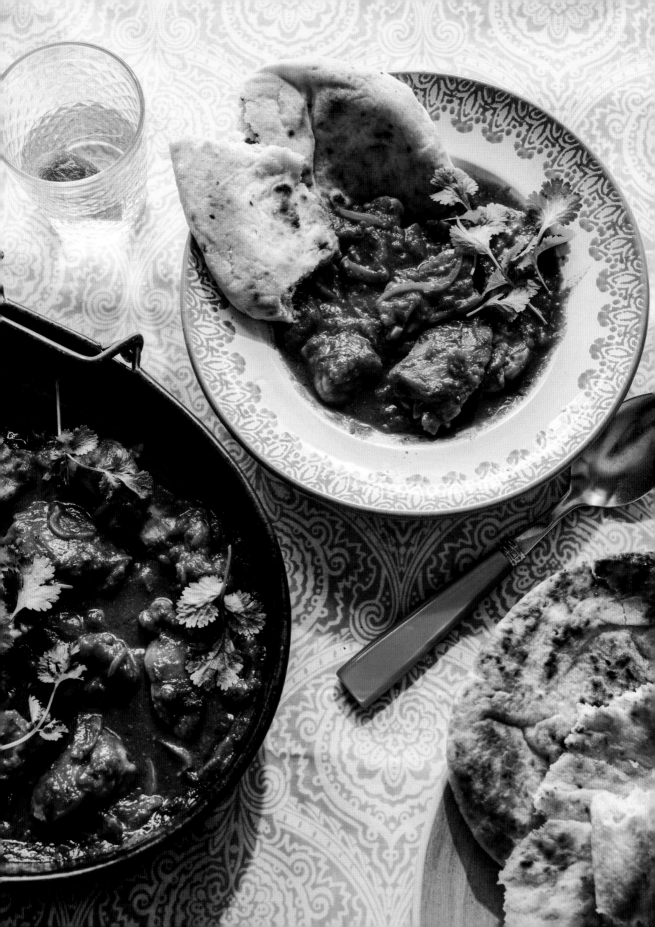

Baked Chicken Pathia

PREP TIME: **10 MINUTES**   COOK TIME: **35 MINUTES**   SERVES: **4**

olive oil spray

650g (23oz) boneless,
skinless chicken thighs,
trimmed of visible fat
and halved

1 large onion, thinly sliced

1 tablespoon grated
fresh ginger

4 garlic cloves, crushed

1½ teaspoons ground cumin

1½ teaspoons ground
coriander

1 teaspoon ground turmeric

1 teaspoon hot chilli powder

1½ tablespoons tomato
purée (paste)

400g (14oz) can plum
tomatoes

1 tablespoon tamarind paste

2 teaspoons light brown sugar

180ml (6fl oz) chicken stock

1 teaspoon dried fenugreek
leaves

1 fresh red chilli, halved
lengthways (optional)

juice of ½ small lime

salt and freshly ground
black pepper

freshly chopped coriander
(cilantro), to serve

Side suggestions:
Great served with rice or
naan bread, or for a low-
carb side serve with some
cauliflower rice.

Chicken pathia is a hugely popular curry, and it's easy to see why. It's a flavour explosion: sweet, spicy and tangy all at once. For my version of this delicious recipe, you simply prepare the base elements on the stove, then bake in the oven until the chicken is tender. A great recipe for a fake-away night.

1. Preheat the oven to 200°C/180°C/400°F/gas 6.

2. Heat a deep, ovenproof frying pan over a medium–high heat and spray with olive oil spray. Once the pan is nice and hot, add the chicken and a pinch of salt and pepper, and fry until the chicken is lightly golden all over. Remove from the pan and set aside on a plate.

3. Spray the empty pan with more olive oil spray, then add the onion and fry for about 4 minutes until really softened and golden. Add the ginger and garlic and fry for a further minute, then add the cumin, ground coriander, turmeric, chilli powder and tomato purée. Stir in a couple of tablespoons of water and cook until paste-like.

4. Add the plum tomatoes, breaking them up with the back of a wooden spoon, then stir in the tamarind paste, brown sugar, chicken stock and fenugreek leaves.

5. Once everything is well combined, return the chicken to the pan, ensuring the meat is coated in the sauce. Add the red chilli (if using), then transfer the pan to the oven and bake, uncovered, for 20–25 minutes until the chicken is cooked through and tender.

6. Squeeze in the lime juice and sprinkle with fresh coriander to serve.

7. Enjoy!

310 kcals per serving

GF

DF

KCALS
310

FAT
11.6g

SAT FAT
3.1g

CARBS
14.0g

SUGARS
12.0g

FIBRE
3.8g

PROTEIN
35.5g

SALT
0.55g

355 *kcals*
per serving

KCALS
355

FAT
12.4g

SAT FAT
3.5g

CARBS
19.5g

SUGARS
14.0g

FIBRE
5.0g

PROTEIN
38.8g

SALT
1.64g

Jamaican Chicken Stew

PREP TIME: **20 MINUTES + MARINATING**   COOK TIME: **50 MINUTES**   SERVES: **4**

8 boneless, skinless chicken thighs, trimmed of visible fat (approx. 720g/1lb 9oz)
olive oil spray
1 onion, sliced
1 tablespoon dark soy sauce
2 tablespoons tomato purée (paste)
1 tablespoon maple syrup
3 garlic cloves, finely sliced
½ tablespoon grated fresh ginger
2 spring onions (scallions), finely chopped
1 Scotch bonnet pepper (you can use jalapeño or another hot chilli if you can't get a Scotch bonnet), chopped
1 red (bell) pepper, sliced into thin strips
½ green (bell) pepper, sliced into thin strips
150g (5½oz) carrot, sliced
300ml (10fl oz) chicken stock
juice of 1 small orange
1 tablespoon cornflour (cornstarch)
fresh thyme, to serve

For the marinade
1 tablespoon dark soy sauce
1 teaspoon garlic powder
1 teaspoon smoked paprika
¾ teaspoon allspice
¾ teaspoon dried thyme
½ teaspoon freshly ground black pepper

If you love jerk chicken, you will love this Jamaican chicken stew: tender oven-baked chicken thighs in a rich gravy sauce with all those yummy Caribbean flavours. It's a delicious meal that you can enjoy with rice or potatoes.

1. Preheat the oven to 180°C/160°C fan/350°F/gas 4.

2. In a bowl, mix together all the marinade ingredients, then add the chicken and mix to cover. Leave to marinate for at least 30 minutes.

3. Heat an ovenproof frying pan or casserole dish over a medium–high heat and spray with olive oil spray. Add the chicken in an even layer and cook for a couple of minutes until deeply golden, then flip and repeat on the other side. Remove the chicken from the pan and set aside on a plate.

4. Add the onion to the empty pan and fry for a couple of minutes, then pour in a little water, just to deglaze anything stuck to the bottom of the dish. Continue to cook for a couple of minutes until softened and golden, then add the soy sauce, tomato purée, maple syrup, garlic, ginger, spring onions and Scotch bonnet. Continue to cook for a few minutes until everything is well softened.

5. Return the chicken to the pan, along with the peppers and carrot. Pour in the stock and juice. In a small bowl or mug, mix the cornflour with a little water to make a slurry, then stir this in as well.

6. Bring to a simmer, then cover with a lid and transfer to the oven. Bake for 20–25 minutes, then remove the lid and continue to bake, uncovered, for another 10 minutes.

7. Serve garnished with fresh thyme and enjoy.

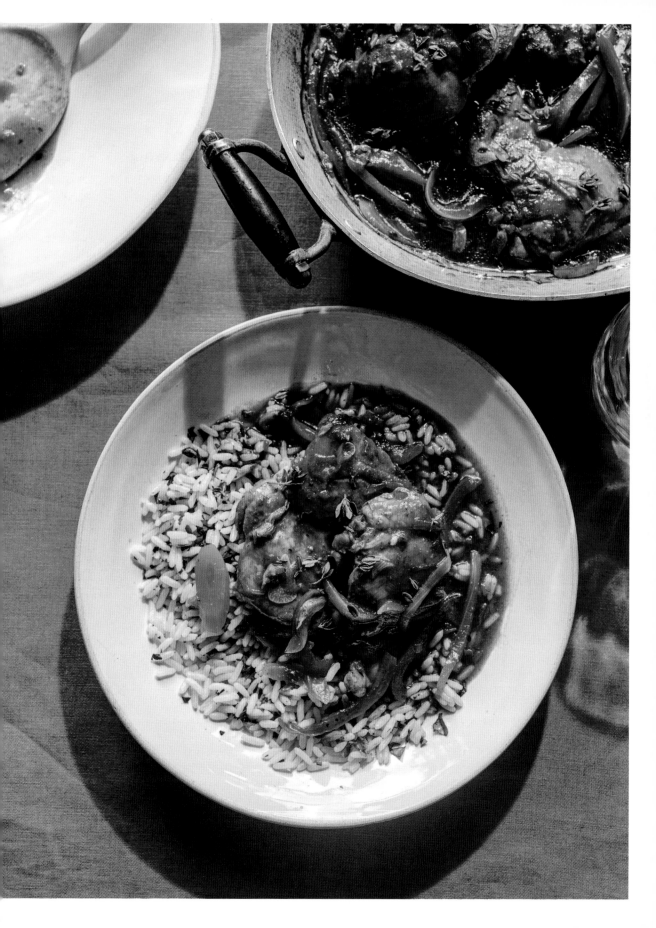

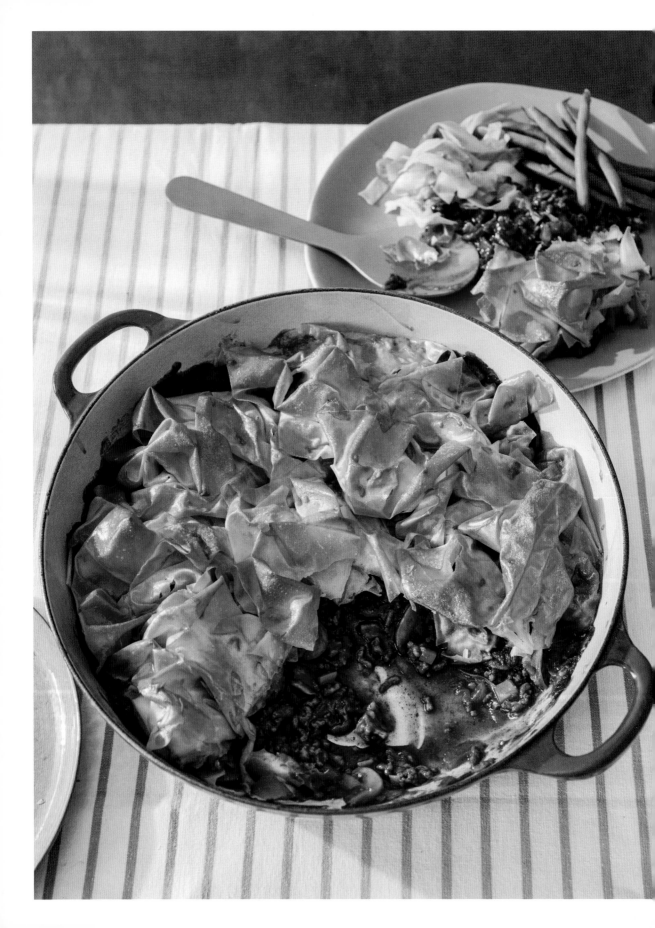

Marmite Minced Beef and Vegetable Filo Pie

PREP TIME: **15 MINUTES**   COOK TIME: **1 HOUR**   SERVES: **4**

379 kcals per serving

455g (1lb) 5% fat beef mince (ground beef)
1 large onion, diced
1 large carrot, peeled and chopped
1 celery stalk, chopped
2 garlic cloves, crushed
200g (7oz) mushrooms, sliced
2 tablespoons tomato purée (paste)
2 teaspoons Marmite
2 tablespoons balsamic vinegar
400ml (14fl oz) beef stock
2 tablespoons cornflour (cornstarch)
4 sheets of filo pastry
olive oil spray
1 large egg, beaten
freshly ground black pepper

Side suggestions:
I serve this with steamed greens, like broccoli or green beans.

Variation:
Stir a few of tablespoons cream cheese into the beef mixture for a creamy version of this pie.

Freezing:
Freeze the filling before topping with filo pastry and baking. Defrost fully before starting step 5.

My family love pies, and crispy golden filo pastry is a great lower-calorie alternative when it comes to pie toppings. This pie has a delicious filling of minced beef with mushrooms and carrots in a rich gravy flavoured with Marmite. It's great paired with some of your favourite vegetables for an easy family meal.

1. Preheat the oven to 200°C/180°C fan/400°F/gas 6.

2. Heat a large frying pan over a medium–high heat. Add the mince and cook for a couple of minutes until lightly browned, breaking it up with your spoon. Add the onion, carrot, celery, garlic and mushrooms, and continue to fry for another 5–6 minutes until the veg has softened.

3. Add the tomato purée, Marmite and balsamic vinegar and stir until coated. Season with a pinch of black pepper, then pour in the stock.

4. In a small mug or bowl, mix the cornflour with a little water to make a slurry, then stir this into the beef mixture. Bring to the boil, then simmer for 15–20 minutes until the gravy is thickened. Transfer to a baking dish.

5. Split the filo sheets in half so you have 8 sheets. Lightly spray each sheet with olive oil spray, then loosely screw into a rough ball and add to the top of the meat mixture until it is covered with the pastry. Brush the beaten egg over the top, then spray with olive oil spray and bake for 30 minutes until golden.

6. Enjoy!

KCALS	**379**
FAT	**8.8g**
SAT FAT	**3.1g**
CARBS	**37.9g**
SUGARS	**8.6g**
FIBRE	**5.1g**
PROTEIN	**34.5g**
SALT	**1.36g**

371 kcals
per serving

Pesto Caprese Chicken Bake

PREP TIME: 5 MINUTES   **COOK TIME: 35 MINUTES**   **SERVES: 4**

GF

❄️

KCALS
371

FAT
16.6g

SAT FAT
5.8g

CARBS
9.0g

SUGARS
7.9g

FIBRE
1.4g

PROTEIN
45.7g

SALT
0.77g

200g (7oz) cherry tomatoes, halved
2 garlic cloves, crushed
2 tablespoons good-quality aged balsamic vinegar
1 tablespoon maple syrup
olive oil spray
4 boneless, skinless chicken breasts (approx. 175g/6oz per breast)
4 tablespoons basil pesto
2 medium-sized tomatoes, sliced into 8 slices
100g (3½oz) mozzarella, grated or sliced
handful of fresh basil leaves, torn
salt and freshly ground black pepper

Side suggestions:

I love serving this with baby potatoes or roasted potato slices, but it's also great with a green salad, roasted green beans or asparagus, long-stem broccoli, grilled courgette (zucchini), spinach or corn on the cob.

Freezing:

The chicken is freezer-friendly without the mozzarella. Defrost the chicken fully before finishing step 4.

Tender, juicy chicken breasts topped with basil pesto, tomato slices and mozzarella, cooked on a bed of roasted balsamic tomatoes: this looks fancy, but is actually a super-simple bake you can whip up any night of the week. It's great served with potatoes or your choice of healthy vegetables.

1. Preheat the oven to 220°C/200°C fan/425°F/gas 7.

2. Place the cherry tomatoes into a baking dish, along with the garlic, balsamic vinegar and maple syrup. Toss to coat, then season with salt and pepper and spray with olive oil spray. Roast for 10 minutes.

3. Season the chicken breasts all over with salt and pepper. Once the tomatoes have been roasting for 10 minutes, remove from the oven and carefully place the chicken breasts on top. Spread 1 tablespoon of pesto over the top of each breast, then top each one with two slices of tomato. Spray with olive oil spray and return to the oven for 15 minutes.

4. Remove from the oven, and top each chicken breast with mozzarella, then return to the oven for another 8–10 minutes, or until the cheese is melted and the chicken is cooked through.

5. Spoon the balsamic tomatoes from the bottom of the dish over the top of the chicken and scatter with the torn basil.

6. Enjoy!

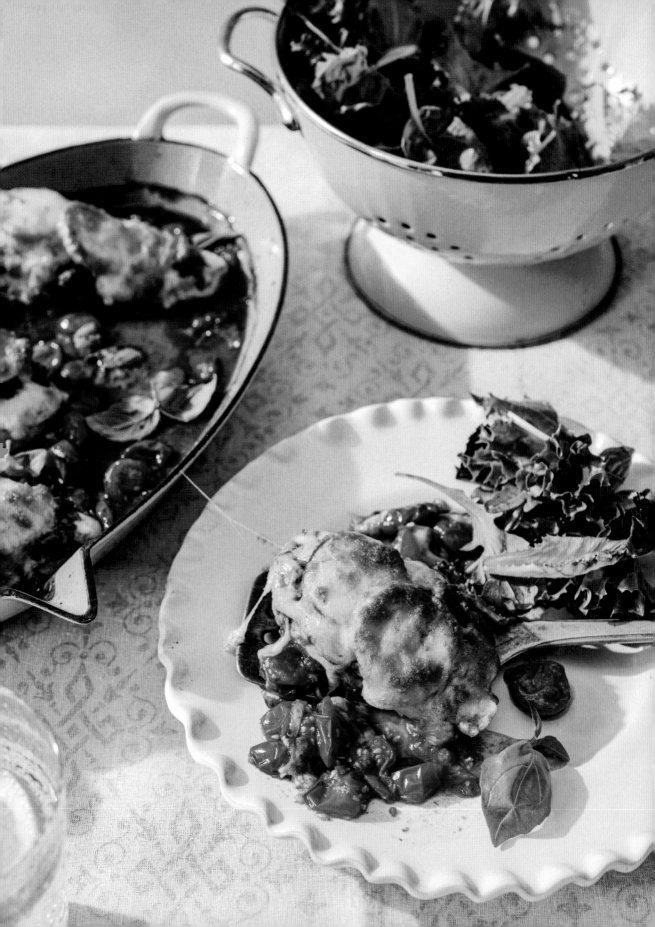

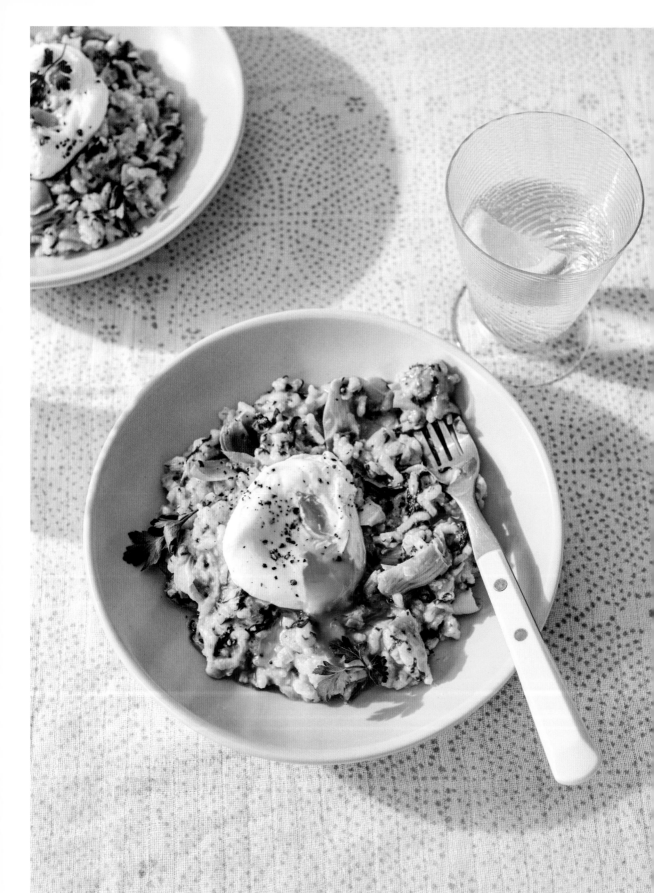

Oven-baked Spinach and Artichoke Risotto with Poached Eggs

PREP TIME: **5 MINUTES**   COOK TIME: **35 MINUTES**   SERVES: **4**

428 kcals per serving

olive oil spray
1 onion, finely chopped
4 garlic cloves, minced
200g (7oz) fresh spinach
400g (14 oz) can artichokes, drained
260g (9oz) arborio rice
1 tablespoon white wine vinegar
600ml (20fl oz) vegetable stock
2 tablespoons light cream cheese
50g (1¾oz) vegetarian Italian-style hard cheese (or use Parmesan if you're not vegetarian)
4 large eggs
salt and freshly ground black pepper

An effortless oven-baked risotto. No standing at the stove stirring constantly for this recipe which is baked in the oven in under 30 minutes. I love the combination of spinach and artichokes and the creamy soft yolk of the poached eggs creates an amazing sauce that compliments all the flavours.

1. Preheat the oven to 200°C/180°C fan/400°F/gas 6.

2. Heat an ovenproof frying pan over a medium–high heat and spray with olive oil spray. Add the onion and fry for a couple of minutes until golden and softened, then add the garlic and spinach and cook for another couple of minutes until the spinach has wilted.

3. Add the artichokes and arborio rice, and stir well to combine, then pour in the white wine vinegar and stock. Stir once more, then cover with a lid and transfer to the oven. Bake for 25 minutes until the rice is cooked and most of the stock is absorbed.

4. Remove from the oven and stir in the light cream cheese and vegetarian Italian-style hard cheese. Taste and season with salt and pepper, then cover and set aside to keep warm while you make the poached eggs.

5. Bring a saucepan of water to the boil, then reduce the heat so it's gently bubbling. Crack one egg into a small, shallow bowl. Lower the edge of the bowl into the water, then carefully tip the egg out. Repeat with the other eggs. Cook for about 3 minutes, then lift the eggs out of the water with a slotted spoon and carefully transfer to a piece of paper towel to absorb any excess water. Finally, serve up the risotto, and top each portion with a poached egg. Enjoy!

KCALS
428

FAT
10.7g

SAT FAT
4.2g

CARBS
60.6g

SUGARS
4.2g

FIBRE
5.2g

PROTEIN
19.6g

SALT
0.87g

V GF ❄

KCAL: **103**

FAT: **6.5g**

SAT FAT: **2.4g**

CARBS: **2.7g**

SUGARS: **0.8g**

FIBRE: **0.6g**

PROTEIN: **8.1g**

SALT: **0.41g**

**Tomato and
pesto muffins**

125 kcals
per serving

GF ❄

KCAL: **125**

FAT: **9.8g**

SAT FAT: **2.1g**

CARBS: **1.6g**

SUGARS: **1.4g**

FIBRE: **0.6g**

PROTEIN: **7.4g**

SALT: **0.44g**

**Bacon, Cheddar,
red pepper and
spring onion
muffins**

155 kcals
per serving

GF ❄

KCAL: **155**

FAT: **11.2g**

SAT FAT: **4.4g**

CARBS: **0.8g**

SUGARS: **0.7g**

FIBRE: **0.5g**

PROTEIN: **12.4g**

SALT: **0.98g**

Frittata Muffins – Three Ways

PREP TIME: **10 MINUTES**   COOK TIME: **25 MINUTES**   MAKES: **12 MUFFINS**

olive oil spray
10 large eggs
salt and freshly ground
   black pepper

**For the feta, spinach
and sweet potato frittata
muffins**

50g (1¾oz) sweet potato,
   peeled and grated
pinch of paprika
pinch of cayenne pepper
30g (1oz) feta cheese,
   crumbled
small handful of spinach
   leaves (approx. 10 leaves),
   roughly chopped

**For the tomato and pesto
frittata muffins**

8 cherry tomatoes, halved
3 tablespoons basil pesto

**For the bacon, Cheddar,
red pepper and spring
onion muffins**

3 slices of lean back bacon,
   cooked and diced small
   (or you can use ham)
4 tablespoons finely diced
   red (bell) pepper
2 spring onions (scallions),
   finely chopped
30g (1oz) Cheddar, grated

Variations:

If you want to make a whole
batch of just one variation,
simply triple the filling
ingredients – or why not try
experimenting with your own
flavour combinations?

**Whether you have them for breakfast, lunch or dinner, these
frittata muffins are great protein bites for the whole family to
enjoy. They're also handy if you're batch-cooking for the week
ahead. This recipe makes 12 frittata muffins with three different
add-ins, so you have a variety to choose from. They are perfect
for popping in a lunchbox to take to work with a salad.**

1. Preheat the oven to 180°C/160°C fan/350°F/gas 4.

2. Grease a 12-hole muffin tray with olive oil spray.

3. In a large bowl or jug, beat the eggs and season with a pinch
of salt and pepper.

4. Divide the egg mixture between all 12 muffin holes; you want
them to be a little over half full. They will rise as they bake, so
don't over-fill. Ten eggs is enough for my muffin tray, but some
may need more or less.

5. In a bowl, toss the grated sweet potato in the paprika and
cayenne, then add this to four of the muffin holes, along with
the feta and spinach leaves.

6. Add the tomatoes and pesto to the next four muffin holes.

7. Add the bacon, red pepper, spring onions and Cheddar to the
final four muffin holes.

8. Give each muffin hole a careful mix to ensure the fillings are
evenly distributed, then bake for 20–25 minutes, or until the eggs
are set. Remove from the oven and allow to cool slightly, then
remove from the muffin tray.

9. These muffins can then be enjoyed hot or cold, and will keep
in the fridge for 3–4 days.

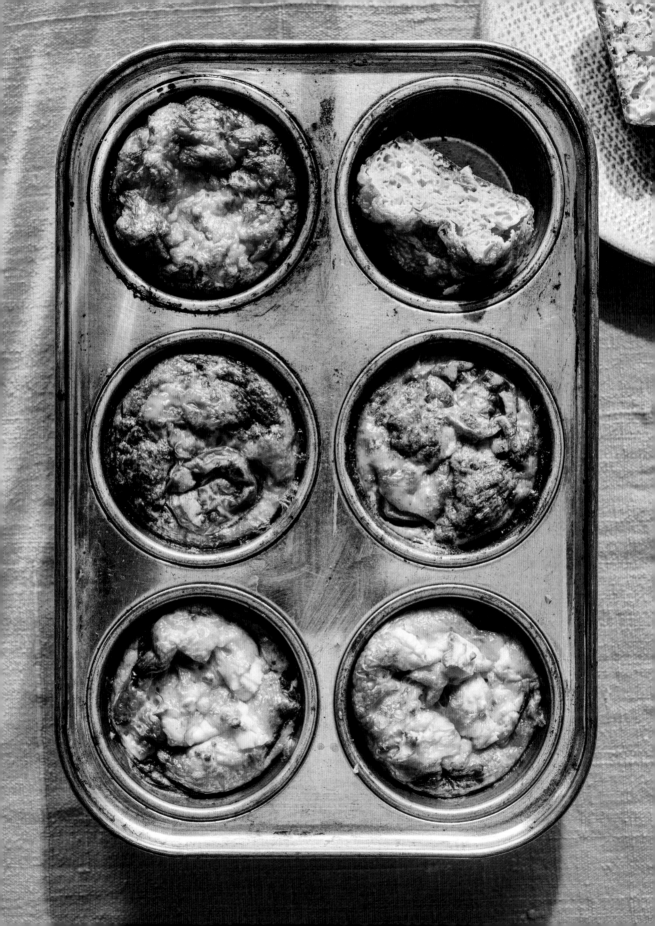

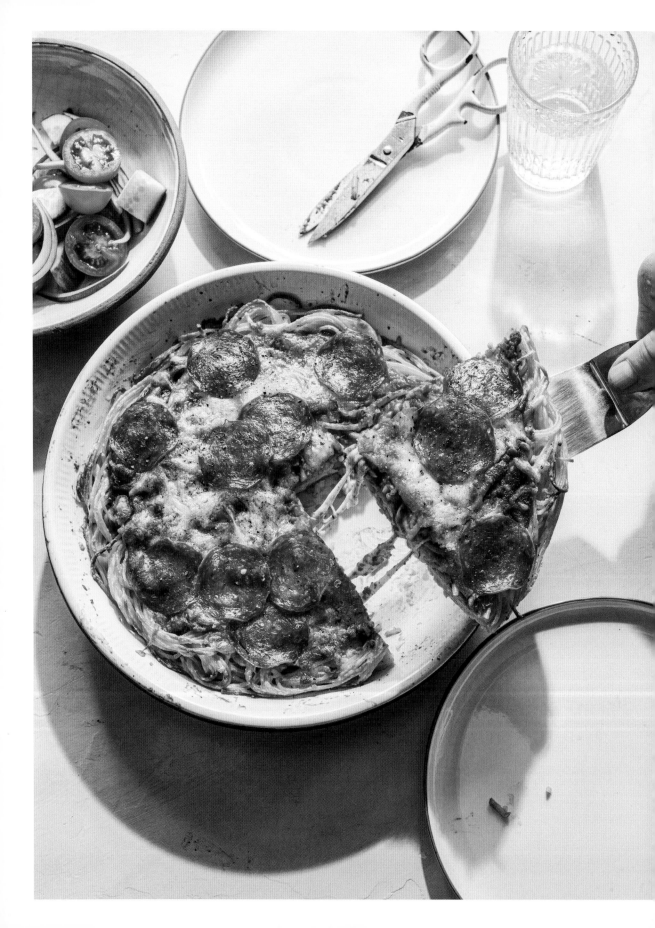

Pizza Spaghetti Pie

PREP TIME: **10 MINUTES**   COOK TIME: **30 MINUTES**   SERVES: **4**

low-calorie cooking spray
250g (9oz) dried spaghetti
50g (1¾oz) light cream
   cheese
½ teaspoon garlic powder
1 large egg, beaten
30g (1oz) Parmesan, grated
100g (3½oz) mozzarella,
   grated
12 pepperoni slices
salt and freshly ground
   black pepper

For the pizza sauce
200g (7oz) passata
4 tablespoons tomato purée
   (paste)
1 teaspoon onion powder
1 teaspoon garlic
½ teaspoon dried parsley
¼ teaspoon dried basil
¼ teaspoon dried oregano
1 teaspoon maple syrup or
   granulated sweetener
½ teaspoon freshly ground
   black pepper

Side suggestions:
Serve with a mixed salad.

Swaps:
Swap the pepperoni for
any toppings you like. Try it
with olives, chicken, ham,
peppers, onions, mushrooms
– whatever you fancy.

Vegetarian:
Use veggie pepperoni slices
and vegetarian Italian-style
hard cheese.

In this recipe, two of the best things in the world – pizza and pasta – are combined to make the ultimate family-friendly meal. It's a cheesy spaghetti base with a pizza sauce filling, all topped with more cheese and your usual pizza topping favourites. You can switch the toppings up each time you make it, for endless variations.

1. Preheat the oven to 190°C/170°C fan/375°F/gas 5 and grease a 23cm (9in) round baking dish with with cooking oil spray.

2. Cook the spaghetti according to the packet directions, then drain and place in a large bowl.

3. Add the cream cheese, garlic powder and a pinch of salt and pepper, and toss until the cream cheese is all melted and coats the pasta. Add the egg and Parmesan and toss again to combine. Press the cheesy spaghetti into the prepared tin to form a crust.

4. Bake for 8–10 minutes to firm up.

5. Meanwhile, in a bowl, combine all the ingredients for the pizza sauce.

6. Remove the spaghetti base from the oven and spoon the pizza sauce over top, leaving the edges uncovered as you would a pizza crust. Top with the mozzarella and pepperoni, then return to the oven and bake for 20 minutes until the cheese is melted and golden. If you want the top to be super-golden, you can place it under the grill for a couple of minutes at the end.

7. Slice and enjoy!

KCALS	
423	
FAT	
13.0g	
SAT FAT	
6.6g	
CARBS	
53.2g	
SUGARS	
7.4g	
FIBRE	
4.2g	
PROTEIN	
21.2g	
SALT	
0.82g	

DF

❄️

KCALS	**498**
FAT	**15.0g**
SAT FAT	**4.0g**
CARBS	**53.9g**
SUGARS	**11.4g**
FIBRE	**4.1g**
PROTEIN	**35.0g**
SALT	**2.35g**

Peanut Chicken Rice Bake

PREP TIME: **10 MINUTES**   COOK TIME: **50 MINUTES**   SERVES: **4**

4 bone-in, skinless chicken thighs, trimmed of visible fat (approx. 125g/4½oz each)
200g (7oz) long-grain rice
100g (3½oz) green cabbage, shredded
60g (2¼oz) carrot, halved lengthways and thinly sliced
½ red (bell) pepper, finely diced
1 spring onion (scallion), chopped
1 tablespoon soy sauce
olive oil spray
500ml (18fl oz) chicken stock

For the marinade
3 tablespoons smooth peanut butter (natural)
1½ tablespoons soy sauce
1½ tablespoons maple syrup
1 tablespoon tomato purée (paste)
½ tablespoon lime juice
½ tablespoon sriracha (you can add more or less, depending on how spicy you like it)
2 garlic cloves, crushed

To serve
1 red chilli, sliced
1 spring onion (scallion), chopped
handful of freshly chopped coriander (cilantro)
lime wedges

This is a fabulous combination: chicken thighs marinated in peanut butter and curry spices, baked until juicy and tender and served on a bed of rice and vegetables. The best part is, the whole thing is cooked in the oven from start to finish, so you can get on with other things while it's cooking. It's a delicious and easy family meal.

1. Preheat the oven to 180°C/160°C fan/350°F/gas 4.

2. In a large, shallow bowl, combine all the marinade ingredients and mix until smooth. Add the chicken and mix to coat, then set aside to marinate while you prep the remaining ingredients.

3. Place the rice, cabbage, carrot, red pepper, spring onion and soy sauce into a shallow casserole dish with a lid. Spray with olive oil spray and mix to combine. Pour in the stock and give everything a little stir.

4. Place the marinated chicken thighs on top, spacing them out evenly, and pour any excess marinade over the chicken. Spray with olive oil spray, then cover with the lid and bake for 30 minutes.

5. Remove the lid and spray with olive oil spray once more, then bake, uncovered, for an additional 20 minutes until the chicken is cooked through and rice is cooked.

6. Serve sprinkled with the chopped red chilli, spring onion and coriander, with lime wedges on the side for squeezing.

Optional add-ons:
Scatter 10g (¼oz) chopped roasted peanuts over the top to serve.

Variation:
For a more indulgent version, swap 250ml (9fl oz) of the stock for the same quantity of light coconut milk.

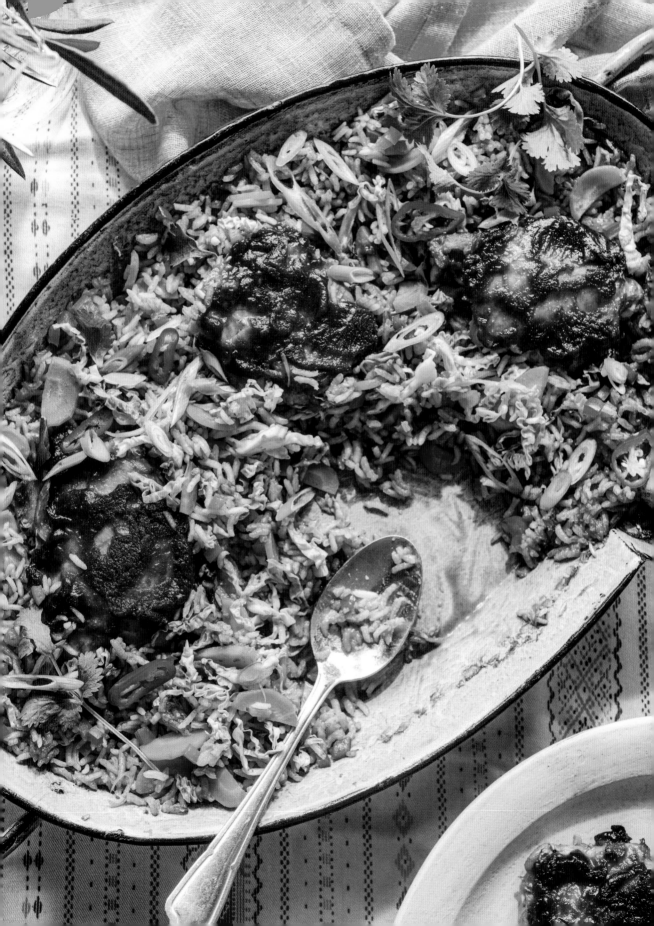

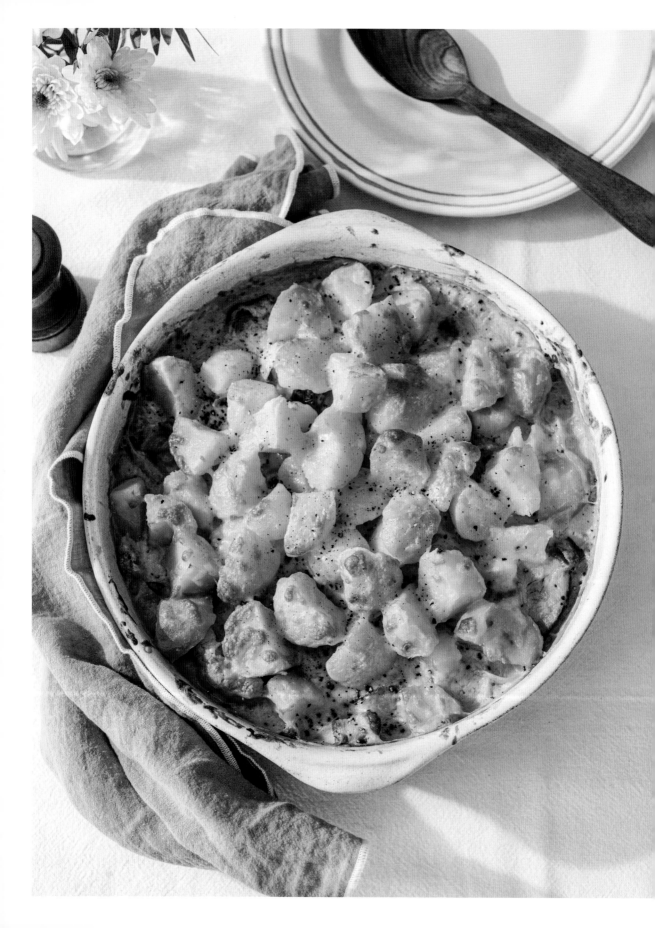

Ham, Leek and Cauliflower Pie with Rustic Cheesy Potato Topping

PREP TIME: **15 MINUTES**   COOK TIME: **1 HOUR**   SERVES: **4**

500 *kcals* per serving

GF

1 tablespoon salted butter
1 onion, finely diced
2 leeks, halved lengthways and sliced
300g (10½oz) cauliflower, broken into small florets
3 garlic cloves, crushed
240ml (8½fl oz) chicken stock
4 tablespoons light cream cheese
240ml (8½fl oz) semi-skimmed milk
1½ tablespoons cornflour (cornstarch)
2 teaspoons wholegrain mustard
325g (11½oz) cooked thick-cut ham or gammon
800g (28oz) potatoes (I use a waxy golden variety), peeled and quartered
olive oil spray
100g (3½oz) Cheddar, grated
salt and freshly ground black pepper

My family loves this simple pie. It's a complete meal in one, although you can pair it with some additional vegetables if you prefer. I like to use waxy potatoes for the topping, as they hold their shape better and tend to have a lovely, natural buttery flavour.

1. Preheat the oven to 200°C/180°C fan/400°F/gas 6.

2. Melt the butter in a large, deep frying pan over a medium–high heat. Add the onion and leeks and fry for a couple of minutes until really softened, then add the cauliflower and garlic and fry for a couple more minutes, just to infuse everything with the garlic. Season with a good pinch of salt and pepper.

3. Add the stock and cream cheese and simmer for about 5 minutes until the cauliflower is tender and the cream cheese has all melted.

4. In a small bowl or mug, mix the milk with the cornflour, then pour this into the pan, along with the mustard. Continue to simmer for 5–8 minutes until the sauce thickens, then add the ham. Taste and adjust the seasoning if needed, then transfer to a pie dish or baking dish and allow to cool slightly.

5. Add the potatoes to the empty frying pan and cover with water. Season the water generously with salt, then bring to the boil and simmer for 8–10 minutes until the potatoes are slightly soft but not mushy.

6. Drain the potatoes and slightly break them up with a wooden spoon, but don't mash them – you want them to still be a bit chunky.

7. Top the pie filling with the potatoes and spray with some olive oil spray. Scatter the cheese over the top and season with a pinch of black pepper, then bake for 30 minutes. At the end, place the pie under the grill for a couple of minutes until the top is lovely and golden, then serve.

Variations:

If you prefer, you can swap the ham for some cooked chicken. You can also omit the Cheddar and just top the pie with the potatoes and bake until lightly golden. This filling also works really well with the filo pastry topping from page 119.

Vegetarian:

Swap the chicken stock for vegetable stock and replace the ham with some more veggies or white beans.

KCALS
500

FAT
17.6g

SAT FAT
9.6g

CARBS
48.1g

SUGARS
11.8g

FIBRE
8.1g

PROTEIN
33.4g

SALT
2.81g

Mediterranean Cod

PREP TIME: **5 MINUTES**   COOK TIME: **35 MINUTES**   SERVES: **4**

KCALS	**236**
FAT	**3.5g**
SAT FAT	**0.6g**
CARBS	**16.4g**
SUGARS	**6.5g**
FIBRE	**6.5g**
PROTEIN	**31.5g**
SALT	**0.51g**

200g (7oz) roasted red peppers in vinegar, drained and rinsed

2 tablespoons tomato purée (paste)

1 onion, finely chopped

3 garlic cloves, minced

300g (10½oz) cherry tomatoes, halved

2 teaspoons extra virgin olive oil

1½ teaspoons sweet paprika

½ teaspoon fennel seeds, crushed

120ml (4fl oz) chicken stock

400g (14oz) can butter beans

4 cod fish fillets (approx. 140g/5oz each)

salt and freshly ground black pepper

freshly chopped parsley, to serve

Freezing:

Only freezer-friendly as long as the fish has not been frozen before.

This one-dish Mediterranean cod can be ready in just under 40 minutes, for a simple meal that is perfect for any night of the week. The lightly seasoned cod is baked in a rich sauce made from roasted tomatoes and red peppers with garlic and butter beans. It pairs well with a variety of sides; we love it with mashed potatoes or rice, but it goes well with pasta too.

1. Preheat the oven to 220°C/200°C fan/425°F/gas 7.

2. Combine the roasted red peppers and tomato purée in a blender and blend until smooth. Set aside.

3. Place the onion, garlic and tomatoes into a baking dish. Drizzle with the olive oil and season with a pinch of salt and pepper. Toss to coat, then bake for 10–13 minutes until the tomatoes are softened and the onions caramelized.

4. Remove from the oven and stir in the blended roasted pepper mixture, along with the paprika, fennel, stock and butter beans. Return to the oven and bake for another 10 minutes.

5. Remove from the oven and add the fish fillets to the baking dish, partially submerging them in the sauce. Reduce the oven temperature to 200°C/180°C fan/400°F/gas 6 and bake for 12 minutes until the fish is tender.

6. Sprinkle with fresh parsley and serve.

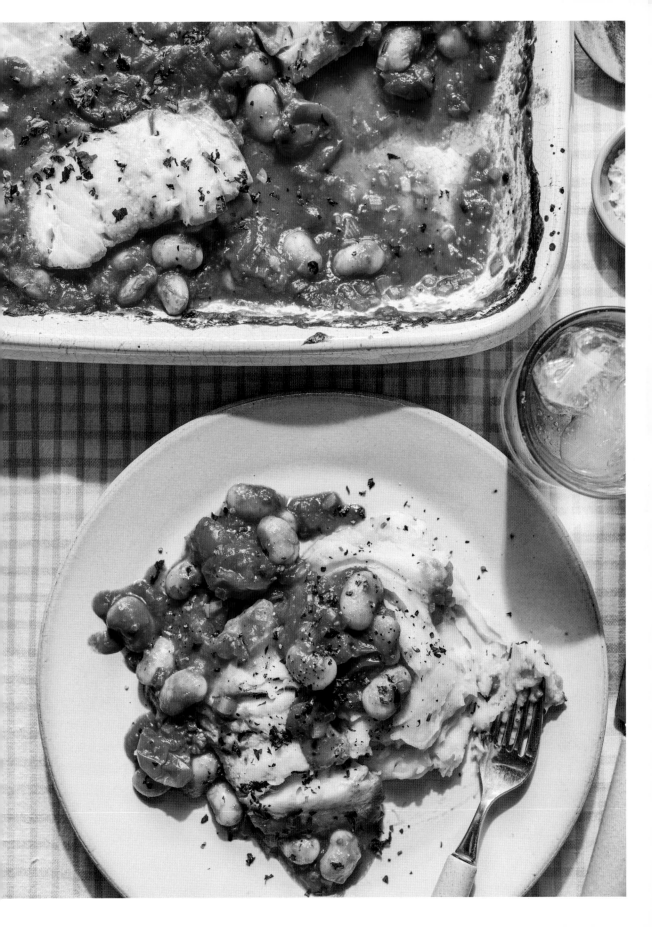

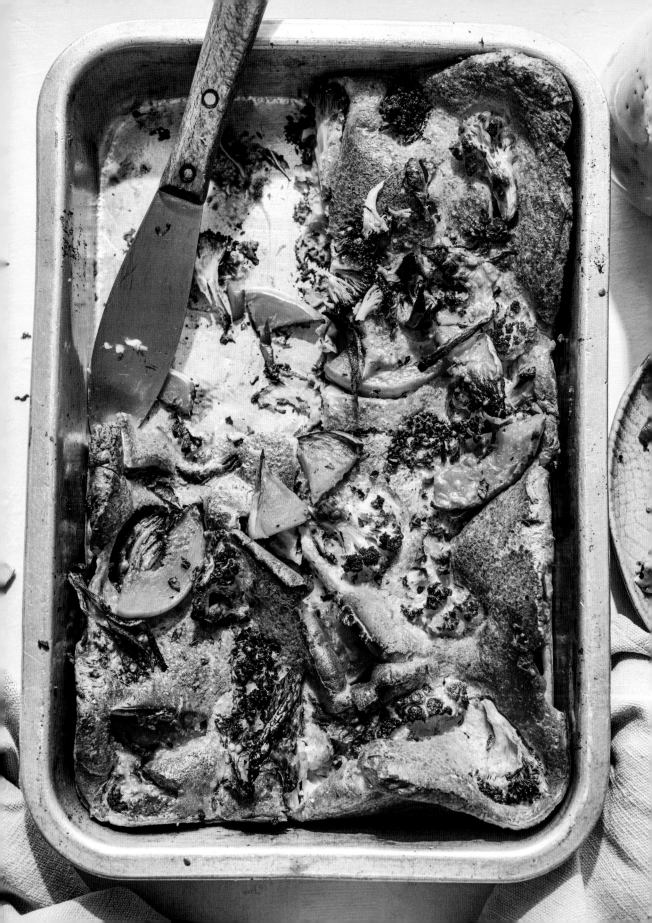

Herby Vegetable Toad-in-the-Hole with Onion Gravy

200g (7oz) cauliflower
  florets
140g (5oz) broccoli florets
140g (5oz) butternut squash,
  peeled and chopped
75g (2½oz) red onion, sliced
2 garlic cloves, crushed
½ tablespoon vegetable oil
½ teaspoon sweet paprika
1½ teaspoons herbes de
  Provence
salt and freshly ground
  black pepper
freshly chopped parsley
  or thyme, to serve

For the batter
120g (4¼oz) plain
  (all-purpose) flour
4 large eggs
200ml (7fl oz) milk

For the onion gravy
olive oil spray
2 onions, sliced (approx.
  200g/7oz)
2 garlic cloves, crushed
1 tablespoon balsamic
  vinegar
pinch of dried thyme
pinch of dried rosemary
600ml (20fl oz) vegetable
  stock
½ tablespoon tomato purée
  (paste)
1 teaspoon Dijon mustard

Freezing:
Freeze the gravy separately.

This is my delicious vegetarian version of the classic toad-in-the-hole, which I make using roasted vegetables like broccoli, cauliflower and butternut squash, flavoured with herbs and garlic. Served with a delicious yet simple homemade onion gravy, it makes a great main meal or can be enjoyed as a side as part of your traditional Sunday dinner.

1. Preheat the oven to 220°C/200°C fan/425°F/gas 6.

2. In a bowl, mix together the ingredients for the batter and set aside.

3. Place the cauliflower, broccoli, squash, onion and garlic in large baking tray. Drizzle over the oil, then sprinkle over the paprika and herbes de Provence. Toss to coat. Season with salt and pepper, then roast for 15 minutes.

4. While the vegetables are cooking, make the gravy. Heat a saucepan over a medium–high heat and spray with olive oil spray. Add the onions and a pinch of salt, and fry for a couple of minutes until golden brown and softened. Add the garlic and fry for a further minute, then add the vinegar and continue to cook until it evaporates off. Next, add the herbs, stock, tomato purée and mustard, then season with black pepper and bring to the boil. Simmer for 15–20 minutes; you want the stock to have reduced down a little to deepen the flavour of the gravy.

5. Once the vegetables have been roasting for 15 minutes, remove from the oven. Spray with olive oil spray and make sure the different veg are scattered evenly across the bottom of the baking tray. Quickly pour in the batter while the pan is still really hot, then return to the oven for 20–25 minutes for the batter to rise and puff up and turn lightly brown.

6. Return your attention to the gravy. Remove about two thirds of the onions from the pan and place in a blender with a little of the stock. Blend until smooth, then return this mixture to the saucepan, mixing it with the rest of the gravy. This will thicken the gravy; if it becomes too thick, you can add a little water to loosen.

7. Remove the toad-in-the-hole from the oven once cooked. Season with salt and pepper and scatter with parsley or thyme, then serve with the gravy and enjoy.

KCALS
338

FAT
10.5g

SAT FAT
3.1g

CARBS
39.8g

SUGARS
12.1g

FIBRE
7.0g

PROTEIN
17.6g

SALT
0.85g

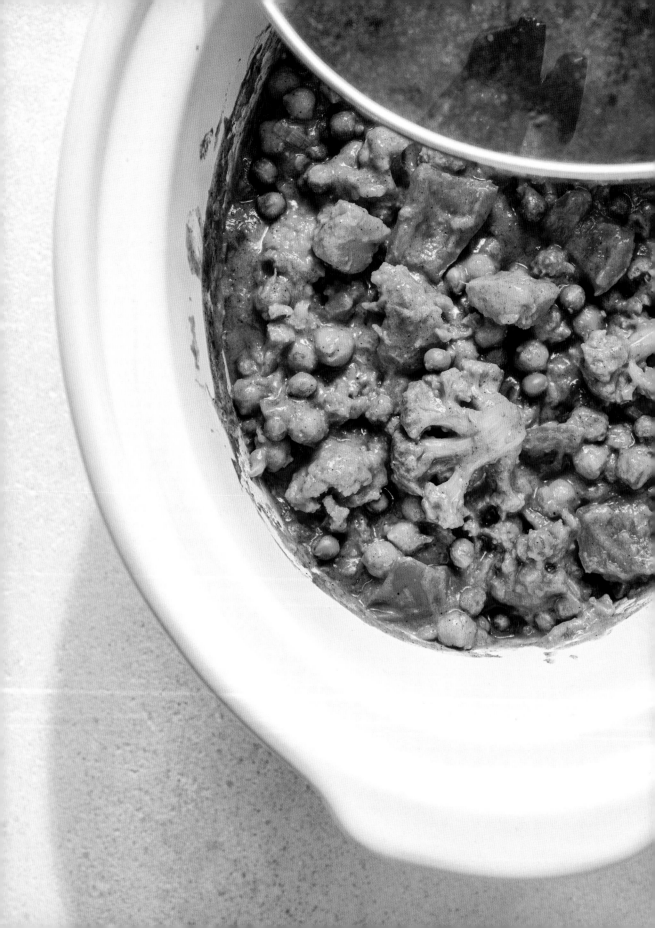

Slow Cooker Recipes

287 kcals
per serving

 GF

DF

KCALS
287

FAT
6.8g

SAT FAT
2.2g

CARBS
23.1g

SUGARS
20.6g

FIBRE
3.7g

PROTEIN
31.5g

SALT
2.29g

Yucatan-style Pulled Pork

PREP TIME: **15 MINUTES**   COOK TIME: **6 HOURS**   SERVES: **4**

600g (1lb 5oz) pork
 tenderloin
1 onion, thinly sliced
3 garlic cloves, crushed
1 tablespoon light brown
 sugar
1 tablespoon apple cider
 vinegar
2 teaspoons sweet paprika
1½ teaspoons ground cumin
1 teaspoon salt
1 teaspoon smoked paprika
1 teaspoon dried oregano
¼ teaspoon freshly ground
 black pepper
½ tsp ground cloves
½ teaspoon ground
 cinnamon
½ teaspoon cayenne pepper
100ml (3½fl oz) orange juice
100ml (3½fl oz) chicken
 stock
1 teaspoon grated orange zest

For the pickled onions
120ml (4fl oz) red wine
 vinegar
3 tablespoons granulated
 sweetener or white sugar
1 teaspoon salt
1 teaspoon whole black
 peppercorns
pinch of red chilli flakes
 (optional)
250g (9oz) red onions,
 thinly sliced
2 cloves
2 garlic cloves, thinly sliced
1 bay leaf

If you love Mexican dishes, you will love this slow-cooker Yucatan-style pork: delicious pork tenderloin braised with a mix of spices and citrusy orange juice for an amazing flavour. Traditionally, it uses annatto seeds, but as those can be hard to source, I use a blend of different spices for the colour instead. There are various yummy ways you can serve it, too. Some of my family's favourite methods are to serve it in tortilla wraps, or as a bowl with some rice, black beans, tomato, avocado, coriander and zingy pickled red onions. It's a great family recipe that you can serve in the middle of the table with various add-ons to build your own creations.

1. To make the pickled red onion, combine the vinegar and 240ml (8½fl oz) water in a small saucepan. Add the sugar, salt, peppercorns and chilli flakes (if using) and place over a medium–high heat until the sugar is fully dissolved. Set aside to cool.

2. Place the onions into a jar with the cloves, garlic and bay leaf. Once the pickling liquid has cooled, pour it into the jar, ensuring the onions are all pushed down and submerged in the liquid. Seal – the jar should be airtight – and keep in the fridge until needed. It's ready to use straight away, but if you like you can make it a day in advance to give the flavours time to develop.

3. To make the pork, add all ingredients to the slow cooker and stir. Cook on low for 6 hours or high for 4 hours, then shred with two forks.

4. If you like your pork crispy at the edges, you can transfer it to a baking tray and then pop it under the grill for a few minutes until the edges are charred; this is my favourite way to serve it.

5. Serve and enjoy with your chosen sides.

Side suggestions:
This is also great served with the guacamole and black bean salsa on page 260.

Freezing:
The pickled onions can't be frozen.

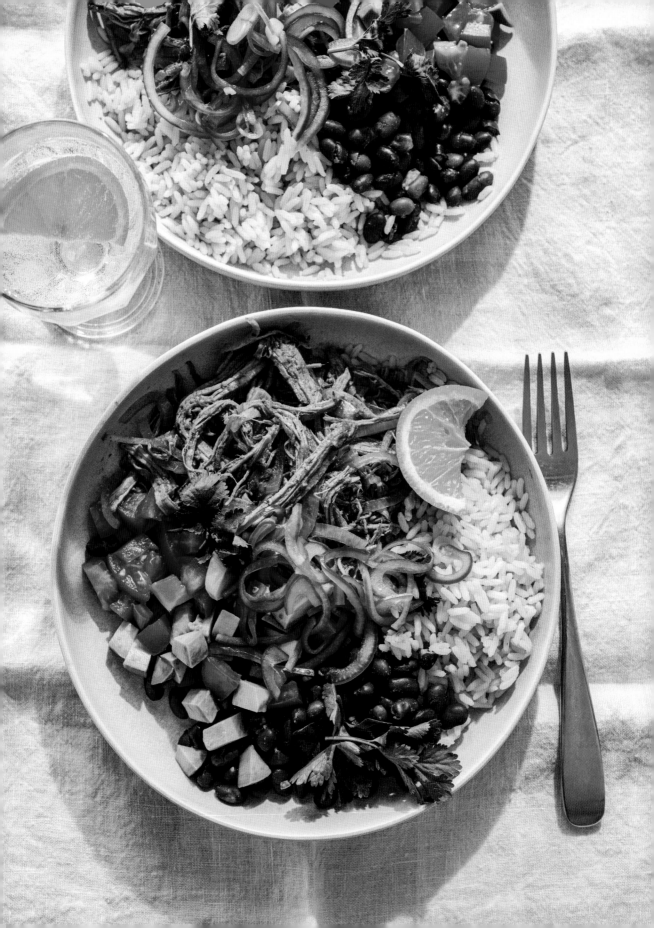

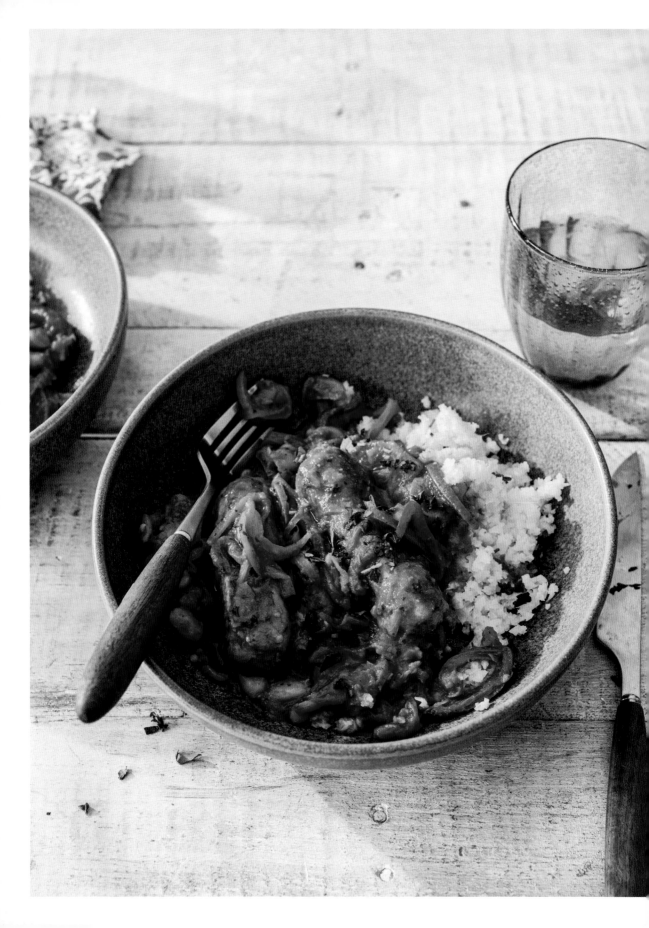

Sausage and Fennel Hot Pot

PREP TIME: **8 MINUTES**   COOK TIME: **8 HOURS**   SERVES: **4**

olive oil spray
1 large onion, sliced
1 small fennel bulb, sliced
2 garlic cloves, crushed
8 low-calorie sausages
1 red (bell) pepper, sliced
1 green (bell) pepper, sliced
1 teaspoon dried parsley
½ teaspoon dried basil
1 tablespoon Worcestershire
 sauce
1 tablespoon balsamic
 vinegar
400g (14oz) can plum
 tomatoes
3 tablespoons tomato purée
 (paste)
180ml (6fl oz) chicken stock
400g can white beans,
 such as cannellini beans
 or white kidney beans
½ tablespoon of maple syrup
 or granulated sweetener

Gluten-free:
Use gluten-free sausages.

An easy slow-cooker sausage casserole with softened peppers and the beautiful flavour of fennel, all cooked in a delicious sauce with white beans. It's perfect over mashed potatoes, or for a low-carb alternative, try it with some cauliflower mash.

1. Heat a frying pan over a medium–high heat. Spray with olive oil spray and add the onion and fennel. Fry for a couple of minutes until lightly golden, then add the garlic and fry for a further minute.

2. Transfer the onion and garlic to the slow cooker, then add the sausages to the empty pan. Fry for a couple of minutes to brown, then transfer to the slow cooker as well.

3. Add all the remaining ingredients to the slow cooker and stir to combine, then cook on high for 4 hours or low for 7–8 hours.

4. Serve and enjoy.

KCALS
299

FAT
5.9g

SAT FAT
2.0g

CARBS
34.2g

SUGARS
18.0g

FIBRE
11.5g

PROTEIN
21.6g

SALT
1.86g

300 kcals
per serving

KCALS
300

FAT
8.8g

SAT FAT
2.3g

CARBS
39.1g

SUGARS
9.6g

FIBRE
9.1g

PROTEIN
11.5g

SALT
0.84g

Lemon, Orzo and Chickpea Soup

PREP TIME: **10 MINUTES**   COOK TIME: **4 HOURS**   SERVES: **4**

½ tablespoon salted butter
½ tablespoon olive oil
200g (7oz) onion,
  finely diced
200g (7oz) carrot,
  finely diced
3 garlic cloves, crushed
½ teaspoon fennel seeds,
  crushed
½ teaspoon dried rosemary
½ teaspoon dried thyme
1 teaspoon dried parsley
2 bay leaves
400g (14oz) can chickpeas
1.2 litres (40½fl oz) vegetable
  stock
100g (3½oz) dried orzo
2 large egg yolks
3 tablespoons lemon juice
salt and freshly ground
  black pepper
freshly chopped parsley,
  to serve

You will love this easy vegetarian version of the Greek soup avgolemono. Traditionally, it's made with chicken, but in this version I've used chickpeas instead. Towards the end, we stir through a mixture of egg yolks and lemon juice, which gives it a silky, creamy appearance.

1. Heat the butter and olive oil in a frying pan over a medium–high heat. Add the onion, carrot and garlic, and fry for a few minutes until softened.

2. Transfer to the slow cooker with the fennel, rosemary, thyme, parsley, bay leaves, chickpeas and stock and stir to combine.

3. Cook on high for 3½ hours, then stir in the orzo. Cook for a further 30 minutes, then turn off the slow cooker.

4. In a bowl, whisk the egg yolks with the lemon juice. Remove 180ml (6fl oz) of the broth from the slow cooker and slowly stir this into the egg and lemon mixture. Now stir this into the soup, along with some fresh parsley.

5. Taste and season with salt and pepper, then serve and enjoy.

Freezing:
Freeze after step 3. Fully defrost before continuing steps 4–5.

Optional add-ins:
If not vegetarian, this is great with some cooked chicken stirred through at the end.

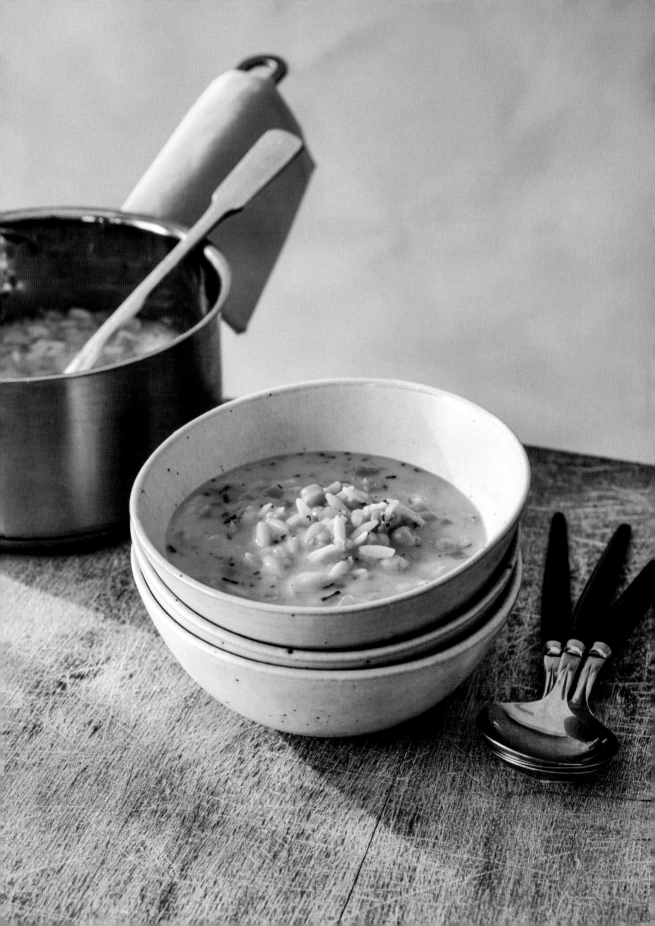

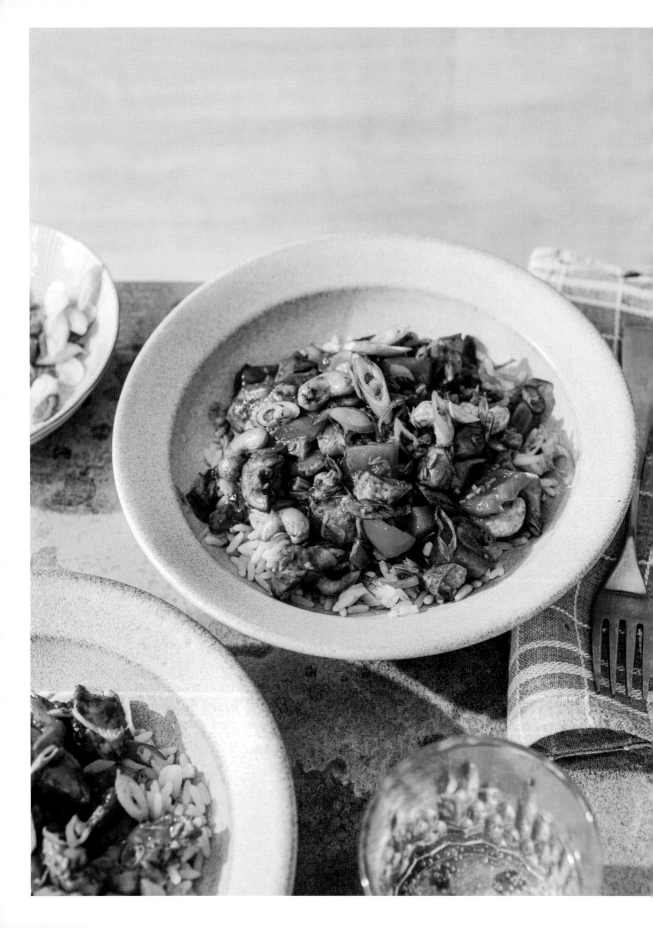

Kung Pao Chicken

PREP TIME: 5 MINUTES   **COOK TIME: 4 HOURS**   **SERVES: 4**

650g (23oz) boneless,
   skinless chicken thighs,
   sliced into bite-sized pieces
1 onion, chopped
2 garlic cloves, thinly sliced
1 thumb-sized piece of fresh
   ginger, peeled and sliced
1 tablespoon light soy sauce
3 tablespoons dark soy sauce
2 tablespoons honey
1 tablespoon balsamic vinegar
1 tablespoon Shaoxing wine
1 teaspoon sesame oil
6–8 dried red chillies
   (depending on how
   spicy you like it)
1 tablespoon cornflour
   (cornstarch)
1 green (bell) pepper,
   chopped
1 red (bell) pepper, chopped
3 spring onions, chopped,
   plus extra to serve
olive oil spray
40 cashews
salt and freshly ground
   black pepper

Side suggestions:
This is great served with rice.
For a low-carb choice, try it
with cauliflower rice.

Freezing:
Freeze before adding the
cashews.

Enjoy a yummy fake-away night with this delicious slow-cooked kung pao chicken. It's a truly effortless recipe: everything is just added to the slow cooker, and several hours later, you have tender pieces of chicken in a yummy, spicy sauce with cashews. Great with rice, noodles and more.

1. Place the chicken into the slow cooker, along with onion, garlic, ginger, soy sauces, honey, vinegar, Shaoxing wine, sesame oil and dried chillies. Stir in 5 tablespoons water and season with black pepper, then cook for 4 hours on low or 2 hours on high.

2. When 1 hour is remaining, mix the cornstarch with a couple of tablespoons of water to make a slurry and stir this into the slow cooker along with the peppers, add back the lid and let it finish cooking for the remaining hour.

3. Meanwhile, heat a large frying pan over a medium–high heat and spray with olive oil spray. Add the cashews, along with a little pinch of salt, and fry until lightly golden. Remove from the pan and set aside.

4. When the chicken is ready, stir the cashews through the sauce, then sprinkle with chopped spring onions and serve.

451 kcals
per serving

DF

KCALS
451

FAT
21.3g

SAT FAT
5.0g

CARBS
25.4g

SUGARS
18.1g

FIBRE
3.7g

PROTEIN
37.6g

SALT
2.21g

329 kcals
per serving

GF

DF

❄

KCALS
329

FAT
11.3g

SAT FAT
3.0g

CARBS
20.3g

SUGARS
18.6g

FIBRE
4.2g

PROTEIN
34.5g

SALT
0.31g

Honey Chipotle Chicken

PREP TIME: **5 MINUTES**   COOK TIME: **4 HOURS**   SERVES: **4**

olive oil spray
1 large onion, sliced
3 garlic cloves, crushed
650g (23oz) boneless,
    skinless chicken thighs
1 green (bell) pepper, sliced
400g (14oz) can plum
    tomatoes or chopped
    tomatoes
2 tablespoons tomato purée
    (paste)
2 tablespoons chipotle paste
    (you can add more if
    you like it really spicy)
2 tablespoons honey
1½ teaspoons sweet paprika
1½ teaspoons ground cumin
½ teaspoon onion powder
½ teaspoon garlic powder
½ teaspoon dried oregano
salt and freshly ground
    black pepper
freshly chopped coriander
    (cilantro), to serve

Optional add-ons:
This is great served with
the black bean salsa and
guacamole on page 260.

Side suggestions:
Serve with rice or cubed
seasoed roasted potatoes or
sweet potato. The chicken
is also great in tortillas
with salad, sour cream and
Cheddar.

Low-carb side:
Serve with some cauliflower
rice or salad.

This smoky slow-cooker chipotle chicken is a great dish for the whole family. It's delicious just as it is with some rice, but if you're feeling creative, you could build the perfect chipotle chicken bowl with some of your favourite toppings, like black beans, Cheddar, sweetcorn, guacamole, coriander and more.

1. Heat a frying pan over a medium–high heat and spray with olive oil spray. Add the onions and garlic and fry for a couple of minutes until golden and softened.

2. Add to the slow cooker, along with all the remaining ingredients (except the coriander). Season with salt and pepper and mix to combine.

3. Cook on high for 4 hours, then roughly shred the meat with two forks.

4. Sprinkle with some fresh coriander, if using, and serve.

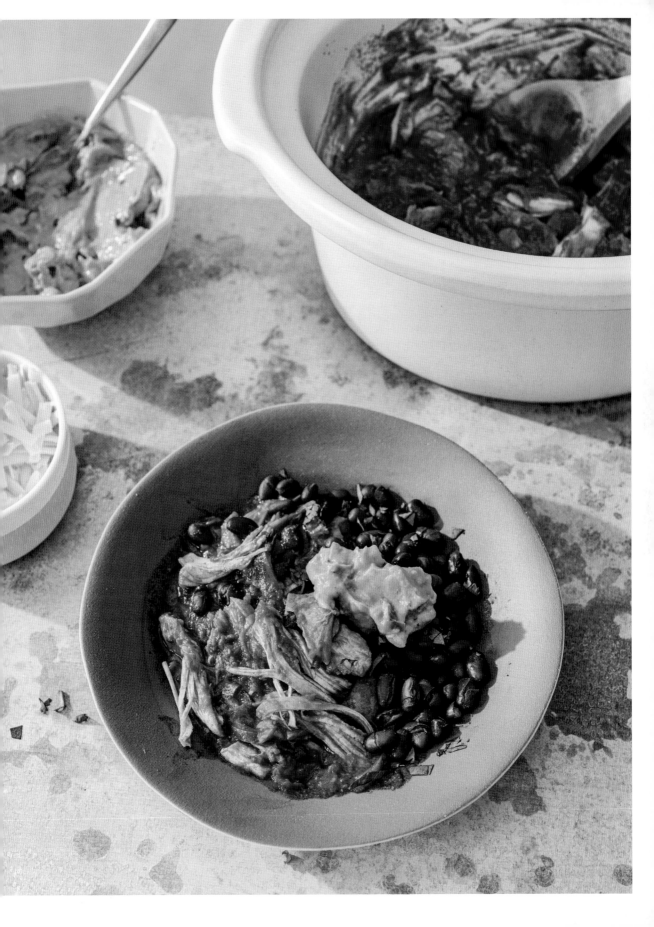

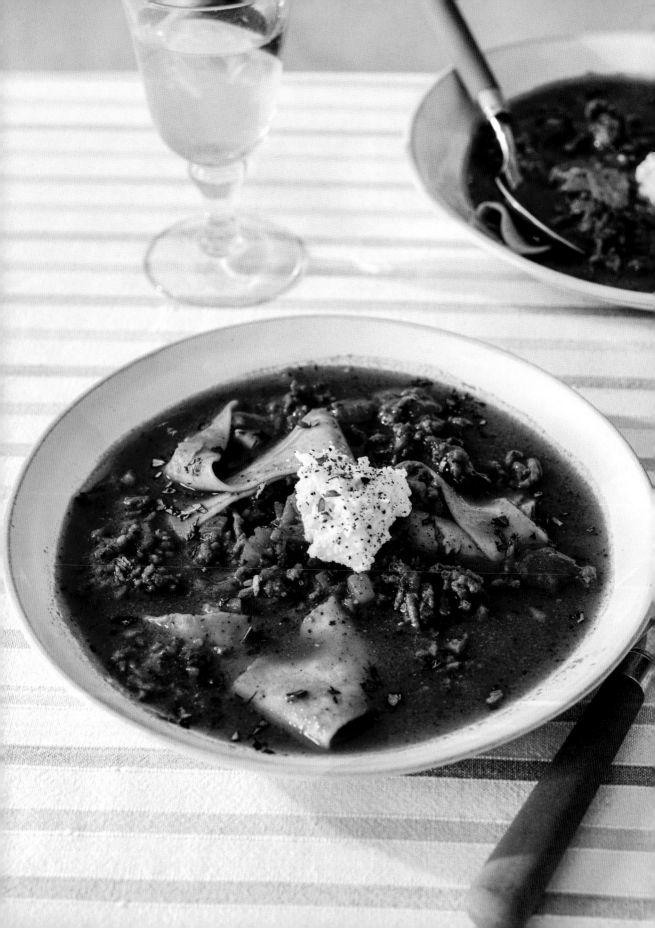

Lasagne Soup with Cheesy Ricotta Balls

328 kcals
per serving

PREP TIME: **5 MINUTES**   COOK TIME: **8 HOURS**   SERVES: **6**

400g (14oz) 5% fat beef mince (ground beef)
2 slices of lean bacon, diced
1 large onion, diced
3 garlic cloves, crushed
1 large carrot, diced
1 teaspoon Italian seasoning
½ teaspoon dried basil
½ teaspoon fennel seeds, crushed
5 tablespoons tomato purée (paste)
400g (14oz) can chopped tomatoes
240g (8½oz) passata
1.2 litres (40½fl oz) chicken stock
1 teaspoon granulated sugar
150g (5½oz) broken dried lasagne sheets
2 tablespoons freshly chopped parsley
salt and freshly ground black pepper

For the cheesy ricotta balls
80g (2¾oz) ricotta
20g (¾oz) Parmesan, grated
40g (1½oz) mozzarella, grated

Freezing:
Freeze after step 4. Defrost fully before starting step 5.

If you love lasagne, you will love lasagne soup. This is a delicious, rich tomato and beef soup with broken lasagne noodles, which I like to serve topped with some cheesy ricotta balls for that ultimate lasagne flavour.

1. Heat a frying pan over a medium–high heat. Add the beef, along with the bacon, onion, garlic and carrot, and fry for a few minutes until browned, breaking up the mince with your spoon as you cook.

2. Transfer to the slow cooker, along with the dried herbs, tomato purée, chopped tomatoes, passata, stock and sugar.

3. Mix to combine and cook on high for 4 hours or low for 8 hours, adding the lasagne sheets for the last 30 minutes.

4. Taste and season with salt and pepper as needed, then stir through the fresh parsley.

5. To make the cheesy ricotta balls, mix together the ricotta, Parmesan and mozzarella in a bowl, then spoon a dollop of the cheesy mixture into each bowl of soup.

6. Enjoy!

KCALS
328

FAT
9.7g

SAT FAT
4.8g

CARBS
28.9g

SUGARS
10.7g

FIBRE
4.5g

PROTEIN
29.2g

SALT
1.70g

DF

KCALS
329

FAT
8.0g

SAT FAT
2.5g

CARBS
23.7g

SUGARS
8.9g

FIBRE
5.1g

PROTEIN
38.1g

SALT
0.75g

Slow Cooker Pot Roast

PREP TIME: **15 MINUTES**   COOK TIME: **8 HOURS**   SERVES: **6**

2 large onions, sliced

4 garlic cloves, crushed

1kg (2.25lb) top sirloin roast

600g (1lb 5oz) baby potatoes, left whole unless they're quite large

2 large carrots, chopped

360ml (12fl oz) beef stock

1 tablespoon tomato purée (paste)

1 tablespoon balsamic vinegar

1 tablespoon dark soy sauce

½ tablespoon Worcestershire sauce

½ teaspoon dried thyme

½ teaspoon dried rosemary

salt and freshly ground black pepper

Variation:

Sometimes I add 6 tablespoons of my favourite barbecue sauce, to add a smoky barbecue taste to the gravy.

Side suggestions:

Delicious served with some additional green vegetables like broccoli, cabbage, green beans etc.

If you love tender, falling-apart pieces of beef with a delicious rich gravy, then wait until you try this pot roast. It's like all the great parts of a roast dinner, but you cook it as a complete meal in your slow cooker. Just pop in all the ingredients in the morning, and by dinnertime, you have a healthy, hearty meal for the whole family.

1. Add the onions and garlic to the base of the slow cooker.

2. Season the outside of the beef with salt and pepper. Heat a frying pan over a medium–high heat and spray with olive oil spray. Add the beef and fry for a few minutes, turning to brown on all sides.

3. Transfer the beef to the slow cooker and place it on top of the onions and garlic. Scatter the potatoes and carrots down the sides of the beef.

4. In a jug, mix together the stock, tomato purée, balsamic vinegar, soy sauce, Worcestershire sauce, thyme and rosemary. Pour this over the beef and veg, then cook on low for 8 hours.

5. Once cooked, carefully remove the beef from the slow cooker and transfer to a large plate, along with the potatoes. Remove enough of the carrots to serve as your vegetable side, but leave a few pieces in the juices with the onions.

6. Using a stick blender, blend the juices, onions and remaining carrots until smooth to create a gravy. Taste the gravy and season as needed with salt and pepper.

7. The beef should be really tender from the slow-cooking and will easily shred into pieces (don't over-shred, though; you just want tender chunks of beef).

8. Slice the baby potatoes in half and serve with the beef and carrots, with the gravy poured over the top.

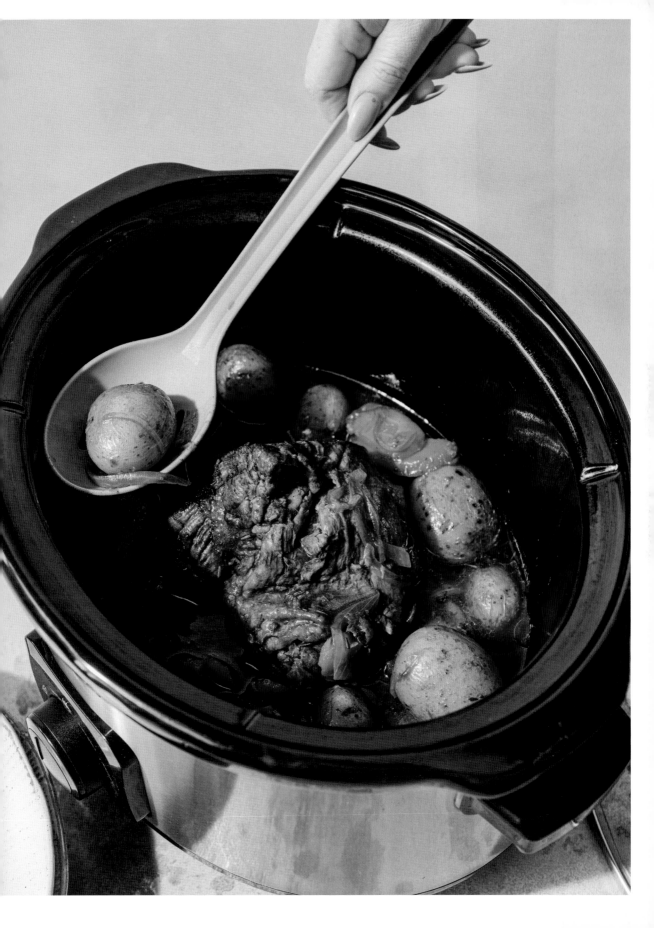

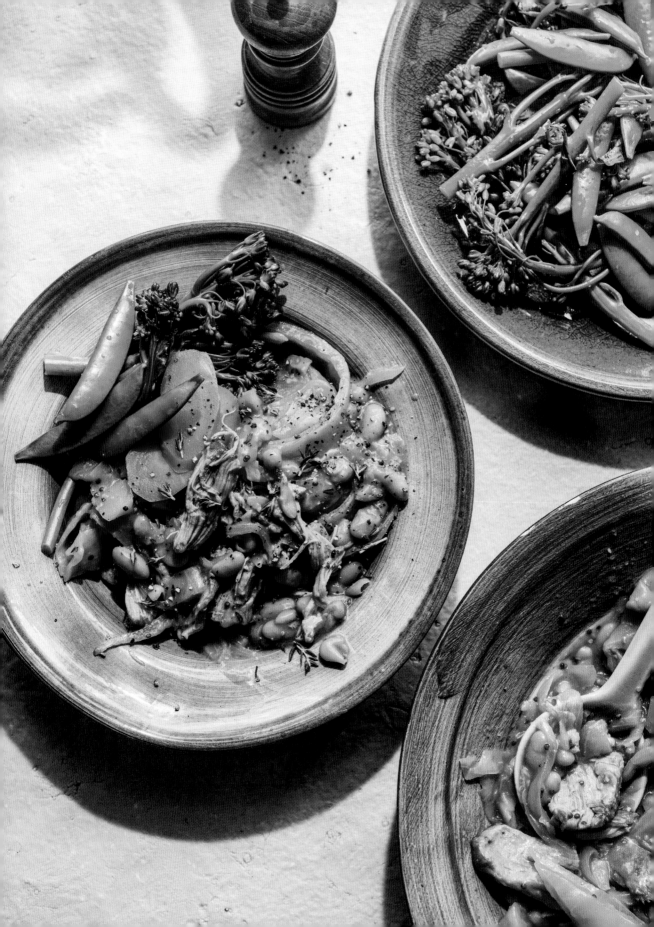

Slow Cooker Pork with Cabbage and White Beans

PRE TIME: 10 MINUTES   **COOK TIME: 8 HOURS**   **SERVES: 6**

550g (1lb 4oz) green cabbage, shredded
400g (14oz) can cannellini beans (or any white beans), drained
1 large onion, thinly sliced
6 garlic cloves, crushed
1kg (2.25lb) pork shoulder, trimmed of visible fat and sliced into 2 big pieces
2 teaspoons sweet paprika
olive oil spray
240ml (8½fl oz) chicken stock
240ml (8½fl oz) fresh apple juice
1 tablespoon wholegrain mustard
2 tablespoons white wine vinegar
2 fresh thyme sprigs
2 tablespoons cornflour (cornstarch)
salt and freshly ground black pepper

Side suggestions:
Serve over mashed potatoes, or for a low-carb option, try it with some cauliflower mash, root veg mash or roasted cubes of butternut squash, or some steamed green vegetables.

Freezing:
Make sure you slice the pork before freezing.

Pork with cabbage has always been my go-to comfort food. It was a dish my mum made regularly, served over mashed potatoes, so I often get cravings for it. My version is slow-cooked until tender with white beans in a delicious broth of apple juice, garlic, mustard and thyme. An effortless meal that you can just prep in the morning and have ready by dinnertime.

1. Add the cabbage, beans, onion and garlic to the slow cooker and mix to combine.

2. Season the pork shoulder all over with the paprika and a good pinch of salt and pepper.

3. Heat a frying pan over a medium–high heat and spray with olive oil spray. Add the pork shoulder and cook for a few minutes, turning to brown on all sides.

4. Transfer the browned pork to the slow cooker, placing it on top of the cabbage and beans.

5. In a jug, mix together the stock, apple juice, mustard and white wine vinegar, then pour it into the slow cooker. Place the sprigs of fresh thyme in the slow cooker and cook on low for 7 hours.

6. In a mug or small bowl, mix the cornflour with a little water to make a slurry. Pour this into the slow cooker and mix to combine. Cover and cook for 1 more hour.

7. Once it's finished cooking, carefully remove the pork to a plate. Carve into slices and return it to the slow cooker. Stir to combine with the cabbage. Season to taste with salt and pepper, then serve.

334 kcals per serving

KCALS
334

FAT
10.5g

SAT FAT
3.2g

CARBS
20.4g

SUGARS
10.3g

FIBRE
8.1g

PROTEIN
35.3g

SALT
0.72g

Slow Cooker Japanese Beef Curry

PREP TIME: 10 MINUTES   **COOK TIME: 8 HOURS**   **SERVES: 4**

KCALS
349

FAT
9.1g

SAT FAT
3.8g

CARBS
34.8g

SUGARS
13.7g

FIBRE
7.0g

PROTEIN
28.5g

SALT
1.26g

455g (1lb) lean stewing beef
300g (10½oz) waxy
    potatoes, peeled
    and halved
200g (7oz) carrots, chopped
1 apple, peeled and finely
    diced
1 tablespoon salted butter
2 onions, chopped
3 garlic cloves, minced
1 thumb-sized piece of fresh
    ginger, grated
2½ tablespoons curry
    powder (mild, medium or
    hot, depending on your
    preferred spice level)
1 teaspoon garam masala
2 tablespoons tomato purée
    (paste)
1½ tablespoons soy sauce
½ tablespoon honey
zest of 1 small orange
320ml (10¾fl oz) beef stock
2 bay leaves
2 tablespoons cornflour
    (cornstarch)
salt and freshly ground
    black pepper

Side suggestions:
Serve over rice or cauliflower
rice for a lower-carb option.

Variations:
You can add other vegetables
to this curry – butternut
squash, sweet potatoes and
green (bell) peppers are great
additions – but you may need
to adjust the stock quantity.

I love Japanese curry; the combination of flavours is just delicious. This is a great recipe for throwing in the slow cooker. Traditional recipes use a Japanese curry roux, but that can be hard to source, so I've created my own mix of ingredients to try and replicate those flavours, and it's become a firm family favourite.

1. Combine the beef, potatoes, carrots and apple in the slow cooker.

2. Melt the butter in a frying pan over a medium–high heat. Add the onions and fry for a couple of minutes until golden, then add the garlic and ginger and fry for a further minute.

3. Now add the curry powder to the pan, along with the garam masala, tomato purée and soy sauce. Add a little water to prevent any sticking, and mix until all the onions are coated.

4. Transfer to the slow cooker and mix until everything is covered in the seasoning.

5. Add the honey and orange zest, then pour in the stock. Top with the bay leaves and cook on low for 7 hours.

6. In a mug or small bowl, mix the cornflour with 3 tablespoons water to make a slurry. Pour this into the slow cooker and mix to combine, then cook for 1 more hour. This will help thicken up the curry sauce.

7. Season to taste with salt and pepper, then serve and enjoy!

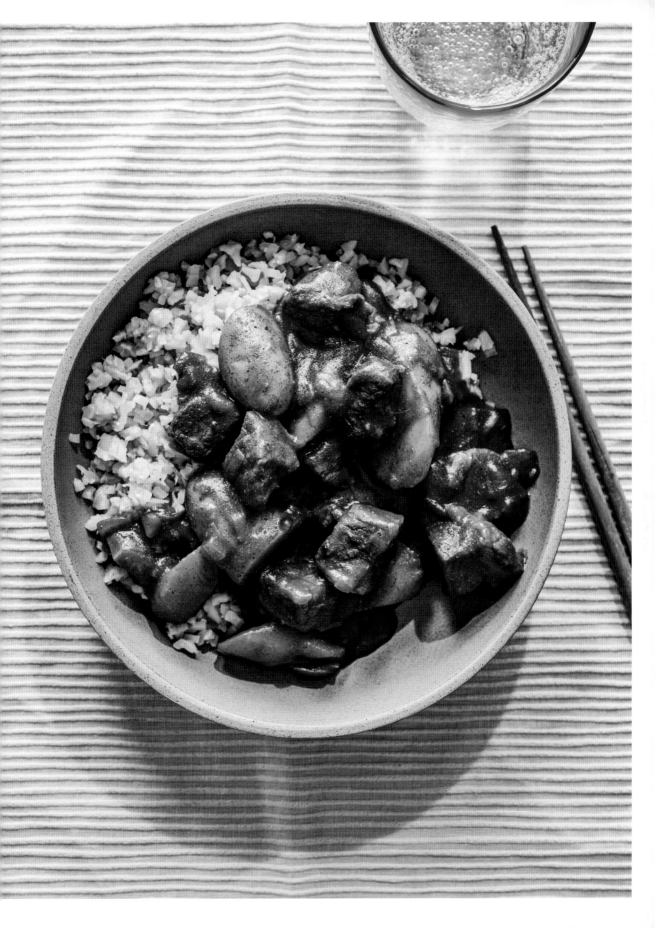

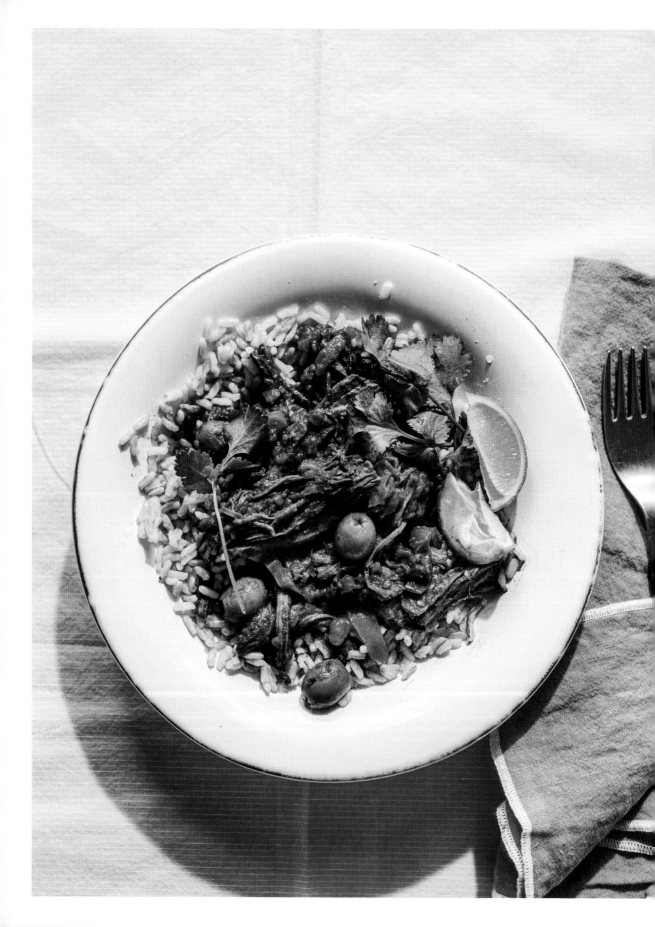

Slow Cooker Ropa Vieja

PREP TIME: 5 MINUTES   **COOK TIME: 8 HOURS**   **SERVES: 4**

358 *kcals* per serving

DF

GF

600g (1lb 5oz) flank steak, trimmed of any visible fat
1 large onion, finely chopped
3 garlic cloves, crushed
1 red (bell) pepper, sliced
1 green (bell) pepper, sliced
20 green olives (I like to use Manzanilla olives)
1½ teaspoons ground cumin
1½ teaspoons sweet paprika
1 teaspoon dried oregano
¾ teaspoon onion powder
¾ teaspoon garlic powder
¾ teaspoon ground turmeric
½ teaspoon ground cinnamon
pinch of red chilli flakes
180ml (6fl oz) beef stock
1 tablespoon apple cider vinegar
400g (14oz) can plum tomatoes
5 tablespoons tomato purée (paste)
2 bay leaves
salt and freshly ground black pepper
handful of freshly chopped coriander (cilantro)
lime wedges, to serve

Side suggestions:
Serve over rice, or choose cauliflower rice for a lower-carb option.

Swaps:
Stewing beef will work as a cheaper substitute for the flank, but for best results, flank is the best cut of meat for ropa vieja.

Ropa vieja is a simple but delicious Cuban stew that is perfectly suited to a slow cooker. This recipe gives you amazingly tender beef, with peppers, onions and olives in a flavour-packed tomato-based sauce with a blend of spices. Serve with some lime wedges and fresh coriander for a fresh, zesty finish.

1. Season the beef all over with salt and pepper. Heat a frying pan over a medium–high heat. Spray with olive oil spray, and add the beef. Fry for a few minutes, turning until lightly browned all over.

2. Transfer to the slow cooker.

3. Spray the empty frying pan with more olive oil spray and add the onions and garlic. Fry for a couple of minutes until lightly golden and softened, then transfer to the slow cooker, along with all the other ingredients (except the coriander). Stir to combine, lightly crushing the tomatoes, and cook on low for 8 hours.

4. Once cooked, roughly shred the beef with two forks. Season to taste with salt and pepper, then sprinkle over the coriander. Serve with your choice of sides and some lime wedges for squeezing.

KCALS
358

FAT
16.2g

SAT FAT
5.9g

CARBS
14.3g

SUGARS
12.3g

FIBRE
6.7g

PROTEIN
35.6g

SALT
0.79g

V

DF

GF

KCALS
213

FAT
2.1g

SAT FAT
0.3g

CARBS
32.1g

SUGARS
10.6g

FIBRE
12.3g

PROTEIN
10.1g

SALT
0.43g

Slow Cooker Bean and Sweet Potato Chilli

PREP TIME: **5 MINUTES**   COOK TIME: **8 HOURS**   SERVES: **8**

olive oil spray
1 large onion, chopped
3 garlic cloves, crushed
400g (14oz) can pinto
    beans, drained
400g (14oz) can kidney
    beans, drained
400g (14oz) can black
    beans, drained
400g (14oz) sweet potato,
    diced
400g (14oz) can chopped
    tomatoes
8 tablespoons tomato purée
    (paste)
1 red (bell) pepper, diced
1 green (bell) pepper, diced
1 jalapeño, deseeded and
    chopped
2 tablespoons sweet paprika
2 tablespoons ground cumin
2 teaspoons mild chilli
    powder
½ tablespoon garlic powder
½ tablespoon onion powder
1 teaspoon dried oregano
¾ teaspoon cayenne pepper
240ml (8½fl oz) vegetable
    stock
salt and freshly ground
    black pepper
freshly chopped coriander
    (cilantro), to serve.

As a family, we love chilli: it's one of those great informal meals that you can serve in the middle of the table, with all your favourite toppings, so that everyone can build their own bowl just the way they like it. I always feel this is a great way to encourage healthy eating for the kids, and it's the perfect way to spend time with your family and chat about your day.

1. Heat a frying pan over a medium–high heat and spray with olive oil spray. Add the onion and fry for a couple of minutes until golden and softened, then add the garlic and cook for a further 2 minutes.

2. Transfer this mixture to the slow cooker. Add all the other ingredients (except the coriander) and mix well to combine. Cook for 8 hours on low or 4 hours on high.

3. Taste and season with salt and black pepper as needed, then serve topped with fresh coriander.

Side suggestions:
Serve over rice, or cauliflower rice for a lower-carb option. Alternatively, set out all your favourite toppings and let everyone build their own bowl. Try guacamole or avocado, soured cream, Cheddar, crumbled tortilla chips, diced tomatoes and sliced jalapeños.

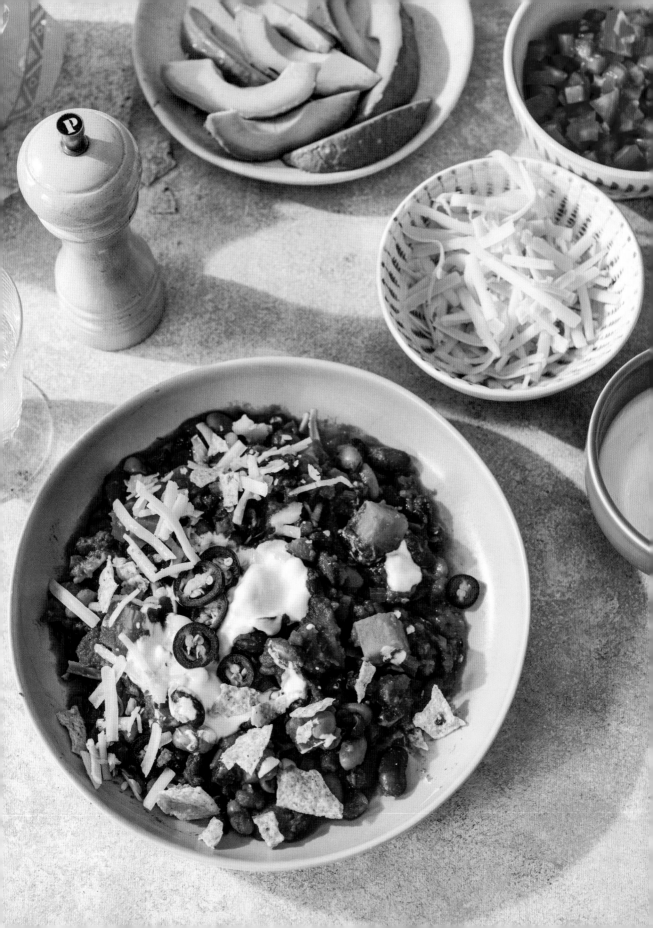

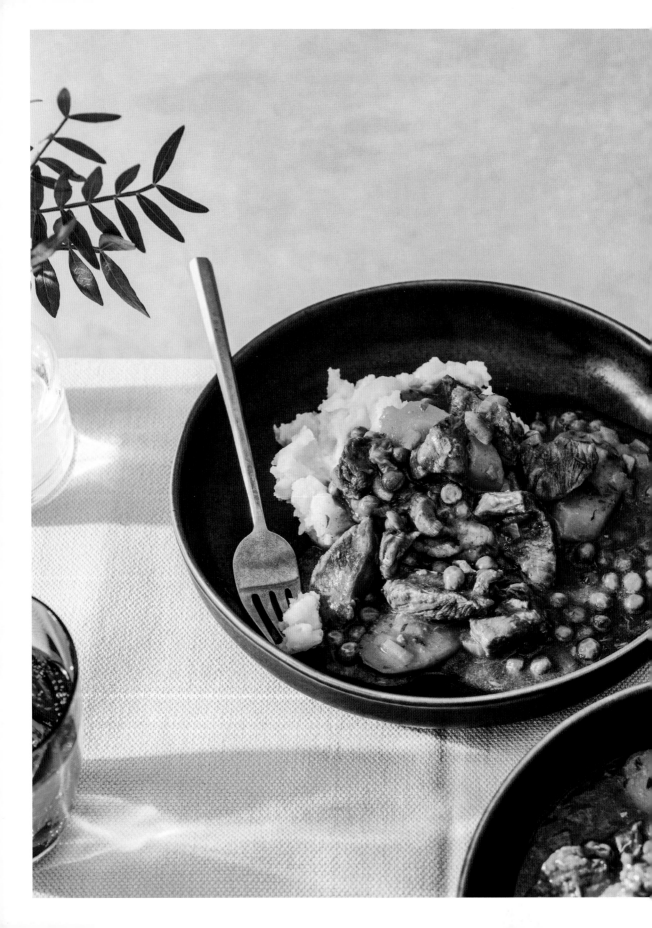

Slow Cooker Lamb and Mint Casserole

PREP TIME: 5 MINUTES + MARINATING   **COOK TIME: 8 HOURS**   **SERVES: 4**

412 kcals per serving

GF

DF

❄

KCALS	**412**
FAT	**17.0g**
SAT FAT	**7.2g**
CARBS	**24.0g**
SUGARS	**15.7g**
FIBRE	**4.5g**
PROTEIN	**38.4g**
SALT	**0.19g**

600g (1lb 5oz) lean stewing lamb, diced
1 large onion, chopped
3 garlic cloves, crushed
2 carrots, chopped
½ teaspoon dried rosemary
¼ teaspoon dried thyme
2½ tablespoons tomato purée (paste)
360ml (12fl oz) lamb stock (or use half chicken and half beef)
1½ tablespoons cornflour (cornstarch)
100g (3½oz) frozen peas
salt and freshly ground black pepper

For the mint sauce
handful of fresh mint leaves, finely chopped (approx. 17g/½oz)
1½ tablespoons granulated sugar or granulated sweetener
2½ tablespoons white wine vinegar
4 tablespoons boiling water

Side suggestions:
This is great served with mashed poatoes or cauliflower mash for a low-carb option and some additional vegetables of your choice.

When I was growing up, my mum would often make lamb with mint gravy on Sundays, and it's always been a bit of a comfort food for me. Lamb can sometimes be hard to source here in Canada, but when I can get some, I always want to make this delicious casserole. It's perfect served with all the usual Sunday dinner favourites, like roasted or mashed potatoes and some your favourite vegetables.

1. To make the mint sauce, simply combine all the ingredients in a jug or bowl. Season with a pinch of salt and allow to marinate for at least 30 minutes. (If you like, you can make this the day before.)

2. Add the diced lamb, onion, garlic and carrots to the slow cooker.

3. Once the mint sauce has finished marinating, add it to the slow cooker and mix to combine, along with the rosemary, thyme and tomato purée. Pour in the stock and cook on low for 7 hours.

4. In a small mug or bowl, mix the cornflour with a couple of tablespoons of water to make a slurry. Add this to the slow cooker, along with the peas. Stir to combine, then cook for 1 more hour to allow the gravy to thicken.

5. Taste and season as needed with salt and pepper, then serve with your favourite sides.

V

DF

GF

KCALS
309

FAT
11.5g

SAT FAT
4.8g

CARBS
33.6g

SUGARS
13.3g

FIBRE
12.2g

PROTEIN
11.8g

SALT
0.26g

Slow Cooker Chickpea and Vegetable Korma

PREP TIME: **20 MINUTES**   COOK TIME: **4 HOURS**   SERVES: **4**

olive oil spray
2 onions, finely chopped
3 garlic cloves, crushed
2 teaspoons freshly
     grated ginger
1 tablespoon mild curry
     powder
2 teaspoons ground cumin
2 teaspoons ground coriander
1 teaspoon ground turmeric
½ teaspoon kashmiri chilli
     powder
25g (1oz) cashews
1 tablespoon tomato purée
     (paste)
240ml (8½fl oz) vegetable
     stock
400g (14oz) can chickpeas,
     drained
300g (10½oz) butternut
     squash, cubed
½ head of cauliflower,
     broken into florets
1 red (bell) pepper, chopped
240ml (8½fl oz) light
     coconut milk
1 tablespoon cornflour
     (cornstarch)
100g (3½oz) frozen peas
salt and freshly ground
     black pepper
handful of coriander
     (cilantro) leaves, to serve

I love cooking Indian food at home. My kids tend to prefer milder curries and they love a korma, so this is the perfect recipe for them: especially as it's a great way to get a good quantity of vegetables into their food! It's so easy to make. For an Indian feast, I love to pair it with my Baked Chicken Pathia (page 115) and some basmati rice.

1. Heat a frying pan over a medium–high heat and spray with olive oil spray. Add the onions, garlic and ginger and fry for a couple of minutes until really golden and softened, then add the spices and mix to coat. Fry for a further 1 minute, then transfer to the slow cooker.

2. In a blender, combine the cashews and tomato purée and blend to form a smooth paste, adding up to 60ml (4 tablespoons) water if needed to blend.

3. Add this to the slow cooker, along with the vegetable stock, then stir in the chickpeas, butternut squash, cauliflower and red pepper. Cook for 3½ hours on high.

4. In a jug or bowl, mix the coconut milk with the cornflour, then add this to the slow cooker, along with the peas. Cook for another 30 minutes.

5. Taste and season with salt and pepper as needed, then sprinkle over the coriander, serve and enjoy.

Side suggestions:

This is great served with basmati rice, or for a low-carb alternative, try it with cauliflower rice. The garlic naan bread from page 171 is also delicious with this.

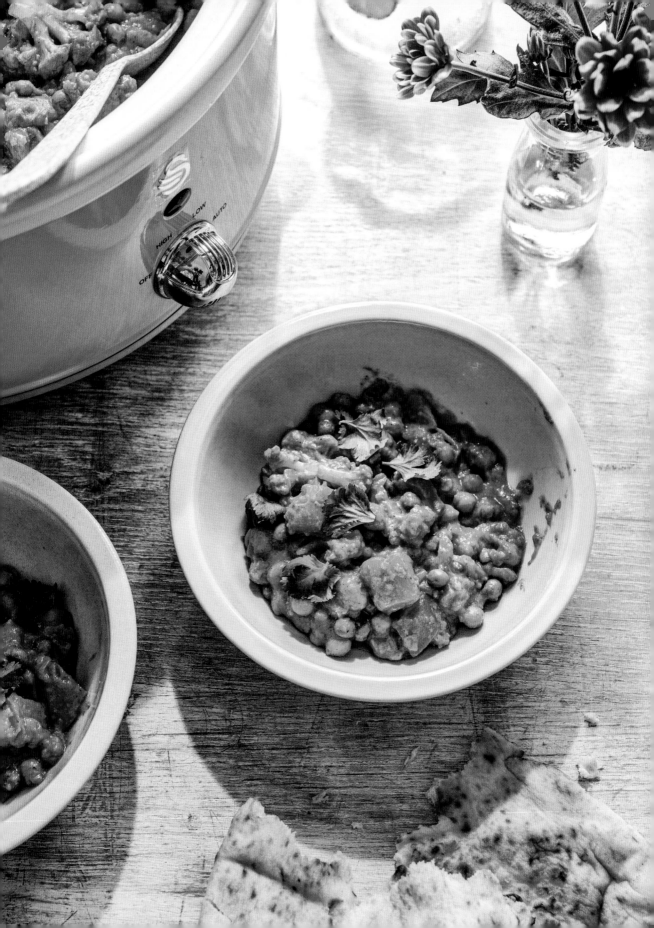

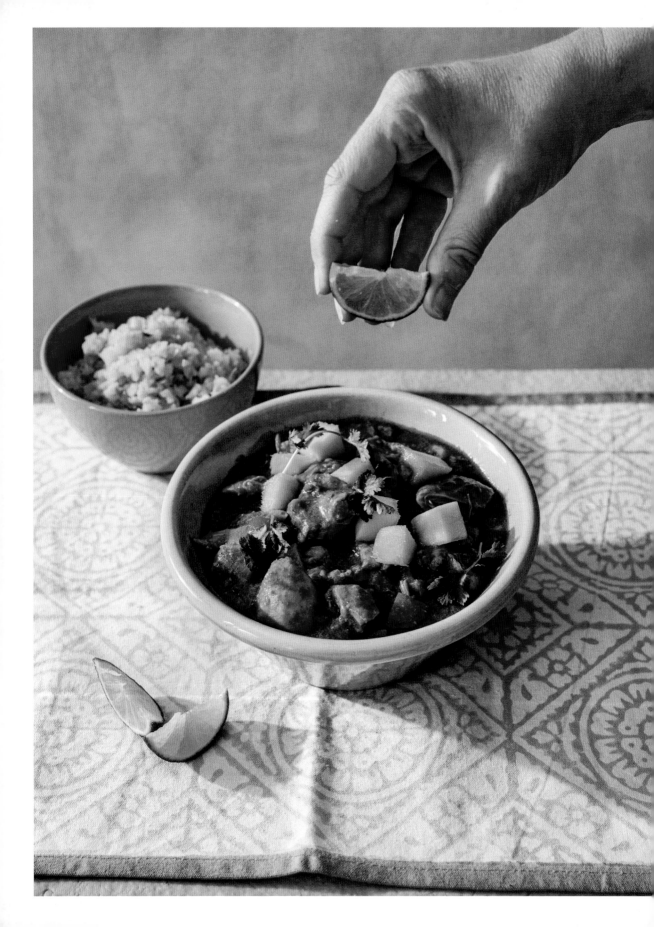

Slow Cooker Chicken and Mango Curry

PREP TIME: **10 MINUTES**   COOK TIME: **6 HOURS**   SERVES: **4**

½ tablespoon ghee or
    vegetable oil
1 onion, chopped
4 garlic cloves, minced
1 thumb-sized piece of
    fresh ginger, grated
1 tablespoon ground cumin
1 tablespoon curry powder
    (see Note)
1½ teaspoons ground
    coriander
1 teaspoon ground turmeric
1 teaspoon hot chilli powder
½ teaspoon garam masala
1 teaspoon salt
100g (3½fl oz) passata
2 tablespoons tomato purée
    (paste)
650g (23oz) boneless
    skinless chicken thighs,
    trimmed of visible fat
    and sliced in half
1 large red (bell) pepper,
    chopped
1 large ripe mango, peeled
    and chopped
400g (14oz) can light
    coconut milk
1 tablespoon cornflour
    (cornstarch)
salt and freshly ground
    black pepper
freshly chopped coriander
    (cilantro), to serve
lime wedges, to serve

Fruit is probably one of my favourite ingredients to add to a curry; it was something my mum always did, adding in some apple or sultanas, and it's perfect for balancing the heat and spices. The mango is not super-sweet in this curry, but really complements all the spices and pairs well with the creaminess of the coconut milk.

1. Melt the ghee or heat the vegetable oil in a frying pan over a medium–high heat. Add the onion and fry for a few minutes until softened and golden, then add the garlic and ginger. Stir in the ground spices and salt and fry for 2 minutes, adding 60ml (4 tablespoons) water to prevent anything from burning or catching on the pan. Stir in the passata and tomato paste, then transfer to the slow cooker.

2. Add the chicken to the slow cooker and stir to coat in the curry mix. Add the red pepper and most of the mango, reserving a little to serve.

3. In a jug, whisk the coconut milk with the cornflour until well combined, then stir this into the slow cooker as well.

4. Cook on low for 6 hours.

5. Taste and season with more salt if needed, then serve, scattered with coriander and topped with the reserved mango, with lime wedges on the side for squeezing.

Note:

Use mild, medium or hot curry powder, depending on your preferred spice level. The chilli powder already packs quite a bit of heat, so if you prefer milder curries, I suggest you opt for a mild curry powder. If you like lots of heat, go for a hotter curry powder. You can even top the curry with some fresh sliced red chilli to really spice things up.

Side suggestions:

Delicious served with rice, or cauliflower rice for a low-carb alternative.

432 kcals per serving

KCALS
432

FAT
21.7g

SAT FAT
10.3g

CARBS
21.3g

SUGARS
15.4g

FIBRE
5.4g

PROTEIN
35.3g

SALT
1.49g

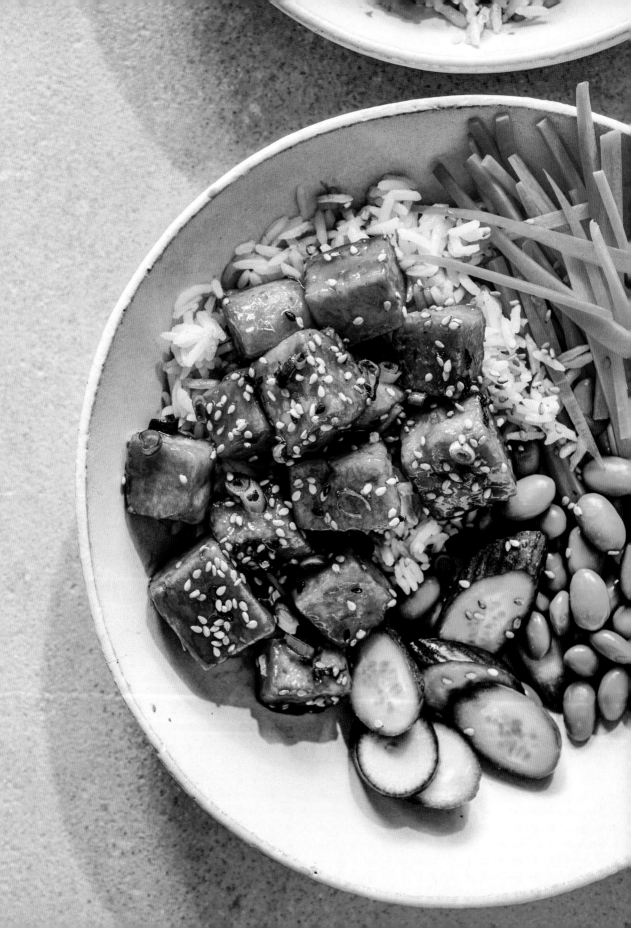

Delicious Bowls

223 kcals per serving

 V

VG

DF

GF

KCALS
223

FAT
3.7g

SAT FAT
0.6g

CARBS
28.3g

SUGARS
13.4g

FIBRE
14.8g

PROTEIN
11.8g

SALT
0.80g

Sun-dried Tomato, Bean and Lentil Soup

PREP TIME: 10 MINUTES   **COOK TIME: 20 MINUTES**   **SERVES: 4**

2 teaspoons extra virgin
   olive oil
80g (2¾oz) onion, diced
150g (5½oz) carrot, diced
3 garlic cloves, minced
60g (2oz) sun-dried
   tomatoes, chopped
2 teaspoons herbes de
   Provence
150g (5½oz) cherry
   tomatoes, chopped
3 tablespoons tomato purée
   (paste)
400g (14oz) can lentils,
   drained
400g (14oz) can haricot
   beans, drained
960ml (32½fl oz) vegetable
   stock
salt and freshly ground
   black pepper
freshly torn basil, to serve

Optional add-ons:
Add 15g (½oz) vegetarian
Italian-style hard cheese or
Cheddar to each bowl of
soup to serve.

This delicious, hearty soup is super-easy and quick to make. It has the beautiful flavour of sun-dried tomatoes, while the filling lentils and beans mean it's a complete meal in a bowl.

1. Heat the olive oil in a large, deep saucepan over a medium–high heat.

2. Add the onion and carrot and fry for a couple of minutes until golden and softened, then add the garlic and sun-dried tomatoes and sauté for another 2 minutes.

3. Add the herbes de Provence, cherry tomatoes and tomato purée, and stir until all combined. Next, add the lentils, beans and stock. Bring to the boil, then reduce the heat and simmer, covered, for 12–15 minutes.

4. Taste and season as needed with salt and pepper, then serve topped with freshly torn basil.

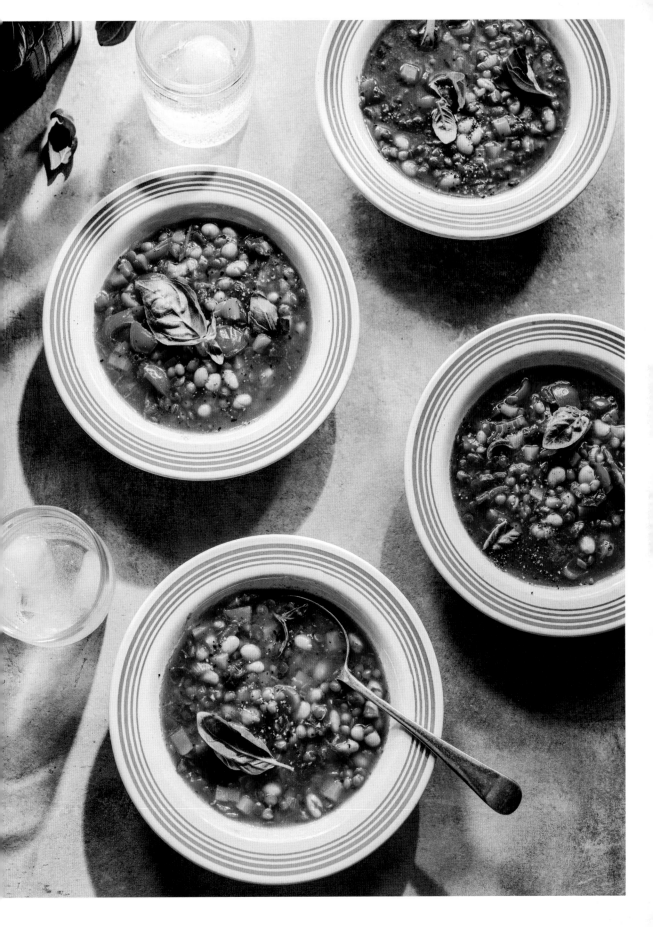

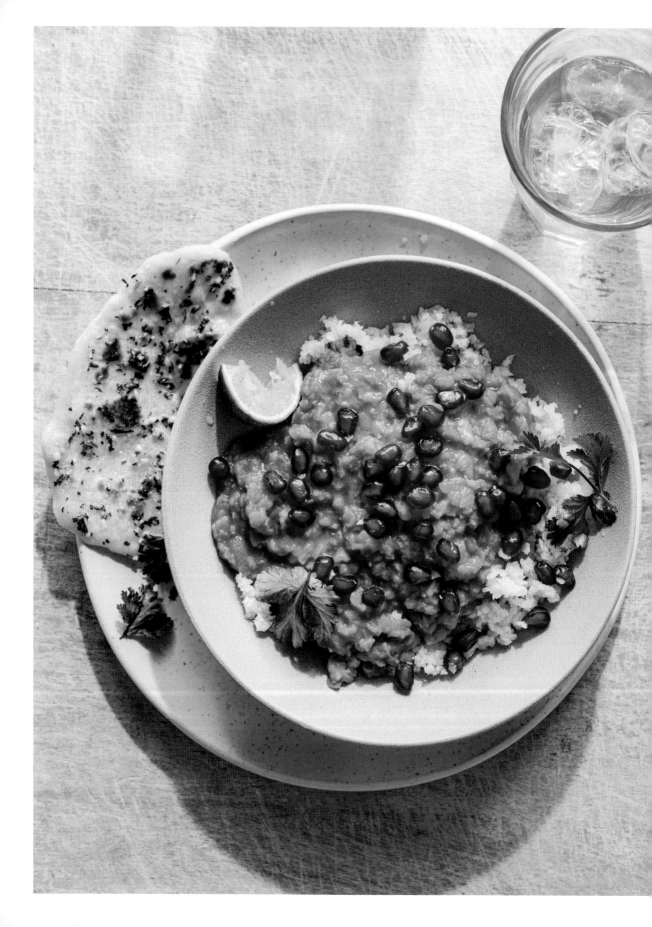

Sweet Potato Lentil Dhal Bowl with Garlic Naan

PREP TIME: **15 MINUTES**   COOK TIME: **30 MINUTES**   SERVES: **4**

olive oil spray
1 onion, finely chopped
4 garlic cloves, crushed
1 tablespoon grated
   fresh ginger
2 teaspoons ground cumin
2 teaspoons ground coriander
1 teaspoon ground turmeric
1 teaspoon chilli powder
1 teaspoon garam masala
2 tablespoons tomato purée
   (paste)
150g (5½oz) dried red lentils
250g (9oz) sweet potatoes,
   peeled and chopped
600ml (20fl oz) vegetable
   stock
120ml (4fl oz) light
   coconut milk
juice of 1 lime

For the garlic naan bread
120g (4¼oz) plain flour,
   plus extra for dusting
1½ teaspoons baking powder
½ teaspoon garlic powder
pinch of salt
150g fat-free Greek yogurt
   (do not use Greek-style!)
olive oil spray
½ tablespoon salted butter,
   melted
1 small garlic clove, minced
1 tablespoon freshly chopped
   coriander (cilantro)

To serve
360g (12¾oz) cooked
   cauliflower rice
freshly chopped coriander
   (cilantro)
8 tablespoons pomegranate
   seeds

Nutritional analysis:
Includes to serve options
as well.

These beautiful dhal bowls are probably one of my favourite things to make – and they're so simple and easy too! The garlic naan is great for dipping and scooping up some of the dhal.

1. Heat a large, deep saucepan or frying pan over a medium–high heat and spray with olive oil spray.

2. Add the onion, garlic and ginger, and fry for a couple of minutes until softened, then add the spices, along with the tomato purée and a little water, and cook until paste-like.

3. Add the lentils and sweet potatoes and stir to coat, then pour in the stock. Bring to the boil, then reduce the heat to medium–low, cover and simmer for 20 minutes until the lentils are cooked (stir occasionally just to ensure the lentils don't stick). Roughly mash the sweet potatoes in the pan using the back of a wooden spoon.

4. Stir in the coconut milk until the dhal is nice and creamy, then add a squeeze of fresh lime juice (the acidity balances the flavour).

5. While the dhal is cooking, make the garlic naan. In a large bowl, mix together the flour, baking powder, garlic powder and salt. Stir in the Greek yogurt with a spatula or wooden spoon; do not touch the mixture with your hands until it all comes together to form a dough. Once this happens, divide into four equal-sized balls.

6. Dust the work surface with some flour, then take one dough ball and use a rolling pin to roll it into a rough oval shape of about 12.5 x 17.5cm (5 x 7in). Set aside and repeat with the other dough balls.

7. Once all the naan breads are shaped, heat a large frying pan over a medium–high heat and spray with olive oil spray. When the pan is hot, add the naan (you can cook 2–3 at a time, depending on the size of your pan). Cook for about 3 minutes on each side until browned or golden in spots.

8. Once all the naan are cooked, mix the melted butter with the minced garlic and coriander, then brush this mixture over the naan.

9. To serve, divide the cauliflower rice between four bowls, then top with the curry. Sprinkle with some fresh coriander and the pomegranate seeds, and serve with the garlic naan.

KCALS	**470**
FAT	**7.1g**
SAT FAT	**3.4g**
CARBS	**73.6g**
SUGARS	**17.5g**
FIBRE	**11.9g**
PROTEIN	**22.1g**
SALT	**1.23g**

470 kcals per serving

Shanghai-style Beef with Egg-fried Cauliflower Rice

PREP TIME: 10 MINUTES　　**COOK TIME: 20 MINUTES**　　**SERVES: 4**

KCALS	**301**
FAT	**11.2g**
SAT FAT	**3.7g**
CARBS	**17.4g**
SUGARS	**11.1g**
FIBRE	**4.3g**
PROTEIN	**30.6g**
SALT	**2.85g**

400g (14oz) sirloin steak, trimmed of visible fat and thinly sliced
1 tablespoon cornflour (cornstarch)
olive oil spray
1 small onion, chopped
200g (7oz) green beans, trimmed and halved
200g (7oz) mushrooms, sliced

For the Shanghai-style sauce
2 tablespoons light soy sauce
1 tablespoon dark soy sauce
1 tablespoon maple syrup (or honey)
2 garlic cloves, crushed
½ teaspoon freshly ground black pepper
2 tablespoon Shaoxing wine
1 teaspoon sesame oil

For the egg-fried cauliflower rice
1 cauliflower, grated
3 spring onions (scallions), sliced
1 garlic clove, crushed
1 teaspoon sesame oil
2 tablespoons light soy sauce
2 large eggs
pinch of freshly ground black pepper

Swaps:
The green beans can be swapped for pak choi, green (bell) peppers or a similar type of veg of your choice.

Tender pan-fried steak with green beans and mushrooms in a delicious Shanghai-style Chinese sauce that is packed with flavour. For a balanced meal I like to serve this over egg-fried cauliflower rice. It's a great lighter alternative to traditional egg-fried rice which is lower in calories but delicious in taste. It's a great way to include more vegetables into a meal too.

1. In a bowl, mix together the steak and cornflour so the meat is coated. Leave to sit for 15 minutes.

2. Meanwhile, make the sauce. In a bowl or jug, whisk together all the ingredients with 60ml (4 tablespoons) water, then set aside.

3. Next, make the rice. Heat a frying pan over a medium–high heat and spray with olive oil spray. Add the cauliflower rice, spring onions and garlic, and stir-fry for about 5 minutes until the cauliflower rice is cooked.

4. Add the sesame oil and soy sauce and stir-fry until coated, then make a space in the middle of the pan and crack in the eggs. Just as they start to set, mix everything together, then season with black pepper and set aside.

5. To prepare the beef, heat a large frying pan over a medium–high heat and spray with olive oil spray. Add the onion, green beans and mushrooms, and fry for about 6 minutes until tender and golden. Remove from the pan and set aside on a plate.

6. Spray the empty frying pan with more olive oil spray, then add the steak and fry for approx 5 minutes, only flipping occasionally so it gets seared a lovely golden brown.

7. Return the veg to the pan, then pour in the sauce. Continue to stir-fry until the sauce slightly reduces and thickens. It should be coating the steak and vegetables.

8. Serve the beef in bowls with the egg-fried cauliflower rice and enjoy!!

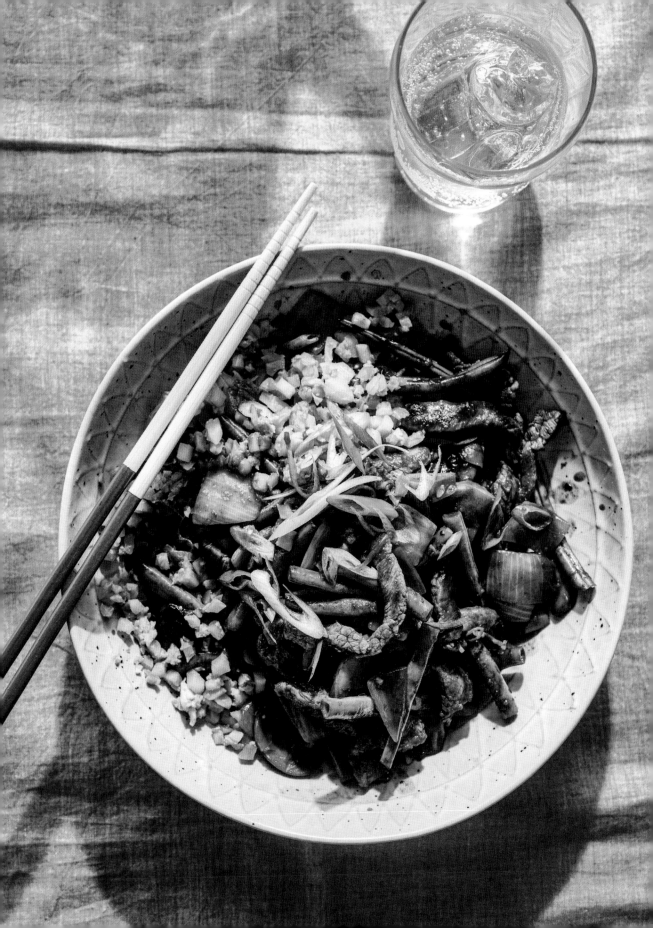

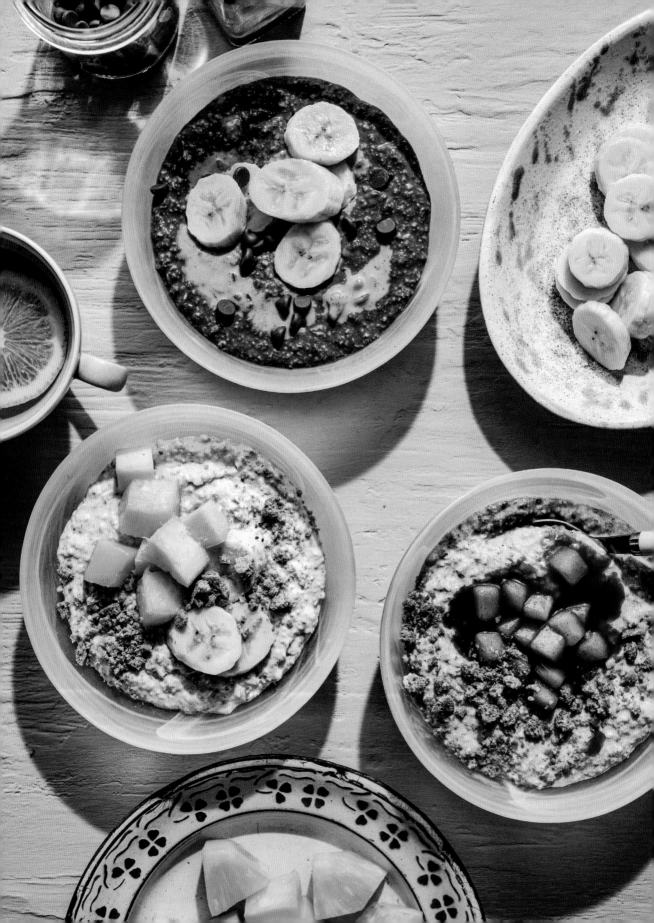

Overnight Oats Bowls – Three Ways

If you find yourself rushed for time in the mornings but still need a filling and delicious breakfast, overnight oats are a great option. Here are three of my favourite versions: Tropical, Caramel Apple Pie (see page 176) and Chocolate Peanut Butter Banana (see page 177). Just mix the base the night before and leave in the fridge, then add your toppings in the morning and it's ready.

Tropical Overnight Oats

PREP TIME: 5 MINUTES   **SERVES: 2**

1 large banana, half mashed, half sliced (see Note)
80g (2¾oz) rolled oats
1 teaspoon chia seeds
100g (3½oz) fat-free Greek yogurt
180ml (6fl oz) coconut milk (from a carton)
1 tablespoon maple syrup or honey
1 small mango, chopped
100g (3½oz) fresh pineapple, chopped
1 coconut biscuit (cookie), crumbled

1. In a bowl, mix together the mashed banana, oats, chia seeds, yogurt, coconut milk and maple syrup or honey. Cover and place in the fridge overnight.

2. When ready to enjoy, divide the overnight oats into two bowls and top with the mango, pineapple, sliced banana, and crumbled coconut biscuit.

KCALS
409

FAT
7.2g

SAT FAT
1.2g

CARBS
69.9g

SUGARS
37.0g

FIBRE
7.2g

PROTEIN
12.4g

SALT
0.17g

Caramel Apple Pie Overnight Oats

PREP TIME: 10 MINUTES   **COOK TIME: 5 MINUTES**   **SERVES: 2**

KCALS
431

FAT
9.9g

SAT FAT
3.1g

CARBS
68.7g

SUGARS
27.2g

FIBRE
7.6g

PROTEIN
11.6g

SALT
0.18g

80g (2¾oz) rolled oats
1 teaspoon chia seeds
100g (3½oz) fat-free
   Greek yogurt
180ml (6fl oz) oat milk
1 teaspoon vanilla extract
½ teaspoon ground
   cinnamon
1 oat biscuit (cookie),
   crumbled

For the caramel apples
½ tablespoon unsalted butter
250g (9oz) apples, peeled
   and diced
1 tablespoon maple syrup
   or honey
1 tablespoon granulated
   brown sweetener
1 tablespoon lemon juice
½ teaspoon ground
   cinnamon
pinch of nutmeg
pinch of ground cloves
½ tablespoon cornflour
   (cornstarch)

1. In a bowl, mix together the oats, chia seeds, yogurt, oat milk, vanilla extract and cinnamon. Cover and place in the fridge overnight.

2. To make the caramel apples, melt the butter in a small saucepan over a high heat. Add the apples and fry for a few minutes until lightly browned, then add the maple syrup, sweetener, lemon juice, cinnamon, nutmeg and cloves, along with 60ml (4 tablespoons) water. Cook for about 10 minutes until the apples are softened and caramelized, and the liquid has been absorbed. Keep stirring to ensure the apples don't burn.

3. In a small mug, mix the cornflour with 4 teaspoons water to make a slurry, then stir this into the apple mixture, still on the heat, until the apples are coated in a thickened sauce. Remove from the heat and allow to cool.

4. When ready to enjoy, divide the overnight oats into two bowls, then top with the caramel apples and crumbled biscuit.

Chocolate Peanut Butter Banana Overnight Oats

PREP TIME: 5 MINUTES   SERVES: 2

80g (2¾oz) rolled oats
10g (¼oz) cocoa powder
100g (3½oz) fat-free
  Greek yogurt
180ml (6fl oz) chocolate milk
  (I use chocolate oat milk)
1 teaspoon vanilla extract
2 tablespoons honey
1 large banana, half mashed,
  half sliced (see Note)
15g (½oz) chocolate chips
1 tablespoon peanut butter

Note:
Slice the banana in half, still in its skin. That way, you can mash the half you need straight away, and wrap the other half. If you keep it in the fridge, it will stay fresh until the morning.

1. In a bowl, mix together the oats, cocoa powder, yogurt, chocolate milk, honey, vanilla extract and mashed banana. Cover and place in the fridge overnight.

2. When ready to enjoy, divide the overnight oats into two bowls, then top with the chocolate chips and sliced banana.

3. Warm the peanut butter in the microwave in 5-second bursts until it reaches a drizzling consistency, then drizzle over the top and enjoy!

KCALS
496

FAT
13.0g

SAT FAT
4.4g

CARBS
73.2g

SUGARS
41.3g

FIBRE
7.2g

PROTEIN
16.5g

SALT
0.28g

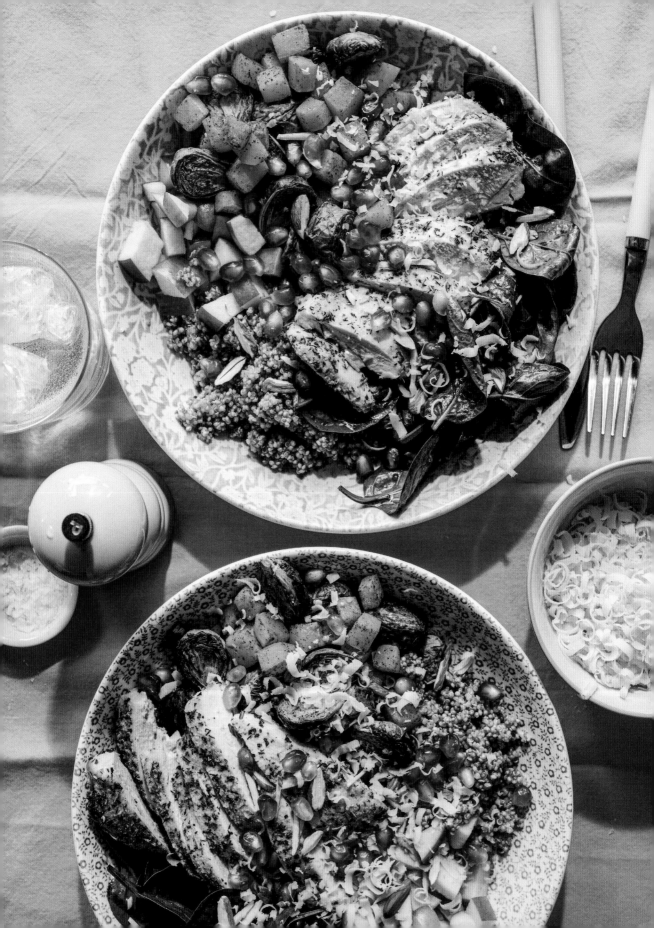

Harvest Chicken Quinoa Bowl

648 kcals
per serving

PREP TIME: 15 MINUTES   **COOK TIME: 40 MINUTES**   **SERVES: 2**

GF

240ml (8½fl oz) chicken
   stock
80g (2¾oz) quinoa, rinsed
200g (8oz) butternut
   squash, diced small
200g (8oz) Brussels sprouts,
   halved
olive oil spray
¾ teaspoon paprika
2 chicken breasts (approx.
   175g/6oz per breast)
1 tablespoon Garlic and Herb
   Seasoning (page 280)
½ tablespoon extra virgin
   olive oil
2 handfuls of mixed baby
   greens or spinach
1 small apple, cored and
   cubed
40g (1½oz) Cheddar, grated
4 tablespoons pomegranate
   seeds
10.5g (1½ teaspoons) flaked
   almonds
salt and freshly ground
   black pepper

For the dressing

1 tablespoon balsamic
   vinegar
½ tablespoon extra virgin
   olive oil,
½ tablespoon maple syrup
pinch of salt and freshly
   ground black pepper

I love bowls like this with lots of different components: deliciously seasoned chicken with roasted Brussels sprouts and butternut squash, along with healthy baby greens tossed in a light balsamic dressing, crunchy apple and sweet bursts of pomegranate, as well as nutty quinoa and an umami hit from the Cheddar. It's a delight in a bowl.

1. Preheat the oven to 220°C/200°C fan/425°F/gas 7 and line a baking tray with baking paper.

2. Place the stock and quinoa in a saucepan over a medium–high heat. Bring to the boil, then reduce the heat to medium and bubble for about 10–12 minutes until the stock is just absorbed. Take off heat and cover with a lid. Leave for 10 minutes, then fluff with a fork.

3. Spread out the diced butternut and Brussels sprouts on the prepared baking tray. Spray with olive oil spray, then sprinkle over the paprika and some salt and pepper. Toss to coat, then roast for 12 minutes.

4. Meanwhile, place the chicken into a bowl with the garlic and herb seasoning and extra virgin olive oil and toss so it's well coated.

5. Remove the baking tray from the oven and add the chicken, then return to the oven and roast for another 15–18 minutes until the chicken is cooked through.

6. Meanwhile, make the dressing. Whisk together the ingredients in a bowl until completely combined and season with salt and pepper. Drizzle the dressing over the mixed greens or spinach in a large bowl and toss to coat.

7. To assemble, slice the cooked chicken breasts and divide them between two bowls, along with the butternut squash, Brussels, quinoa, apple and Cheddar. Add the dressed baby greens and sprinkle with the pomegranate seeds and almond slices.

8. Enjoy!

KCALS	648
FAT	19.6g
SAT FAT	6.3g
CARBS	47.5g
SUGARS	22.0g
FIBRE	13.9g
PROTEIN	63.5g
SALT	2.59g

DF

Pork Potsticker Noodle Bowl

PREP TIME: **5 MINUTES**   COOK TIME: **20 MINUTES**   SERVES: **4**

400g (14oz) 5% fat pork mince (ground pork)
1 tablespoon grated fresh ginger
3 garlic cloves, finely chopped
4 tablespoons soy sauce
1 teaspoon sesame oil
1 tablespoon maple syrup
1 tablespoon oyster sauce
3 spring onions, chopped
250g (9oz) green cabbage, shredded
1 carrot, sliced into thin sticks
150g (5½oz) flat rice noodles
handful of freshly chopped coriander (cilantro)
pinch of red chilli flakes (optional)
salt and freshly ground black pepper

Swaps:
This also works well with chicken or turkey mince.

Ever had potstickers, also known as Chinese dumplings? This is a delicious deconstructed version in a bowl: seasoned ground pork in a flavour-packed sauce with shredded cabbage, carrots and flat rice noodles. Super-quick and easy to make, too, so it's perfect for those busy days.

1. Heat a large frying pan over a medium–high heat. Add the pork mince, ginger and garlic and fry for a few minutes until browned, breaking up the mince with your spoon.

2. Add the soy sauce, sesame oil, maple syrup, oyster sauce and spring onions and fry for a further 2 minutes, adding a couple of tablespoons of water to prevent the pork from becoming too dry.

3. Push the pork to one side of the pan and add the cabbage and carrot to the other side. Season with salt and pepper and sauté for 5–6 minutes until tender.

4. Meanwhile, cook the rice noodles according to the packet instructions, then drain.

5. To assemble, divide the pork, cabbage, carrots and noodles between four bowls. Top with the coriander and a pinch of chilli flakes (if using).

6. Enjoy!

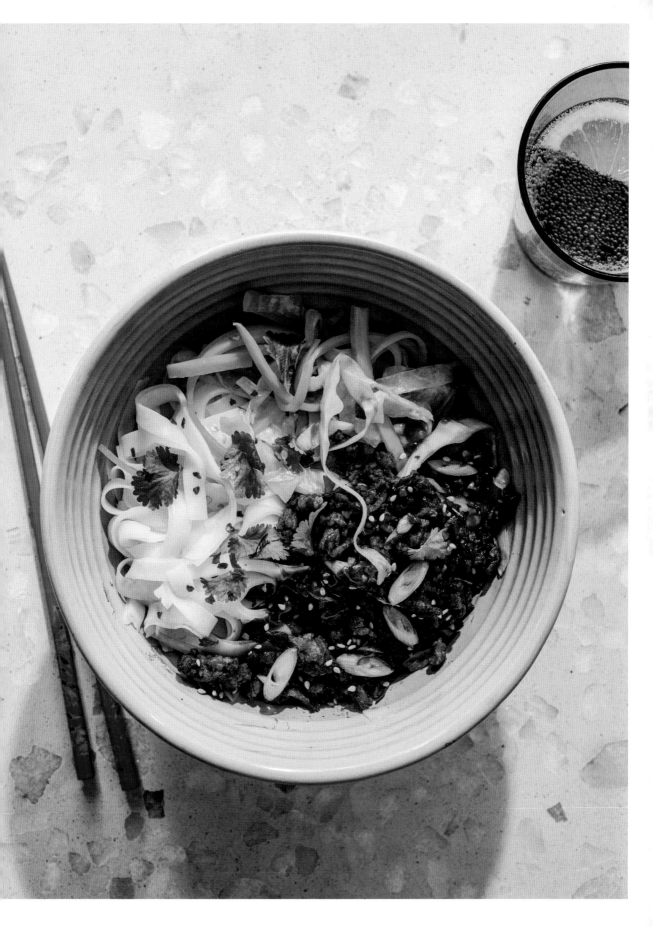

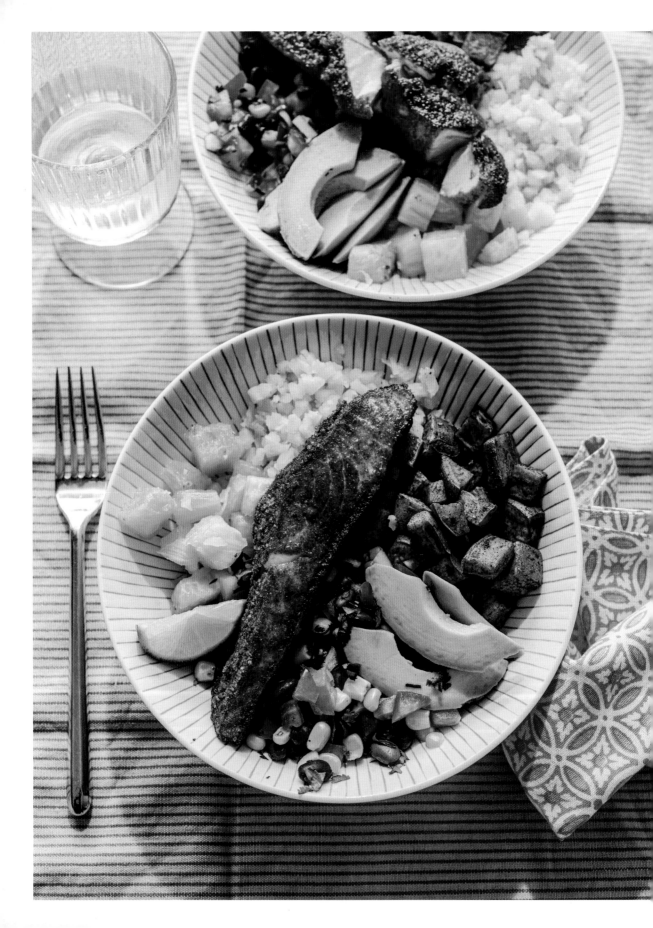

Barbecue Salmon Cauliflower Rice Bowl

PREP TIME: 10 MINUTES   **COOK TIME: 30 MINUTES**   **SERVES: 2**

562 *kcals* per serving

DF

GF

250g (9oz) sweet potatoes, cubed (skin left on)
1 teaspoon sweet paprika
olive oil spray
2 teaspoons light brown sugar
½ teaspoon smoked paprika
¼ teaspoon onion powder
2 fresh salmon fillets (approx. 125g/4½oz each)
pinch of sea salt
200g (7oz) cooked cauliflower rice
½ portion Black Bean Salsa (page 261)
100g (3½oz) pineapple, chopped
50g (1¾oz) avocado, sliced
lime wedges, to serve

Swaps:
If you prefer, you can swap the cauliflower rice for some cooked white rice or brown rice.

This beautiful bowl features perfectly cooked barbecue-seasoned salmon, served with cauliflower rice, black bean salsa, pineapple and avocado. It's an easy, quick dinner and full of flavour.

1. Preheat the oven to 220°C/200°C fan/425°F/gas 7 and line a baking tray with baking paper.

2. Spread out the sweet potato cubes on the prepared tray and sprinkle with ½ teaspoon of the sweet paprika. Spray with olive oil spray, then toss to coat. Spread out once more and bake for 18 minutes.

3. Meanwhile, mix the brown sugar with the remaining sweet paprika, along with the smoked paprika and onion powder. Rub this spice mix into the top of the salmon fillets, then spray each one with olive oil spray. Season each fillet with a pinch of sea salt.

4. When the sweet potato has been cooking for 18 minutes, remove from the oven and push the sweet potato cubes to one side of the tray. Place the salmon fillets on the other side, then return the tray to the oven and bake for 12–15 minutes until the salmon and sweet potato cubes are cooked through.

5. To assemble, warm up your cauliflower rice and divide it between two bowls, along with the black bean salsa, pineapple, avocado and sweet potato. Add the salmon (all in one piece, or you can roughly flake if you prefer) and serve with lime wedges for squeezing.

KCALS
562

FAT
22.7g

SAT FAT
4.4g

CARBS
48.7g

SUGARS
21.4g

FIBRE
12.7g

PROTEIN
34.3g

SALT
0.29g

Easy Cheat's Beef Pho Bowls

PREP TIME: 5 MINUTES   **COOK TIME: 15 MINUTES**   **SERVES: 2**

DF

KCALS
432

FAT
6.5g

SAT FAT
2.3g

CARBS
51.4g

SUGARS
7.6g

FIBRE
5.6g

PROTEIN
39.1g

SALT
4.28g

200g (7oz) sirloin steak,
    trimmed of visible fat
olive oil spray
1 small onion, finely sliced
2 garlic cloves, finely sliced
thumb-sized piece of
    fresh ginger, sliced
1 star anise
1 cinnamon stick
2 whole cloves
1 litre (33¾fl oz) beef broth
    (or stock)
1 tablespoon fish sauce
2 tablespoons hoisin sauce
100g (3½oz) flat rice noodles
80g (2¾oz) beansprouts
handful of fresh coriander
    (cilantro)
1 spring onion (scallion)
    sliced
1 red chilli, sliced
freshly ground black pepper
lime wedges, to serve

Notes:

I don't add any salt to the pho, as I find the balance of flavours here doesn't need it, but as with any dish, always taste and season more if needed.

I typically use fat-free beef broth from a carton for this recipe as it tastes much fresher than stock made with cubes. Stock cubes are fine to use, of course, but make sure you choose your favourite brand to get the best possible taste for this dish.

We love pho, but making the amazing flavoursome broth for a traditional pho can take quite a few different steps and processes. So, when I am rushed for time, this is my go-to quick method: it's all cooked in one pot and so easy to prepare. It's a favourite recipe with my kids, and one they request regularly.

1. Freeze the steak for about 15 minutes: this will firm it up, making it easier to slice thinly (a must for pho). Once the steak is slightly firm, use a very sharp knife to slice it into very thin slices. Set aside.

2. Heat a large, deep saucepan over a medium–high heat and spray with olive oil spray. Add the onion, garlic and ginger, and fry for a couple of minutes to soften, then add the star anise, cinnamon and cloves, and fry for another minute or so.

3. Pour in the stock, along with the fish sauce, hoisin sauce and a pinch of black pepper. Bring to the boil, then reduce the heat to medium and simmer for 10 minutes. Remove the star anise, cloves and cinnamon stick (you can also remove the onions if you prefer to have just broth, but we like to leave them in).

4. Add the rice noodles to the pan and continue to simmer for about 4 minutes until the noodles are cooked.

5. Using tongs, divide the noodles between two bowls, then top the noodles with the raw thinly sliced beef. Ladle the hot broth over the beef (the broth will be hot enough to cook the meat in the bowls; don't be tempted to add the meat to the pan and boil on the stove, or it will become tough and overcooked).

6. Top each bowl with beansprouts, coriander, chopped spring onion and red chilli, and serve with a wedge of lime for squeezing.

7. Enjoy!

Variation:

This can also be made with chicken. Swap the beef stock for chicken stock and cook the chicken in the broth from the beginning. A small chicken breast is normally enough for two people.

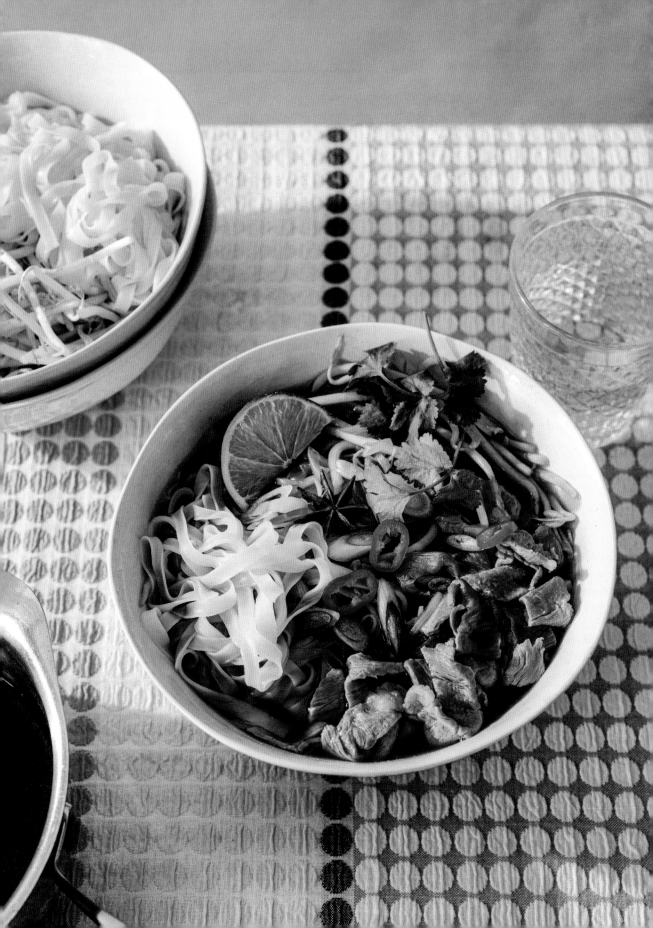

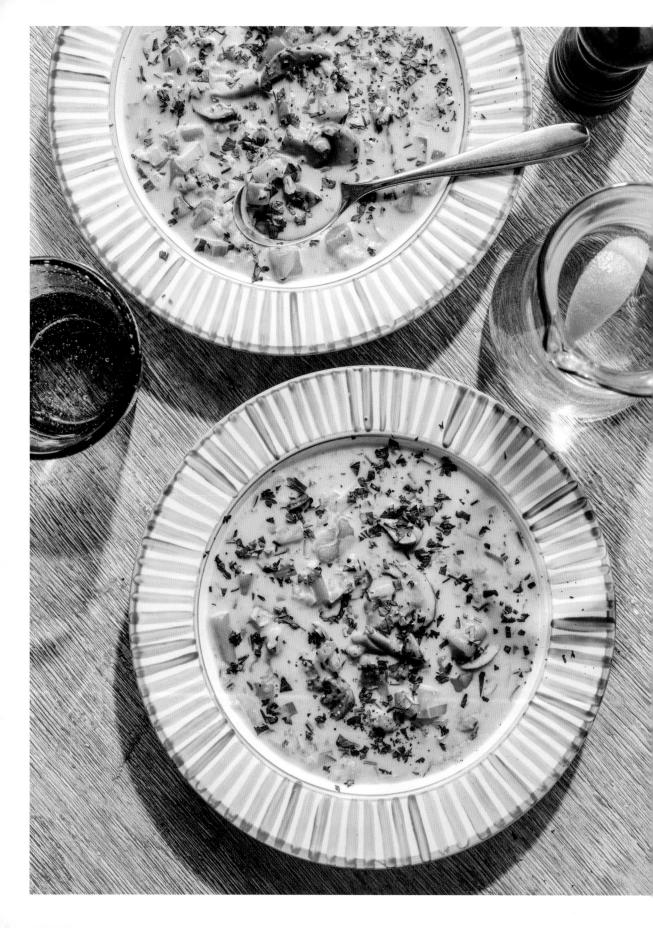

Creamy Mushroom and Vegetable Barley Soup

PREP TIME: 15 MINUTES   **COOK TIME: 50 MINUTES**   **SERVES: 4**

olive oil spray

1 small onion, diced

2 garlic cloves, minced

1 carrot, diced

1 celery stalk, diced

200g (7oz) butternut
squash, peeled and diced

200g (7oz) chestnut
mushrooms, sliced

1 litre (33¾fl oz) vegetable
stock

¼ teaspoon dried thyme

¼ teaspoon dried rosemary

¼ teaspoon dried sage

75g (2½oz) dried barley

1 tablespoon cornflour
(cornstarch)

240ml (8½fl oz) semi-
skimmed milk

75g (2½oz) light cream
cheese

2 tablespoons freshly
chopped parsley

salt and freshly ground
black pepper

Note:
Do not use skimmed milk for
this recipe, or you will not get
the same creamy finish.

Dairy-free:
The milk can be replaced
with light coconut milk, but
make sure you don't forget
the cornflour, or it won't
thicken.

**My whole family loves soup, which is lucky, because it's always
a great way to include lots of veggies in a meal. This creamy
soup, made with mushrooms, vegetables and barley, is simple,
delicious, hearty and filling. Occasionally when I have some
leftover roast chicken, I will throw some of that in at the end,
for a complete meal in a bowl.**

1. Heat a large saucepan over a medium–high heat and spray with
olive oil spray.

2. Add the onion and fry for a couple of minutes to soften, then add
the garlic, carrot, celery, butternut squash and mushrooms and fry
for a further 5 minutes until golden. Add a splash of stock if needed
to prevent anything catching on the bottom of the pan.

3. Stir in the herbs, then add the stock and barley and stir to combine.
Bring to the boil, then reduce the heat to medium. Cover and
simmer for 40 minutes until the barley is cooked through.

4. In a small mug or bowl, mix the cornflour with a little water to
make a slurry. Stir this into the pan, along with the milk and cream
cheese. Keep stirring until the cream cheese is all melted and the
soup thickens and is creamy.

5. Taste and season with salt and pepper, then stir in the chopped
parsley and serve.

195 kcals
per serving

KCALS
195

FAT
3.0g

SAT FAT
1.2g

CARBS
31.2g

SUGARS
9.8g

FIBRE
4.0g

PROTEIN
8.9g

SALT
0.85g

Bibimbap Bowls

PREP TIME: 15 MINUTES   **COOK TIME: 15 MINUTES**   **SERVES: 4**

DF

KCALS
522

FAT
13.5g

SAT FAT
4.2g

CARBS
59.4g

SUGARS
13.3g

FIBRE
5.0g

PROTEIN
38.3g

SALT
2.53g

175g (6oz) jasmine rice
low-calorie cooking oil spray
200g (7oz) mushrooms,
   thinly sliced
2 teaspoons soy sauce
250g (9oz) beansprouts,
   soaked in boiling salted
   water for a couple of
   minutes, then drained
200g (7oz) courgette
   (zucchini), halved
   lengthways and thinly sliced
150g (5½oz) carrot, sliced
   into thin sticks
250g (9oz) spinach,
   chopped into strips
½ teaspoon garlic powder
4 medium eggs
salt and freshly ground
   black pepper
sesame seeds, to serve
   (optional)

For the beef
400g (14oz) 5% fat beef
   mince (ground beef)
2 garlic cloves, minced
1 tablespoon light soy sauce
1 tablespoon dark soy sauce
1 tablespoon gochujang
½ tablespoon maple syrup
   or honey
1 teaspoon sesame oil

For the bibimbap sauce
3 tablespoons gochujang
1 tablespoon maple syrup
½ tablespoon rice wine
   vinegar
1 garlic clove, crushed

Bibimbap is a Korean dish that most of us have probably heard of, and it's up there with one of my family's all-time favourites. Don't be put off by the long list of ingredients; it's actually pretty easy to make. The key is getting all your ingredients ready in advance, and then as you cook each component, you can add them to a large plate, ready to assemble in the bowl.

1. Cook the rice according to the packet instructions and set aside.

2. In a bowl or jug, mix together the ingredients for the bibimbap sauce with 1 tablespoon water until well combined, then set aside.

3. To prepare the beef, heat a frying pan over a medium–high heat. Add the mince and garlic and fry for a couple of minutes until browned. Next, add the soy sauces, gochujang, maple syrup and sesame oil, and fry for another few minutes until slightly caramelized. Reduce the heat to low to keep the beef warm while you prepare the vegetables.

4. Heat another large frying pan over a medium–high heat and spray with low-calorie cooking oil spray. Add the mushrooms and fry for a couple of minutes until golden, then add 1 teaspoon of the soy sauce and stir-fry until the soy sauce evaporates, giving the mushrooms a nice colour. Transfer the mushrooms to a large plate.

5. Add the beansprouts to the empty frying pan, along with the remaining 1 teaspoon soy sauce and a pinch of black pepper. Fry for about a minute until just tender (don't overcook), then set aside on the plate with the mushrooms.

6. Spray the empty frying pan with low-calorie cooking oil spray then add the courgette and carrots. Fry for a couple of minutes until tender, seasoning with a little pinch of salt. Set aside on the plate.

7. Add the spinach and garlic powder to the empty pan and cook until wilted. Set aside on the plate.

8. Spray the frying pan with low-calorie cooking oil spray, then crack the eggs into the empty frying pan and fry to your preference.

9. Warm up four serving bowls and portion the cooked rice into the bottom of each bowl. Divide the meat mixture between the bowls, then top with the vegetables from the plate, arranging them in sections in the bowls. Top with the fried egg and sprinkle each bowl with a pinch of sesame seeds. Serve with the bibimbap sauce.

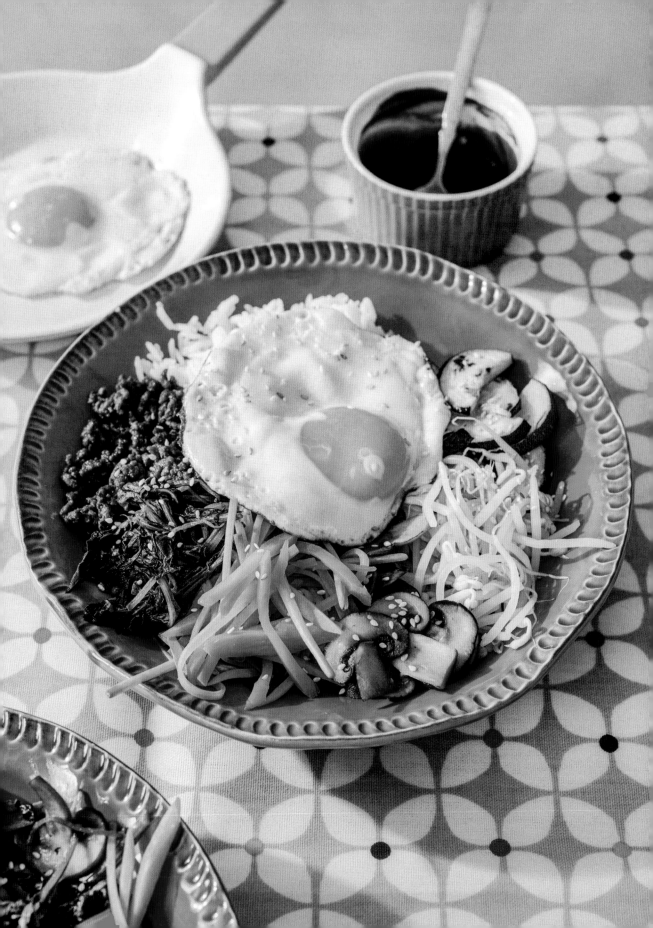

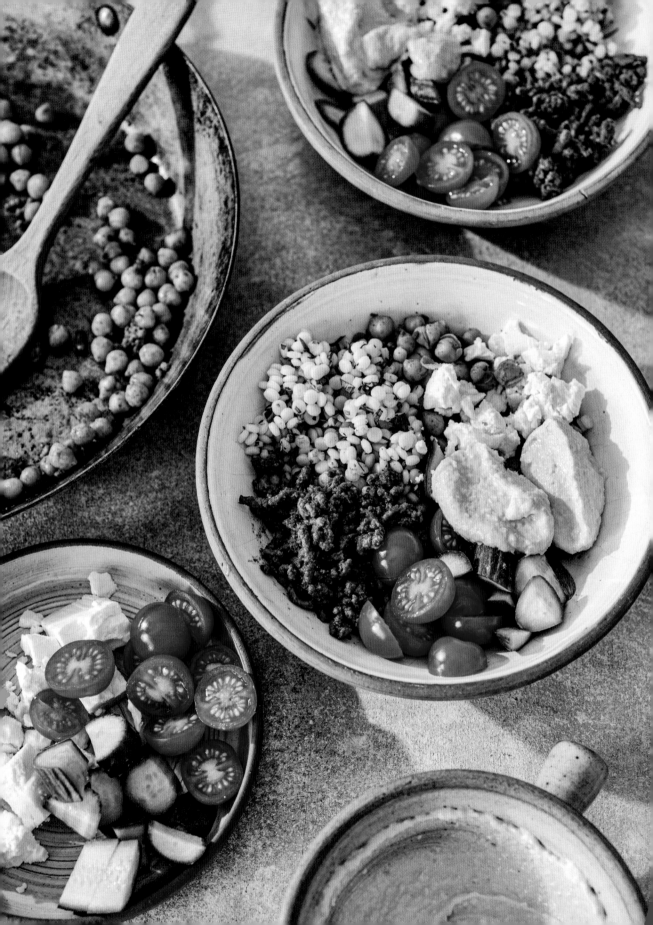

Middle Eastern-style Lamb Bowls

PREP TIME: **5 MINUTES**   COOK TIME: **12 MINUTES**   SERVES: **4**

400g (14oz) 10% fat lamb
mince (ground lamb)
1 teaspoon ground cumin
1 teaspoon ground coriander
1 teaspoon sweet paprika
½ teaspoon garlic powder
½ teaspoon onion powder
½ teaspoon dried oregano
¼ teaspoon ground
cardamom
pinch of red chilli flakes
2 tablespoons tomato
purée (paste)
125g (4½oz) canned
chickpeas, drained
pinch of paprika
olive oil spray
salt and freshly ground
black pepper

To serve
Lemon and Herb Israeli
Couscous (page 266)
80g (2¾oz) reduced-fat
feta, crumbled
8 tablespoons reduced-fat
hummus
20 cherry tomatoes,
halved
4 baby cucumbers,
halved lengthways
and sliced

**Where I live in Canada, there are some great choices for Lebanese
and Middle Eastern places to eat, and when I am not out for lunch
with a friend at one of the amazing restaurants, I am often
creating my own Middle Eastern-inspired dishes at home. These
bowls – made with lamb and lemon-and-herb couscous, paired
with hummus, chickpeas, salty feta, cucumbers and tomatoes –
are delicious. They're so quick and easy to make, too.**

1. Heat a large frying pan over a medium–high heat. Add the lamb
and fry for a few minutes until browned, breaking up the mince with
your spoon as it cooks. Add the cumin, coriander, sweet paprika,
garlic powder, onion powder, oregano, cardamom, chilli flakes and
tomato purée, and mix to coat, adding a splash of water to prevent
it drying out too much. Continue to fry for a few minutes until fully
cooked, then season to taste with salt and pepper.

2. Push the lamb to one side of the frying pan and add the chickpeas
to the other side. Season with the pinch of paprika and some salt,
then spray with olive oil spray and fry for about a minute just until
the chickpeas take on a lovely colour from the paprika.

3. To assemble, build your bowls with the lamb, couscous, feta,
hummus, chickpeas, tomatoes and cucumbers, and enjoy!

KCALS	484
FAT	17.2g
SAT FAT	6.3g
CARBS	42.2g
SUGARS	6.1g
FIBRE	8.7g
PROTEIN	35.7g
SALT	0.83g

Swaps:
If you like, you can swap the
lamb for 5% fat beef mince.

Optional add-ins:
Warmed toasted pitta cut
into triangles is a great
addition to these bowls.

Make your own hummus:
If you want to make your own
hummus, just tip 400g (14oz) canned
chickpeas into a food-processor
along with 1 garlic clove, 1 tablespoon
tahini, ¾ teaspoon ground cumin
and the juice of ½ lemon. Pulse until
the mixture reaches your preferred
consistency (you can add chickpea
juice from the can if needed), then
season to taste with salt.

Arroz Con Albondigas Bowls

PREP TIME: **20 MINUTES**   COOK TIME: **40 MINUTES**   SERVES: **4**

KCALS
470

FAT
10.8g

SAT FAT
2.4g

CARBS
51.5g

SUGARS
12.3g

FIBRE
7.3g

PROTEIN
37.9g

SALT
2.10g

1 onion, finely chopped
4 garlic cloves, crushed
½ red (bell) pepper,
    finely chopped
½ green (bell) pepper,
    finely chopped
50g (1¾oz) carrot, finely grated
1½ teaspoons sweet paprika
1 teaspoon ground cumin
½ teaspoon ground turmeric
½ teaspoon dried oregano
½ teaspoon cayenne pepper
    (optional)
1 bay leaf
180g (6½oz) long-grain rice
120g (4¼oz) passata
480ml (16¼fl oz) chicken stock
85g (3oz) frozen peas
salt and freshly ground
    black pepper
1 lime, cut into 4 wedges, to serve

For the meatballs
455g (1lb) turkey mince
    (ground turkey)
1 tablespoon freshly
    chopped parsley
1 teaspoon salt
1 teaspoon paprika
pinch of freshly ground
    black pepper
olive oil spray

For the herby dressing
3 tablespoons light mayonnaise
3 tablespoons fat-free
    Greek yogurt
¾ tablespoon finely
    chopped parsley
¾ tablespoon finely chopped
    coriander (cilantro)
½ teaspoon garlic powder
juice of ½ lime

For the salad
½ red (bell) pepper, thinly sliced
½ small red onion, thinly sliced
12 baby plum tomatoes,
    halved
70g (2½oz) baby salad leaves

If you love arroz con pollo, you will love these delicious bowls. This is a popular recipe with my kids: they love the combination of the rice with meatballs. Paired with a simple salad, with lime wedges and a light, herby dressing, it is a complete meal in a bowl.

1. In a large bowl, mix together the ingredients for the meatballs (except the olive oil spray) until well combined. Spray your hands with olive oil spray and use them to form the mixture into 16 equal-sized meatballs.

2. Heat a frying pan over a medium–high heat and spray with olive oil spray. Add the meatballs and fry for a few minutes until lightly golden, then remove from the pan and set aside on a plate.

3. Add the onion, garlic, peppers and carrot to the empty pan and fry for a few minutes to soften. Next add the herbs and spices and season with salt and pepper. Fry for a further minute, adding a splash of water to deglaze any bits stuck to the bottom of the pan, then return the meatballs to the pan, along with the rice, and stir to coat in all the seasoning.

4. Pour in the passata and stock and stir again, then bring to the boil. Reduce the heat to medium–low, then cover and simmer for about 12 minutes until the stock is just absorbed. Now stir in the frozen peas. Turn off the heat but leave the lid on, and leave to rest for 10–12 minutes; the residual heat will finish cooking the rice perfectly.

5. Meanwhile, mix together all the dressing ingredients in a small bowl and season with salt and pepper.

6. In a large bowl, combine the ingredients for the salad and mix together, then divide between four serving bowls. When the arroz con albondigas is ready, add it to the bowls, then drizzle over the dressing. Serve with the lime wedges for squeezing.

Swaps:
You can also use chicken mince if you prefer – and if you like additional heat, add some sliced fresh jalapeño to the salad for an extra kick.

Freezing:
Only the meatballs can be frozen.

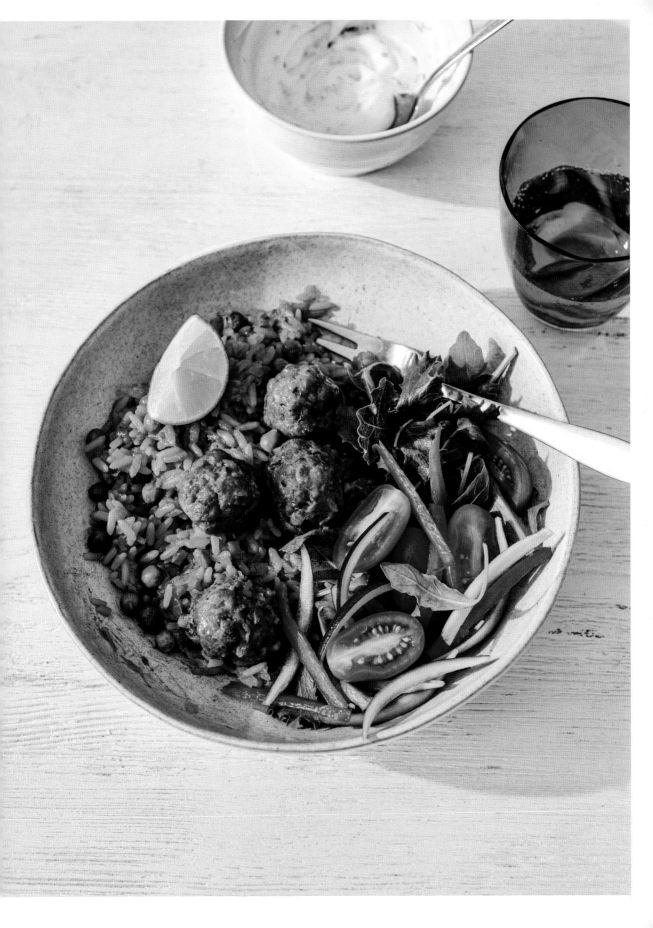

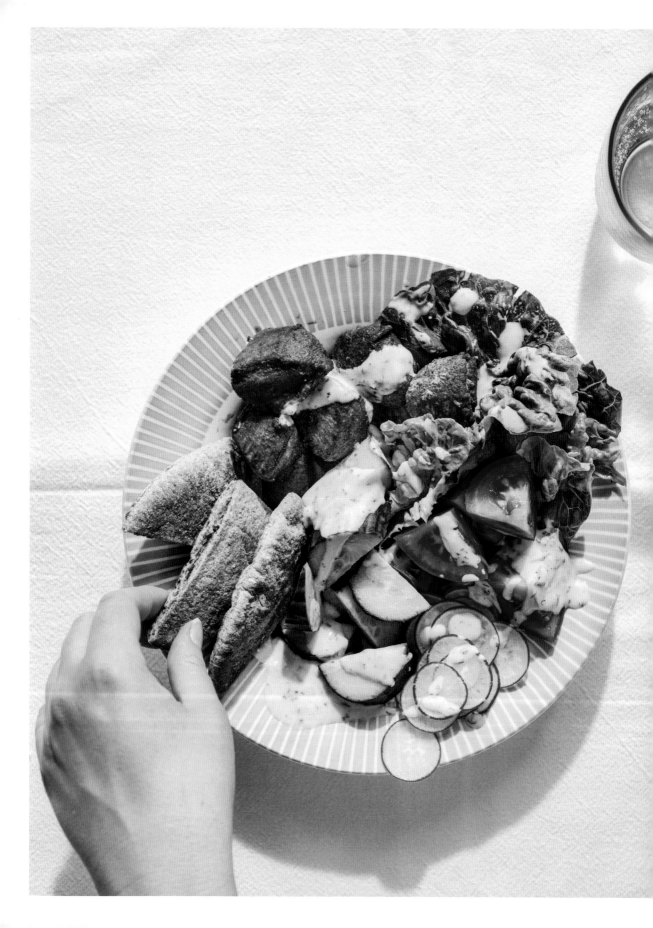

Spiced Chicken Salad Bowls

PREP TIME: 5 MINUTES **COOK TIME: 8 MINUTES** **SERVES: 2**

488 kcals
per serving

70g (2½oz) romaine
  lettuce, chopped
2 ripe tomatoes, quartered
100g (3½oz) cucumber,
  halved lengthways
  and chopped
¼ red onion, thinly sliced
3 radishes, thinly sliced
2 small low-calorie
  wholemeal pitta breads,
  warmed
fresh lemon wedges, to serve

**For the mint and
mango raita**
6 tablespoons fat-free
  Greek yogurt
1½ tablespoons very finely
  chopped fresh mint
1 tablespoon mango chutney
1 tablespoon lemon juice
½ teaspoon garlic powder
salt and freshly ground
  black pepper

For the chicken
300g (10½oz) boneless,
  skinless chicken breast,
  diced into cubes
2 teaspoons curry powder
  (mild, medium or hot,
  depending on your
  preferred spice level)
1 teaspoon paprika
¼ teaspoon chilli powder
1 tablespoon lemon juice
1 garlic clove, crushed
1 teaspoon grated
  fresh ginger
olive oil spray
1 tablespoon honey

When I want a quick lunch or dinner, these spiced chicken salad bowls are my go-to: super-quick to make, but oh so tasty. You can use the wholemeal pitta for scooping up little bits of everything, as well as dipping in the mint and mango raita.

1. In a bowl, combine all the ingredients for the mint and mango raita and mix to combine. Set aside.

2. In a separate bowl, mix the chicken with the curry powder, paprika, chilli powder, lemon juice, garlic and ginger. Season with salt and pepper and toss until well coated in all the spices.

3. Heat a frying pan over medium–high heat and spray with olive oil spray. Once the pan is hot, add the seasoned chicken and fry for 6–7 minutes until really golden, then add 1 tablespoon water and the honey and allow to reduce around the chicken for about 1 minute.

4. Divide the chicken between two bowls, along with the lettuce, tomatoes, cucumber, onion and radishes. Serve with the warmed pittas and raita, with lemon wedges on the side for squeezing.

KCALS
488

FAT
4.2g

SAT FAT
0.7g

CARBS
51.7g

SUGARS
23.3g

FIBRE
8.4g

PROTEIN
56.5g

SALT
1.20g

V

DF

KCALS
499

FAT
13.6g

SAT FAT
1.8g

CARBS
69.1g

SUGARS
17.7g

FIBRE
5.8g

PROTEIN
22.1g

SALT
1.51g

Sticky Sriracha Tofu Bowls

PREP TIME: **15 MINUTES**   COOK TIME: **15 MINUTES**   SERVES: **4**

180g (6½oz) white
  jasmine rice
4 baby cucumbers,
  sliced diagonally
160g (5¾oz) cooked
  edamame beans
1 large carrot, julienned
  or grated
pinch of sesame seeds
  (I use black and toasted
  sesame seeds)

**For the spicy sriracha
sauce**
2 tablespoons soy sauce
3 tablespoons maple syrup
  or honey
1 tablespoon sriracha
  (see Note)
1½ tablespoons rice wine
  vinegar
2 garlic cloves, finely
  chopped
1½ teaspoons grated
  fresh ginger
1 tablespoon cornflour
  (cornstarch)

For the tofu
400g (14oz) extra-firm tofu
1½ tablespoons cornflour
  (cornstarch)
pinch of salt
4 teaspoons vegetable oil
2 spring onions (scallions),
  sliced

These spicy sriracha tofu bowls make a great meat-free meal: golden pan-fried cubes of tofu in a sticky sriracha sauce, with white jasmine rice, edamame, carrot and cucumber creating the perfect contrast to the spicy tofu. I know tofu isn't for everyone, but cooked correctly it can be really tasty, especially in a flavoursome sauce like this – so give it a try! You won't regret it.

1. Cook the jasmine rice according to the packet instructions.

2. Meanwhile, make the sauce by whisking together all the ingredients in a bowl with 120ml (4fl oz) water until well combined.

3. To prepare the tofu, press it between two paper towels to absorb any excess moisture, then slice into 2cm (¾in) cubes. Add to a large bowl with the cornflour and salt and toss to coat.

4. Heat 2 teaspoons of the oil in a large non-stick frying pan over a medium–high heat. Once hot, add half the tofu cubes and fry for about 6 minutes until golden and crispy on all sides, then remove and set aside on a plate. Repeat with the remaining oil and tofu and again set aside on the plate.

5. Add the sauce to the empty pan and allow to bubble until it thickens, then return the tofu to the pan and toss until coated. Sprinkle with the chopped spring onions.

6. Divide the spicy tofu between four bowls, along with the cooked rice, baby cucumber, edamame beans and grated carrot. Sprinkle over a pinch of sesame seeds and enjoy!

Low-carb side suggestions:
Swap the rice for cauliflower rice, or use the egg-fried cauliflower rice from page 172. You could also skip the rice and serve with additional stir-fried vegetables.

Note:
If you don't like your food too spicy, you may want to start with less sriracha and adjust to your preferred level.

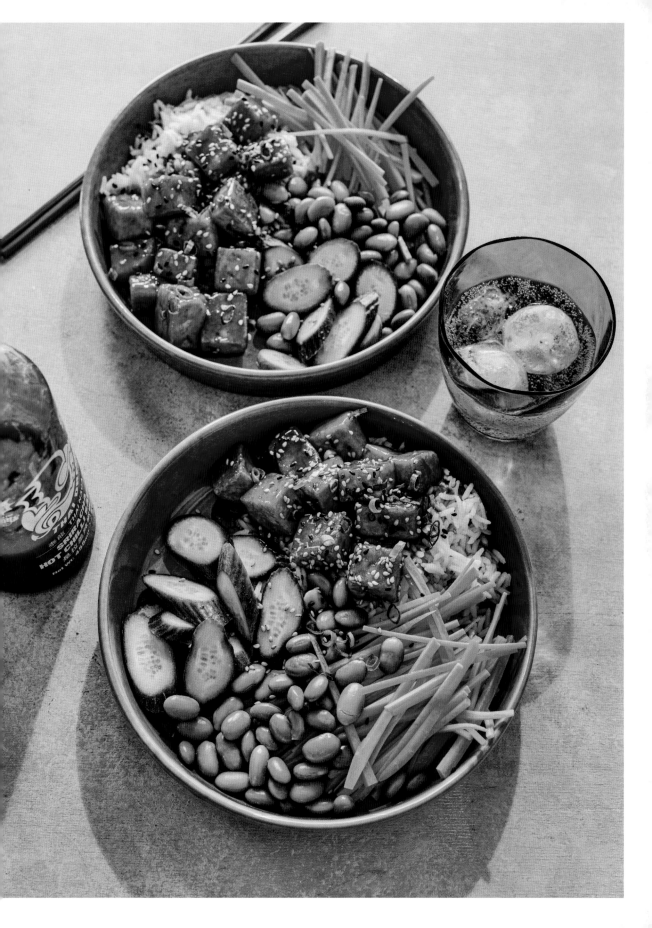

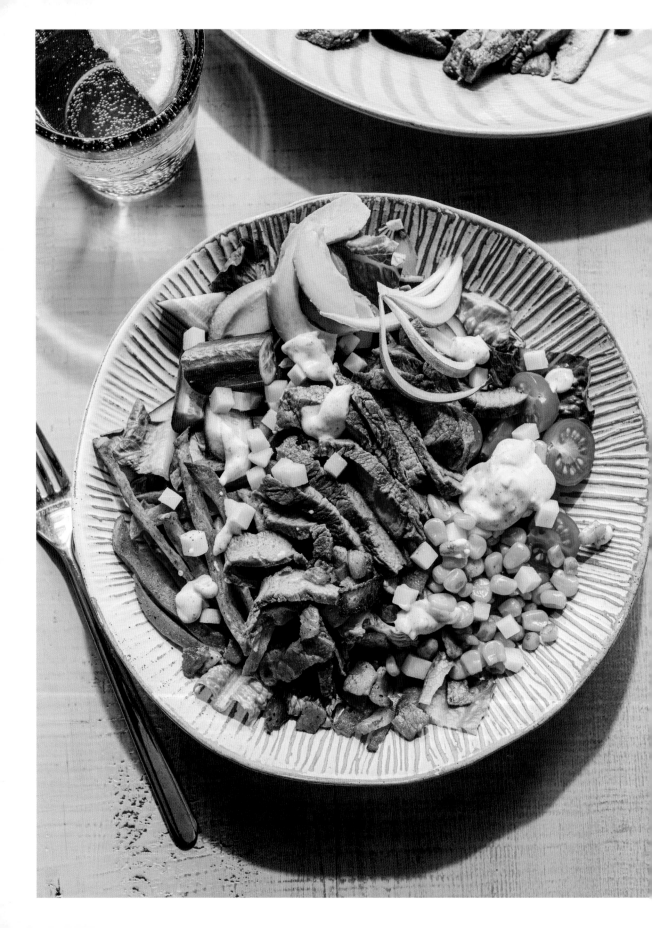

Steak Salad Bowl with Sweet Potato Fries and Creamy Cajun Dressing

PREP TIME: 10 MINUTES   **COOK TIME: 30 MINUTES**   **SERVES: 2**

250g (8½oz) sirloin steak, (or any steak of your preference), trimmed of all visible fat

1 sweet potato (approx. 200g/7oz), peeled and sliced into thin fries

olive oil spray

2 pinches of paprika

1 tablespoon Cajun Seasoning (page 281)

pinch of coarse sea salt

85g (3oz) frozen or canned sweetcorn

100g (3½oz) romaine lettuce, chopped

2 baby cucumbers, sliced

¼ small red onion, sliced

10 cherry tomatoes, halved

60g (2oz) avocado, sliced

3 cooked lean bacon medallions, chopped

50g (1¾oz) Cheddar, cubed

salt and freshly ground black pepper

For the creamy Cajun dressing

4 tablespoons light mayonnaise

½ teaspoon Cajun Seasoning (page 281)

1 teaspoon lime juice

Swaps:
You can swap the Cheddar for blue cheese or feta.

This is the ultimate steak salad bowl: perfectly cooked Cajun-seasoned steak with salad, golden paprika sweet potato fries, charred corn, golden bacon and Cheddar, all finished off with a spicy creamy Cajun mayo.

1. Preheat the oven to 220°C/200°C fan/425°F/gas 7 and line a baking tray with baking paper.

2. Remove the steak from the fridge about 30 minutes before cooking.

3. Place the sweet potato fries on the prepared tray and spray with olive oil spray. Sprinkle over the paprika and a pinch of salt and pepper. Toss to coat, then spread out the fries and spray with olive oil spray once more. Bake for 25–30 minutes until golden, tossing halfway through and giving them another spray of oil.

4. Meanwhile, mix together the ingredients for the Cajun dressing in a small bowl. Add a little water to loosen until you have a drizzling consistency, then set aside.

5. Season the steak all over with the Cajun seasoning and add a pinch of coarse sea salt to both sides.

6. Heat a frying pan over a medium–high heat and spray with olive oil spray. Once hot, add the steak and sear for 3–4 minutes on each side (depending on thickness). If you like your steak well done, it will take a little longer. Once it's cooked to your liking, remove from the pan and set aside on a plate to rest.

7. Add the sweetcorn to the empty pan and sprinkle with another pinch of paprika. Move the corn around the pan so it takes on all the flavour from the steak and gets slightly blackened.

8. To assemble, divide the sweet potato fries between two bowls, along with the lettuce, cucumber, red onion, tomatoes, avocado, bacon and Cheddar. Add the charred corn, then slice the steak and layer this on top. Drizzle with the creamy Cajun dressing and enjoy.

KCALS	657
FAT	33.0g
SAT FAT	10.8g
CARBS	34.9g
SUGARS	15.1g
FIBRE	10.0g
PROTEIN	50.3g
SALT	3.09g

454 kcals
per serving

GF

KCALS
454

FAT
15.2g

SAT FAT
6.7g

CARBS
36.3g

SUGARS
12.6g

FIBRE
5.3g

PROTEIN
40.4g

SALT
2.77g

Zuppa Toscana Soup Bowls

PREP TIME: **15 MINUTES**   COOK TIME: **25 MINUTES**   SERVES: **4**

olive oil spray
3 slices of lean back bacon, fat removed, diced small
½ tablespoon olive oil
1 large onion, diced
4 garlic cloves, crushed
400g (14oz) potatoes, peeled and roughly chopped into large cubes (don't chop too small)
720ml (24¾fl oz) chicken stock
475ml (16fl oz) semi-skimmed milk
50g (1¾oz) light cream cheese
2 tablespoons cornflour (cornstarch)
100g (3½oz) fresh kale, stem removed, roughly chopped
40g (1½oz) Parmesan, freshly grated
pinch of red chilli flakes (optional)
salt and freshly ground black pepper

For the Italian sausage
400g (14oz) 5% fat pork mince (ground pork)
1 tablespoon red wine vinegar
½ tablespoon maple syrup or honey
1½ teaspoons Italian seasoning
1 teaspoon garlic powder
1 teaspoon onion powder
¾ teaspoon paprika
½ teaspoon fennel seeds, crushed
¾ teaspoon red chilli flakes (optional)
½ teaspoon salt
pinch of freshly ground black pepper

Traditionally, Zuppa Toscana uses Italian sausage, but I make my own using lean pork mince and seasonings. The classic version also contains cream, but here I've used a mixture of milk and stock, with some starch to thicken. The result is still a delicious, creamy soup.

1. Heat a large, deep saucepan over a medium–high heat and spray with olive oil spray. Add the bacon and fry for a few minutes until really golden. Remove from the pan and set aside on a plate.

2. In a large bowl, mix together all the ingredients for the Italian sausage until just combined.

3. Add to the saucepan and cook for about 6 minutes until golden around the edges. Once brown, remove from the pan and set aside.

4. Add the olive oil to the empty pan. Once hot, add the onion and fry for a couple of minutes until golden and softened, then add the garlic and fry for a further minute to infuse the flavour.

5. Add the potatoes, along with a pinch of salt and pepper. Pour in the stock and bring to the boil, then reduce the heat to medium–low and simmer for 14–15 minutes until the potatoes are just tender.

6. Stir in the milk and cream cheese, then add the sausage to the soup.

7. In a small bowl or mug, mix the cornflour with a couple of tablespoons water to make a slurry. Add this to the soup, then allow to bubble, stirring until the cream cheese melts and the soup thickens and becomes creamy.

8. Stir in the kale until just slightly wilted down, then taste the soup for seasoning and adjust if needed.

9. To serve, ladle the soup into bowls and sprinkle with the bacon, parmesan and pinch of chilli flakes.

Side suggestion – garlic bread:
This is great served with an optional side of garlic bread for dipping. To make, mix together 40g (1½oz) Parmesan (or Cheddar) with 1 crushed garlic clove and 1 teaspoon dried parsley. Slice 2 low-calorie bread rolls in half and rub the garlic mix into the cut side of the rolls. Place on a baking tray, spray with olive spray oil and bake for 10–12 minutes at 200°C/180°C fan/400°F/gas 6 until the cheese is melted and bread is lightly golden.

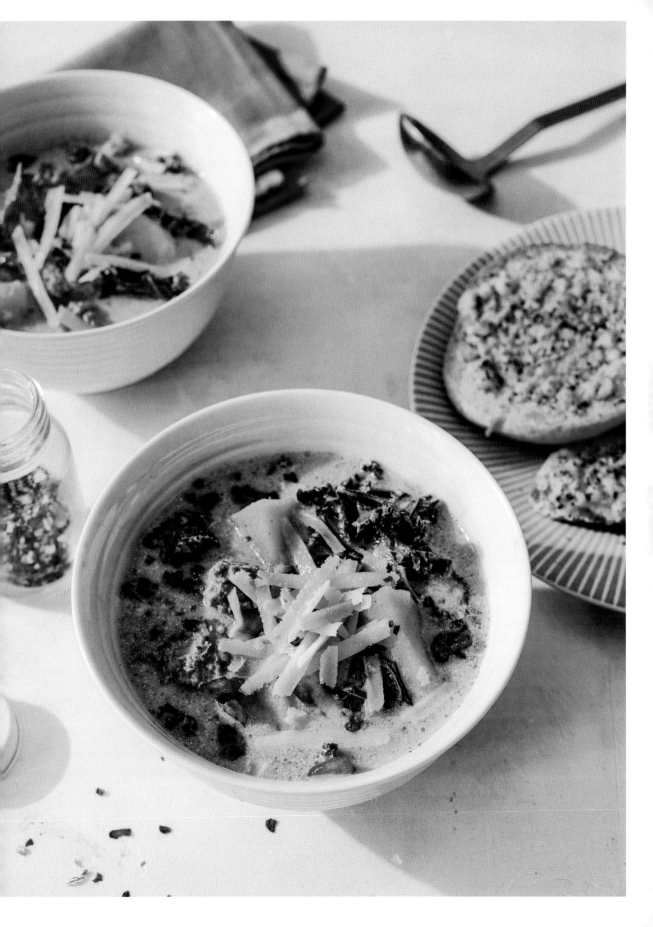

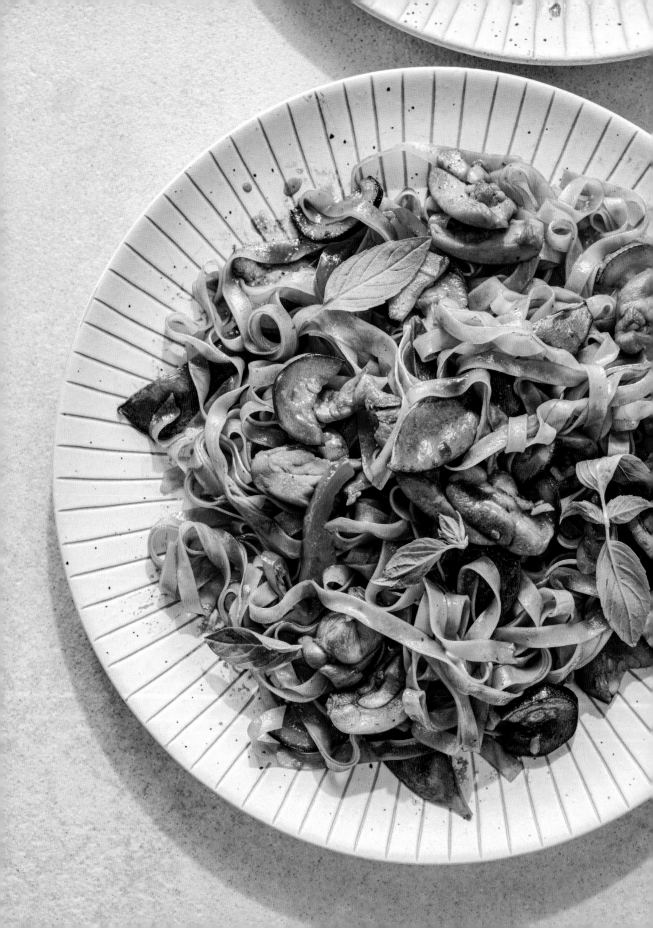

Blog
Favourites

One-pot Cheeseburger Pasta

PREP TIME: **10 MINUTES**   COOK TIME: **20 MINUTES**   SERVES: **4**

KCALS
596

FAT
17.9g

SAT FAT
9.4g

CARBS
60.6g

SUGARS
6.7g

FIBRE
6.3g

PROTEIN
45.1g

SALT
2.00g

1 teaspoon paprika

½ teaspoon onion powder

½ teaspoon garlic powder

½ teaspoon mustard powder

olive oil spray

450g (1lb) 5% fat beef mince (ground beef)

1 onion, finely chopped

2 tomatoes, peeled and chopped

2 tablespoons tomato purée (paste)

½ tablespoon Worcestershire sauce

1 tablespoon brown granulated sweetener (optional)

300g (10½oz) dried penne pasta (or other pasta of choice)

720–960ml (24¾–32½fl oz) chicken stock

2–3 tablespoons chopped gherkins (pickles)

120g (4¼oz) Cheddar

salt and freshly ground black pepper

freshly chopped parsley, to serve

The most-loved recipe on Slimming Eats, One-pot Cheeseburger Pasta is everyone's favourite all-in-one dish. It's a super-simple recipe that has all the best parts of a cheeseburger – plus, of course, it has pasta! It's got a few more calories than the usual Slimming Eats recipes, but it's worth it for that occasional indulgence. This recipe is always a winner with my kids, too. Keep it simple with the basic pasta dish, or make the burger sauce drizzle and serve it alongside a mixed salad for the perfect fake-away night.

1. In a small bowl, mix together the paprika, onion powder, garlic powder and mustard powder. Season with salt and pepper and set aside.

2. Heat a frying pan over a medium–high heat and spray with olive oil spray. Add the beef mince and onion and cook for couple of minutes until brown, breaking up the beef with your spoon as it cooks.

3. Add the spice mix, tomatoes, tomato purée, Worcestershire sauce and sweetener and mix well to combine.

4. Stir in the pasta, then pour in 720ml (24¾fl oz) of the stock. Bring to the boil, then reduce the heat to medium and allow to bubble for 12–14 minutes until the pasta is cooked, adding more stock if needed.

5. Add the chopped gherkins and most of the Cheddar (reserve a little for later), and stir until the sauce is velvety and cheesy and coats everything in the pan.

6. To serve, sprinkle with freshly chopped parsley and the remaining cheese. Enjoy!

Side suggestions:
I always pair this with a big mixed salad containing all my favourites: crisp lettuce, red onion, tomatoes, cucumber and shredded carrot.

Swaps:
For the best results, I prefer to use fresh tomatoes in this recipe, but if you prefer, you can used canned chopped tomatoes (about 200g/7oz).

Optional add-on – homemade burger sauce:
Mix together 3 tablespoons light mayonnaise, 1 tablespoon fat-free Greek yogurt, 1 teaspoon tomato purée (paste), 1 teaspoon American yellow mustard, ½ teaspoon paprika, ¼ teaspoon garlic powder, ¼ teaspoon onion powder, a pinch of black pepper, 1 teaspoon granulated sweetener (optional), and 2 finely diced gherkin (pickle) slices. Loosen with a little water until you have a drizzling consistency, then drizzle this over the top of the pasta for the perfect burger sauce.

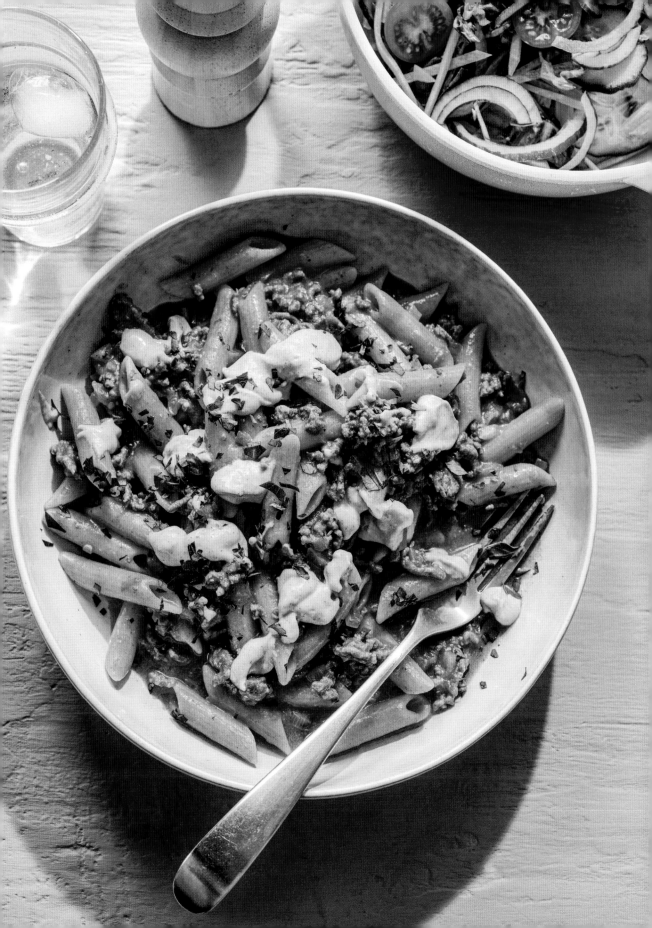

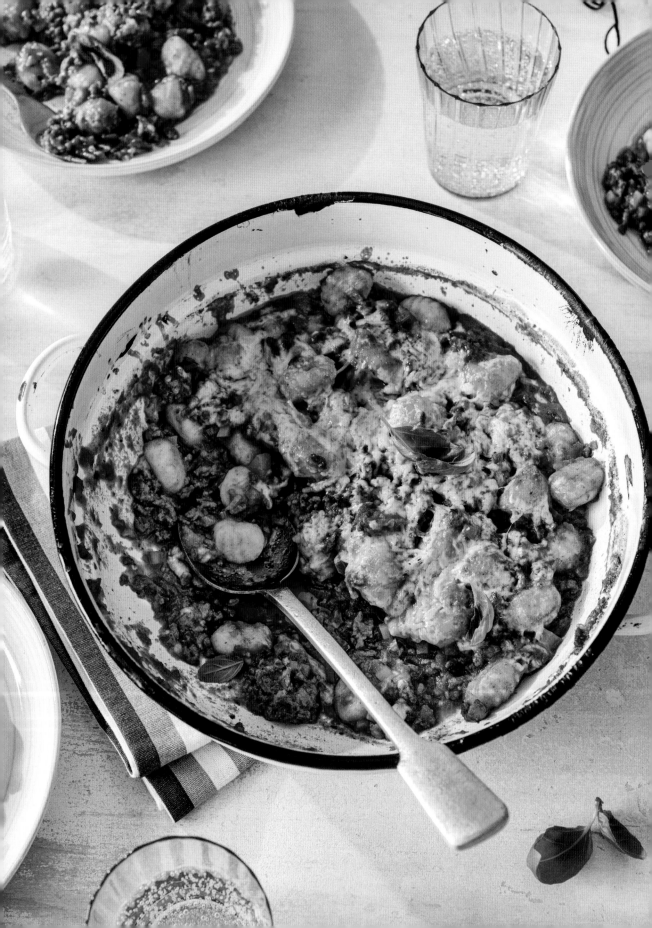

Cheesy Bolognese Gnocchi Bake

PREP TIME: 10 MINUTES   **COOK TIME: 40 MINUTES**   **SERVES: 4**

olive oil spray

2 slices of lean back bacon, fat removed, chopped

3 shallots, finely diced

1 carrot, finely diced

2 small celery stalks, finely diced

3 garlic cloves, crushed

400g (14oz) 5% fat beef mince (ground beef)

½ tablespoon dried mixed herbs

400g (14oz) can chopped tomatoes

3 tablespoons tomato purée (paste)

1 teaspoon granulated sweetener or sugar (optional)

240ml (8½fl oz) chicken or beef stock

1 tablespoon balsamic vinegar

500g (1lb 2oz) gnocchi

120g (4¼oz) Cheddar, freshly grated

salt and freshly ground black pepper

a few fresh basil leaves, torn, to serve

Swaps:

You can swap the beef for a leaner turkey or chicken mince if you want to bring the calories down a little further.

Side suggestions:

I like to pair this with a mixed side salad, but it also goes well with whatever greens you like best, such as broccoli, asparagus or green beans.

A rich, delicious bolognese meat sauce with gnocchi, all finished off with melted cheese. If you love a traditional spaghetti bolognese and love gnocchi, then this is the dish for you.

1. Heat a frying pan over a medium–high heat and spray with olive oil spray. Add the bacon and fry for a few minutes until golden, then remove from the pan and set aside on a plate.

2. Spray the empty pan with some more olive oil spray and add the shallots, carrot and celery. Fry for a couple of minutes to soften, adding a little water or a splash of stock to prevent it sticking, if needed.

3. Now add the garlic and beef and cook for a few minutes until browned, breaking up the mince with your spoon as it cooks.

4. Return the bacon to the pan, along with the mixed herbs, chopped tomatoes, tomato purée, sweetener or sugar (if using), stock and balsamic vinegar. Stir and bring to the boil, then cover and simmer for 20 minutes; the sauce should be rich and thickened.

5. Drop in the gnocchi and stir to combine, then cover once more and simmer for 5–8 minutes until the gnocchi is cooked, stirring occasionally to ensure the gnocchi doesn't stick to bottom of the pan. You can add a little more stock if the gnocchi absorbs too much liquid.

6. Taste the sauce and season with salt and pepper as needed, then transfer the contents of the pan to a baking dish. Scatter the Cheddar over the top and place under the grill for about 4 minutes until the cheese is melted and golden.

7. Scatter with some freshly torn basil and enjoy!

KCALS	**528**
FAT	**18.8g**
SAT FAT	**10.0g**
CARBS	**49.0g**
SUGARS	**8.0g**
FIBRE	**5.1g**
PROTEIN	**38.3g**
SALT	**3.50g**

488 kcals per serving

Bang Bang Chicken Pasta

PREP TIME: 10 MINUTES   **COOK TIME: 25 MINUTES**   **SERVES: 4**

KCALS
488

FAT
3.6g

SAT FAT
1.0g

CARBS
67.7g

SUGARS
12.4g

FIBRE
5.4g

PROTEIN
43.5g

SALT
1.32g

olive oil spray
500g (1lb 2oz) chicken breasts, thinly sliced
1 teaspoon paprika
½ teaspoon onion powder
½ teaspoon garlic powder
1 small onion, sliced
240ml (8½fl oz) chicken stock
2 garlic cloves, crushed
1 small courgette (zucchini), diced
1 red (bell) pepper, diced
300g (10½oz) dried spaghetti
2 teaspoons sriracha (see Note)
4 tablespoons low-fat cream cheese
4 tablespoons shop-bought sweet chilli sauce
salt and freshly ground black pepper
freshly chopped parsley or coriander (cilantro), to serve (optional)

This recipe is a huge favourite among Slimming Eats blog readers, and it's easy to see why! It's such a simple and quick dish to make, but packs in so much flavour. With tender pieces of chicken, tasty spaghetti and delicious vegetables all coated in creamy, spicy sauce, it is sure to become a regular feature on your meal plan.

1. Heat a deep frying pan over a medium–high heat and spray with olive oil spray.

2. Add the chicken, paprika, onion powder and garlic powder, and season with salt and pepper. Fry for a couple of minutes until lightly browned, then remove from the pan and set aside on a plate.

3. Spray the frying pan with some more olive oil spray, then add the onion and a little splash of the stock to deglaze the pan. Fry the onion for a few minutes until translucent and softened, then add the garlic and continue to fry for a further 1 minute. Add the courgette and red pepper and cook for a couple of minutes, stirring to combine.

4. Return the chicken to the pan, along with the remaining stock, then leave to simmer and reduce down while you cook the pasta.

5. Cook the pasta according to the packet instructions until al dente, then drain and set aside.

6. Add the sriracha to the chicken and vegetables, and stir to combine, then add the cooked spaghetti, along with the cream cheese and sweet chilli sauce. Toss for a couple of minutes until everything is combined and the sauce is creamy and velvety.

7. Season with salt and pepper if needed, then stir through some chopped parsley or coriander (if using), and serve. Enjoy!

Swaps:
Feel free to swap the vegetables in this dish for any you like; it's a great dish for using up any veg you have in the fridge. You can also swap the chicken for pork or prawns, or keep it completely meat-free with some vegetables of your favourite veggie protein.

Note:
The spice level can be adjusted by adding more or less sriracha. If you don't like much heat, I recommend adding just a little sriracha at a time, until it reaches a heat you are comfortable with.

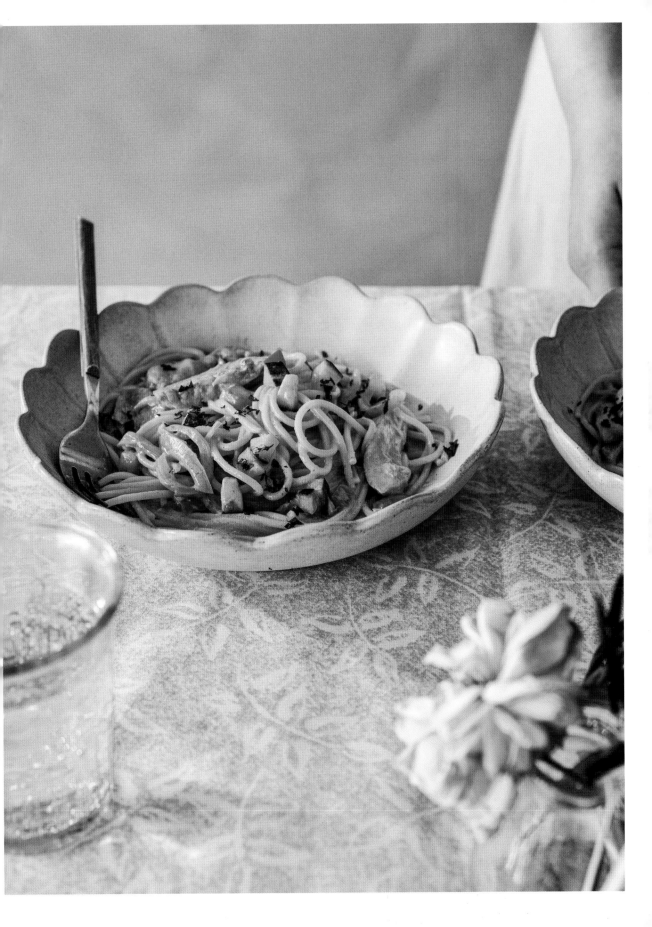

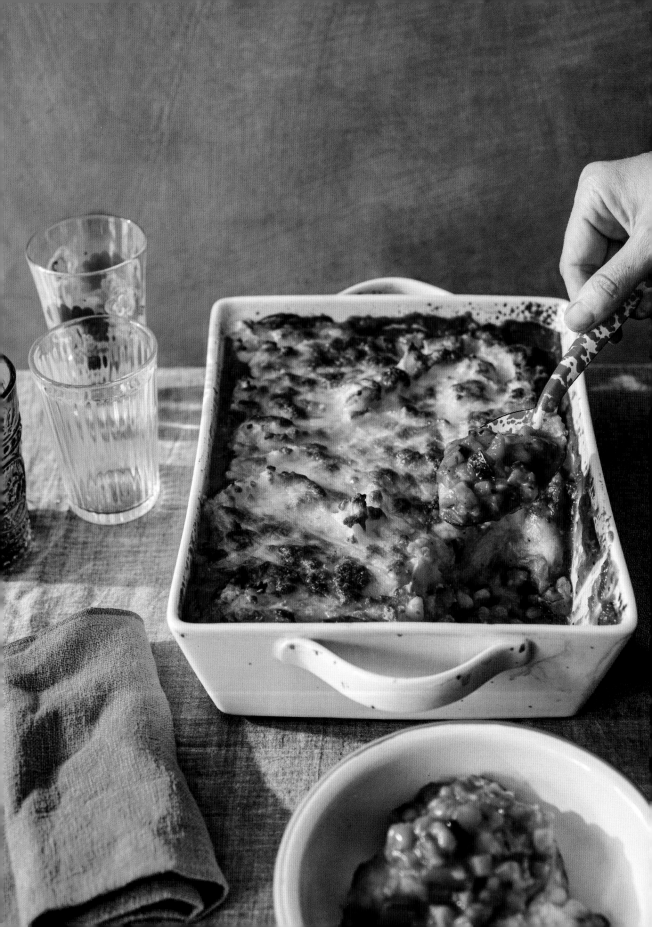

Baked Bean Cheesy Potato-topped Pie

PREP TIME: 15 MINUTES　　**COOK TIME: 50 MINUTES**　　**SERVES: 6**

For the cheesy mashed potato topping

1kg (2lb 4oz) yellow-fleshed potatoes, such as Desiree or Yukon Gold, peeled and chopped into cubes

960ml (32½fl oz) vegetable stock

120ml (4fl oz) semi-skimmed milk

2 tablespoons salted butter

75g (2½oz) mozzarella, grated or torn

45g (1½oz) Cheddar, grated

1 spring onion (scallion), finely sliced (optional)

salt and freshly ground black pepper

For the filling

olive oil spray

1 onion, diced

1 carrot, finely diced

1 red (bell) pepper, diced

2 garlic cloves, crushed

400g (14oz) can baked beans in tomato sauce

1 courgette (zucchini), diced

240g (8½oz) passata

2 teaspoons paprika

1 teaspoon dried parsley

1 teaspoon dried basil

few dashes of Tabasco sauce (optional)

120ml (4fl oz) vegetable stock

A delicious tomatoey baked bean and vegetable filling with a beautiful cheesy mashed potato topping. This is a perfect meat-free recipe for the whole family, and it's always a popular choice on the Slimming Eats blog.

1. Preheat the oven to 200°C/180°C fan/400°F/gas 6.

2. To make the mashed potato topping, put the potatoes into a saucepan and cover with the stock. Place over a high heat and bring to the boil, then simmer for about 12 minutes until the potatoes are very soft and most of the stock has been absorbed.

3. Drain any excess liquid (there should be very little), then add the milk and butter and mash until really smooth. Season to taste, then set aside.

4. To make the filling, heat a frying pan over a medium–high heat and spray with some olive oil spray. Add the onion, carrot, pepper and garlic, and fry for a couple of minutes until softened.

5. Add the baked beans, courgette, passata, paprika, herbs and Tabasco (if using). Season with salt and pepper, then stir in the stock. Bring to the boil, then reduce the heat to medium. Cover and simmer for 15 minutes, stirring occasionally, until the vegetables are nice and tender. Season if needed.

6. Transfer the filling to a large oven dish and top with the mashed potatoes, leaving the edges clear. Scatter the mozzarella and Cheddar over the top and bake for about 30 minutes, or until the cheese is all melted and lightly golden on top.

7. Sprinkle with the chopped spring onion (if using), serve and enjoy!

Optional add-ins:
If you're not vegetarian, this is also great with some cooked beef, turkey or chicken mince added into the bean mixture. If you have some leftover roast chicken, some of that stirred into the sauce is a great option too.

Variations:
If you like it spicy, try adding some curry powder to the bean mixture, or a pinch of cayenne or red chilli flakes.

Freezing:
Freeze this before adding the cheese.

345 kcals per serving

KCALS	**345**
FAT	**10.9g**
SAT FAT	**6.3g**
CARBS	**43.6g**
SUGARS	**12.3g**
FIBRE	**9.4g**
PROTEIN	**13.3g**
SALT	**1.29g**

287 kcals
per serving

GF

KCALS
287

FAT
4.7g

SAT FAT
1.7g

CARBS
14.5g

SUGARS
13.4g

FIBRE
4.1g

PROTEIN
44.7g

SALT
1.43g

Creamy Honey Mustard Chicken

PREP TIME: 5 MINUTES   **COOK TIME: 25 MINUTES**   **SERVES: 4**

250g (9oz) carrots, sliced
olive oil spray
1 onion, finely chopped
600g (1lb 5oz) boneless,
  skinless chicken breast,
  diced into cubes
360ml (12fl oz) hot chicken
  stock
180g (6½oz) low-fat
  cream cheese
1 tablespoon honey
4 teaspoons wholegrain
  mustard
1–2 teaspoons yellow
  American mustard
salt and freshly ground
  black pepper
freshly chopped parsley,
  to serve

Side suggestions:
We love this with rice or
mashed potatoes, but it is
equally good with some
cauliflower rice or cauliflower
mash for a low-carb alternative.
For some additional veggie
hit, I love to serve it with
some courgettes sautéed in
a pan with olive oil spray,
salt, black pepper and garlic
powder, but any greens
are great.

Creamy honey mustard chicken has always been a true comfort food for me. But back in the days before I became a mum and ventured into healthy home cooking, it would simply have been a case of browning some chicken and opening up a jar of ready-made sauce. But then I created this healthier version back in 2013, and it's been a well-loved recipe on Slimming Eats ever since.

1. Put the sliced carrots into a steamer set above a pan of boiling water and steam for about 4 minutes until slightly tender. Take off the heat and plunge into a bowl of cold water to prevent them from cooking any further.

2. Heat a frying pan over a medium–high heat and spray with olive oil spray. Add the onion and chicken and fry for a few minutes until lightly golden.

3. In a jug, whisk together the stock, cream cheese, honey and both types of mustard until combined. Pour this mixture into the frying pan. Slowly bring to the boil, then reduce the heat to medium. Add the carrots and simmer for about 15 minutes until the sauce thickens. If it gets too thick, you can stir in a little more stock.

4. Taste and season with salt and pepper, then sprinkle with chopped fresh parsley and serve.

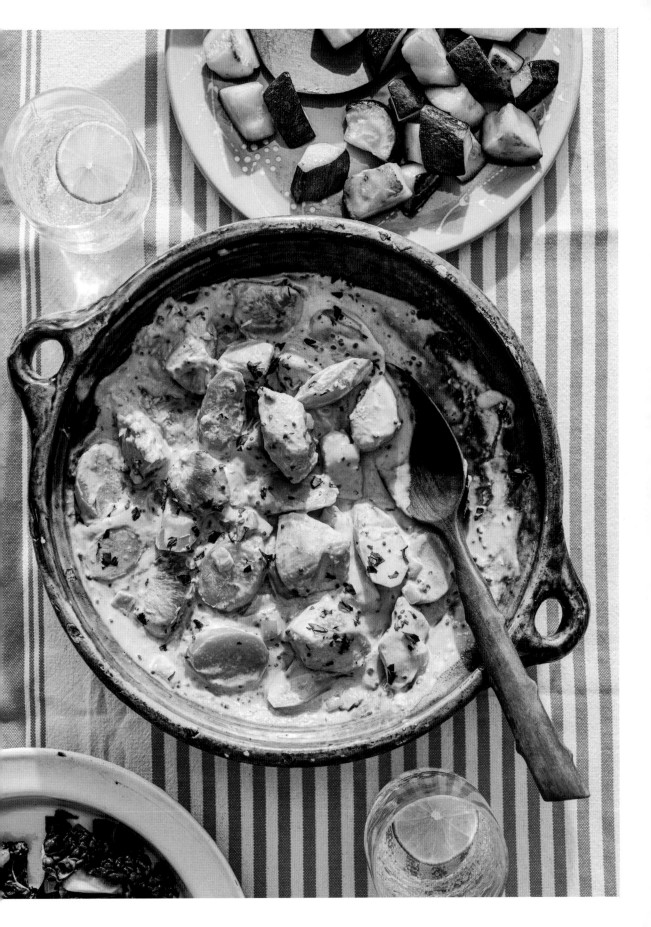

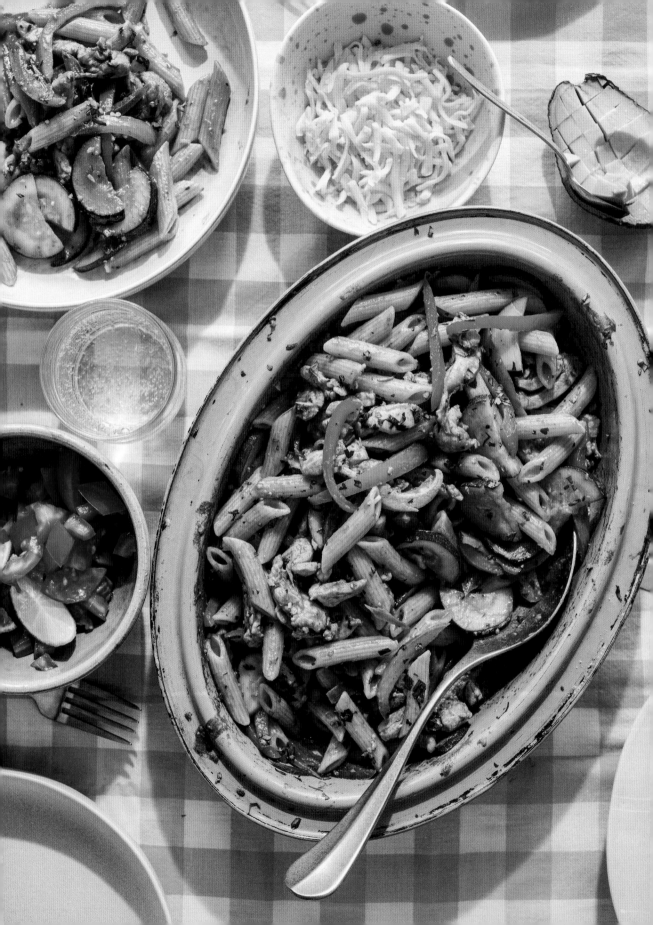

Fajita Chicken Pasta

PREP TIME: 5 MINUTES + MARINATING   COOK TIME: 20 MINUTES   SERVES: 4

446 kcals
per serving

DF

500g (1lb 2oz) boneless, skinless chicken thighs, sliced into bite-sized pieces
260g (10½oz) dried penne pasta
low-calorie cooking oil spray
1 red onion, sliced
1 red (bell) pepper, sliced
1 green (bell) pepper, sliced
1 courgette (zucchini), halved lengthways and sliced
2 tablespoons tomato purée (paste)
freshly chopped coriander (cilantro)

For the marinade
juice of 1 small lime
1 teaspoon olive oil
1 tablespoon ground cumin
1 tablespoon paprika
2 garlic cloves, crushed
1 jalapeño, deseeded and finely chopped
1 teaspoon dried oregano
1 teaspoon salt
1 teaspoon brown granulated sweetener
¼ teaspoon cayenne (optional)

Side suggestions:
All your fajita favourites! Salad, avocado, diced tomatoes or salsa, soured cream or fat-free Greek yogurt with some lemon juice, grated Cheddar... the list goes on!

Swaps:
You can use chicken breast instead of thighs if you prefer. This is also delicious with beef, prawns or pork.

Here we have everything you love about fajitas, all combined into a delicious pasta dish that will be loved by the whole family. I love to place this in the middle of the table with some sides and toppings, so the whole family can dig in and build their own fajita pasta bowls.

1. Combine all the marinade ingredients in a mini food-processor or blender and blitz a few times until you have a paste. Transfer to a bowl. Add the chicken and mix to coat thoroughly, then leave to marinate for a few hours in the fridge.

2. When you're ready to cook, cook the pasta according to the packet instructions until al dente. Reserve 120ml (4fl oz) of the pasta water, then drain and set aside.

3. Heat a frying pan over a medium–high heat and spray with low-calorie cooking oil spray. Add the marinated chicken and cook, stirring occasionally, for about 5 minutes, until the chicken is browned and cooked through. Remove from the pan and set aside on a plate.

4. Add the onion, peppers and courgette to the empty pan and cook for a couple of minutes, stirring constantly, until the vegetables are nice and tender, but still crisp. Return the chicken to the pan and stir to combine, then stir in the tomato purée and the reserved pasta water.

5. Add the cooked pasta and mix everything together thoroughly until the sauce lightly coats the pasta and everything is heated through.

6. Season with salt and pepper and top with some freshly chopped coriander, then serve with your choice of sides/toppings.

KCALS	446
FAT	6.6g
SAT FAT	1.4g
CARBS	55.4g
SUGARS	8.3g
FIBRE	8.0g
PROTEIN	37.1g
SALT	1.55g

KCALS
365

FAT
17.7g

SAT FAT
6.8g

CARBS
5.6g

SUGARS
2.4g

FIBRE
1.3g

PROTEIN
45.2g

SALT
1.74g

Smothered Garlic Chicken

PREP TIME: 5 MINUTES   COOK TIME: 60 MINUTES   SERVES: 4

8 small skinless, bone-in chicken thighs, trimmed of all visible fat (approx. 125g/4½oz each)
olive oil spray
300g (10½oz) white mushrooms, thinly sliced
8 garlic cloves, halved
360ml (12fl oz) low-sodium chicken stock
120g (4¼oz) light cream cheese
70g (2½oz) light mozzarella, grated or broken into small pieces
30g (1oz) Parmesan, grated
1 tablespoon freshly chopped parsley

For the seasoning mix

1 teaspoon paprika
1 teaspoon dried mixed herbs
¾ teaspoon coarse sea salt
½ teaspoon onion powder
½ teaspoon black pepper

Freezing:
Freeze before step 6. Defrost fully and add to a pan before starting step 6.

This delicious dish of juicy chicken thighs smothered in a creamy garlic sauce with mushrooms and topped with melted, golden cheese feels like it should contain a lot more calories than it actually does, just because it tastes so good! Blog readers often comment that this is a huge hit with their entire family. Once you make it, it's sure to become a regular on your table, too.

1. Preheat the oven to 220°C/200°C fan/425°F/gas 7.

2. Place the chicken into a bowl with all the ingredients for the seasoning mix and toss to evenly coat.

3. Heat a large, deep ovenproof frying pan over a medium–high heat and spray with olive oil spray. Add the chicken pieces, arranging them all in one layer in the pan, and brown for 4–5 minutes on each side until nice and golden. Remove from the pan and set aside on a plate.

4. Spray the empty pan with a little more olive oil spray and add the mushrooms. Fry for a couple of minutes, scraping up all the flavour that's been left at the bottom of the pan from the chicken. Add the garlic and stir to combine, then gradually add 120ml (4fl oz) of the chicken stock, letting it reduce down between each addition, until the garlic has really softened and has a lovely golden colour. This will make the garlic deliciously sweet. Don't rush this process, or you will burn the garlic and cause it to become bitter.

5. Add the cream cheese and pour in the remaining stock, then allow to bubble away, gently stirring, until the cream cheese is all melted and the sauce is thickened and creamy.

6. Return the chicken pieces to the pan in an even layer and spoon the sauce all over the top so they are well covered.

7. Scatter the mozzarella and Parmesan over the top, then cover with a lid and place in the oven. Bake for 25–30 minutes, then remove the lid and bake, uncovered, for another 10 minutes. The cheese should be all melted and lightly golden, and the chicken cooked through.

8. Sprinkle with freshly chopped parsley and serve.

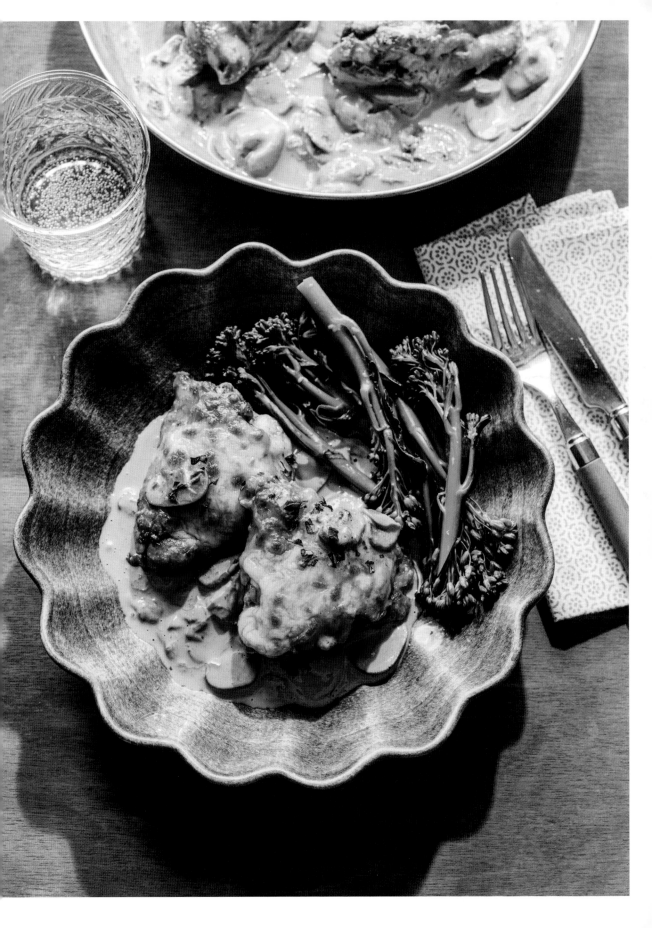

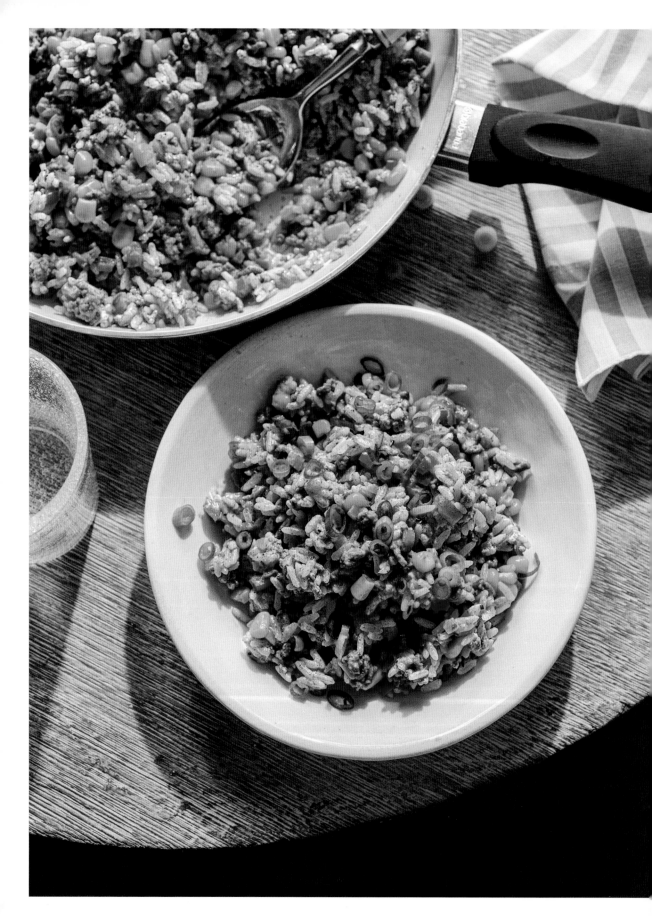

One-pot Taco Beef Rice Skillet

PREP TIME: 10 MINUTES   **COOK TIME: 30 MINUTES**   **SERVES: 4**

450g (1lb) 5% fat beef mince
   (ground beef)
1 onion, finely diced
1 red (bell) pepper, diced
1 green (bell) pepper, diced
180g (6½oz) passata
175g (6oz) frozen sweetcorn
180g (6½oz) long-grain rice
600ml (20fl oz) chicken
   stock or water
5 tablespoons reduced-fat
   soured cream
120g (4¼oz) Cheddar, grated
4 spring onions (scallions),
   diced

**For the taco seasoning
(see Note)**
1½ teaspoons ground cumin
1½ teaspoons paprika
1½ teaspoons chilli powder
½ teaspoon dried oregano
¼ teaspoon garlic powder
¼ teaspoon onion powder
¼ teaspoon cayenne pepper
   (you can add more or
   less, depending on your
   preferred spice level)

Note:
If you already have some of
my Taco Seasoning from page
281 made up, you can use
2 tablespoons of that instead
of the seasoning in this recipe.

Freezing:
Freeze after step 4.

**Here we have delicious spicy, cheesy taco beef, all cooked in
one pan with rice and vegetables. Mexican-inspired food is
always a big favourite with my family, especially beef tacos,
but for variety, I often swap out a typical ingredient (like
switching corn tacos for rice or pasta) to transform it into
an easy one-pot recipe.**

1. Heat a large frying pan over a medium–high heat. Add the beef
and onion and fry for a few minutes until browned, breaking up
the mince with your spoon as you cook.

2. Add all the ingredients for the taco seasoning and stir until the
meat mixture is all coated, then add the red and green peppers,
passata, sweetcorn and rice and mix to combine.

3. Pour in the stock or water and give everything a little stir. Bring
to the boil, then reduce the heat to a simmer for about 12 minutes
until the liquid is almost absorbed.

4. Turn off the heat, and leave, covered, for 10–12 minutes. The
steam trapped underneath the lid will continue to cook the rice
to perfection.

5. Once ready, stir in the soured cream and Cheddar until melted,
then sprinkle with chopped spring onions.

6. Serve and enjoy!

531 kcals
per serving

GF

KCALS
531

FAT
17.9g

SAT FAT
9.4g

CARBS
47.9g

SUGARS
8.2g

FIBRE
6.4g

PROTEIN
41.4g

SALT
1.84g

Buffalo Chicken Pasta Bake

PREP TIME: 10 MINUTES   **COOK TIME: 40 MINUTES**   **SERVES: 4**

olive oil spray
1 onion, diced
400g (14oz) boneless,
     skinless chicken thighs),
     sliced into thin bite-sized
     strips
1 teaspoon paprika
1 garlic clove, minced
240ml (8½fl oz) canned
     chopped tomatoes
80ml (2¾fl oz) hot sauce
     (I used Frank's Red Hot
     Sauce)
350g (12oz) fresh tomatoes,
     diced
240g (8½oz) dried penne
     pasta
salt and freshly ground
     black pepper

For the topping
100g (3½oz) light
     cream cheese
½ teaspoon garlic powder
½ teaspoon onion powder
1 teaspoon dried parsley
1 teaspoon dried dill
240ml (8½fl oz) chicken
     stock
1 tablespoon cornflour
     (cornstarch)
30g (1oz) Cheddar, grated
50g (1¾oz) mozzarella,
     grated
2 spring onions (scallions),
     thinly sliced

Side suggestions:
Buffalo chicken is not
complete without some
ranch dressing: see page
280 for my recipe.

This delicious pasta bake is super-easy to make, combining chicken in hot sauce with penne pasta, topped with a cheesy, creamy ranch topping and melted cheese. If you love buffalo hot sauce, you will love this dish. Although I only added it to Slimming Eats at the beginning of 2022, it has fast become a blog favourite.

1. Preheat the oven to 200°C/180°C fan/400°F/gas 6.

2. Heat a frying pan over a medium–high heat and spray with olive oil spray. Add the onion and fry for a couple of minutes until lightly golden and softened.

3. Spray with a little more olive oil spray, then add the chicken, paprika and garlic, along with a pinch of salt and pepper. Fry for a few minutes until the chicken is browned and has a lovely colour from the paprika.

4. Add a little splash of water to deglaze the pan of anything stuck to the bottom, then stir in the canned tomatoes, hot sauce and fresh tomatoes. Allow to simmer for a few minutes until the tomatoes are slightly softened.

5. Meanwhile, cook the pasta according to the packet instructions until al dente.

6. Add the cooked pasta to the pan with the chicken and sauce and mix to combine, then transfer into an ovenproof dish.

7. To make the topping, combine the cream cheese, garlic powder and onion powder in a saucepan or frying pan over a medium–high heat. Add the parsley and dill, along with the stock, and whisk until the cream cheese is all melted and no lumps are visible.

8. In a small bowl or mug, mix the cornflour with a couple of tablespoons of water to make a slurry. Add this to the cream cheese mixture and allow to bubble, stirring every now and then, until it thickens.

9. Once thickened, spread the cream cheese mixture over the top of the pasta bake, then scatter over the grated cheeses. Bake for about 20 minutes until the cheese has melted and is lightly golden on top.

10. Sprinkle with the chopped spring onions, and it's ready to enjoy.

KCALS
491

FAT
10.7g

SAT FAT
5.0g

CARBS
56.5g

SUGARS
10.0g

FIBRE
6.1g

PROTEIN
39.0g

SALT
1.77g

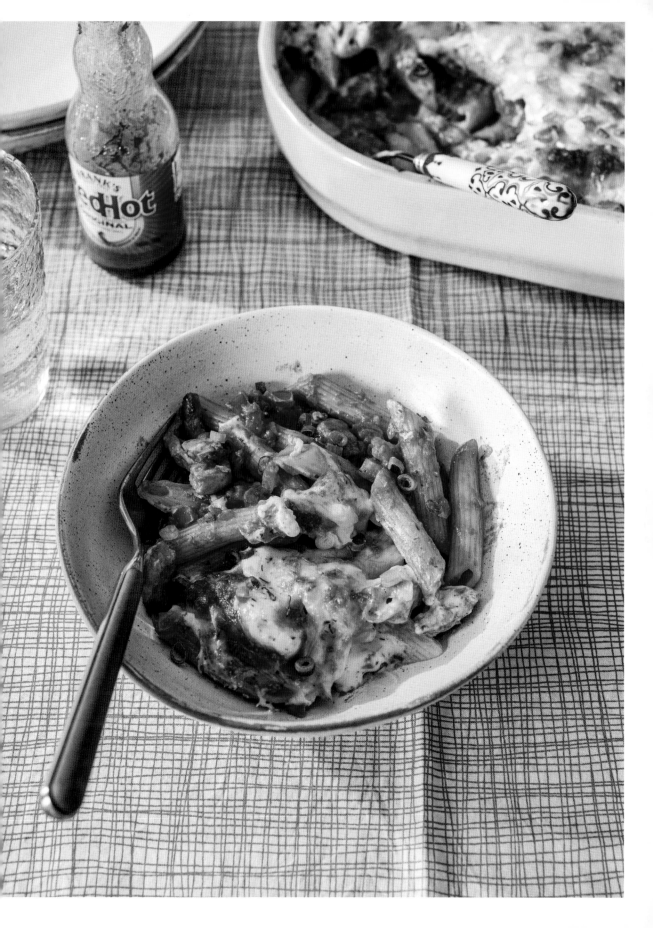

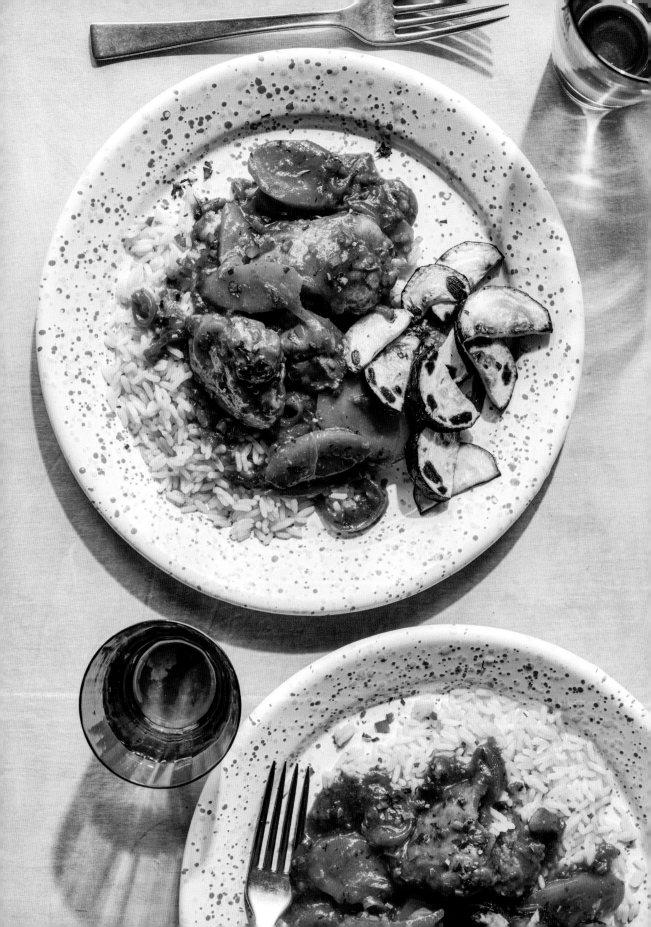

Spicy Ginger Chicken

PREP TIME: 10 MINUTES **COOK TIME: 35 MINUTES** **SERVES: 4**

8 skinless, boneless chicken
   thighs (approx. 720g/1lb
   9oz)
1 onion, sliced
2 garlic cloves, minced
1 tablespoon finely chopped
   fresh ginger
1 teaspoon ground coriander
1 teaspoon ground cumin
2 teaspoons paprika
olive oil spray
1 red chilli, chopped, or
   ½ teaspoon red chilli flakes
2 tablespoons apricot jam
2 large carrots, sliced
360ml (12fl oz) chicken stock
1 tablespoon cornflour
   (cornstarch)
salt and freshly ground
   black pepper
freshly chopped coriander
   (cilantro), to serve

Side suggestions:
This is delicious served
with rice or your favourite
potatoes – or, for a low-carb
option, some cauliflower rice.
A side of green vegetables
makes a great addition, too:
I like it with grilled courgette
(zucchini).

**If you love simple recipes with delicious sauces, then this one
is for you! The sweet, spicy sauce is bursting with flavour, and
it's an easy meal the whole family will love. It's really versatile,
too, as you can mix it up with a variety of sides – see my
suggestions below.**

1. In a large bowl, combine the chicken thighs with the onion,
garlic, ginger and ground spices, and mix to evenly coat.

2. Heat a frying pan over a medium–high heat and spray with olive
oil spray. Add the chicken and onion mixture and fry for a couple
of minutes until lightly golden, then stir in the chilli, apricot jam,
carrots and chicken stock.

3. Bring to the boil, then reduce the heat to medium–low and
simmer for 30 minutes until the chicken is lovely and tender.

4. In a small bowl or mug, mix the cornflour with a little water to
make a slurry. Add this to the pan and stir until the sauce thickens.

5. Season to taste, then stir through the fresh coriander to serve.

316 kcals
per serving

DF

GF

KCALS
316

FAT
11.7g

SAT FAT
3.2g

CARBS
15.6g

SUGARS
11.0g

FIBRE
4.2g

PROTEIN
35.1g

SALT
0.68g

GF

KCALS
216

FAT
7.1g

SAT FAT
3.2g

CARBS
8.4g

SUGARS
6.6g

FIBRE
2.8g

PROTEIN
27.6g

SALT
0.90g

Beef Stroganoff

PREP TIME: 10 MINUTES　　**COOK TIME: 25 MINUTES**　　**SERVES: 4**

fresh thyme sprig (or
　½ teaspoon dried thyme)
400ml (14 oz) beef stock
olive oil spray
400g (14oz) lean beef fillet
　(tenderloin) or lean sirloin
　steak, sliced into thin strips
1 large onion, thinly sliced
3 garlic cloves, crushed
10 mushrooms, thinly sliced
splash of Worcestershire
　sauce
splash of balsamic vinegar
2 tablespoon tomato purée
　(paste)
2 teaspoons Dijon mustard
½ teaspoon sweet paprika
5 tablespoons light
　cream cheese
salt and freshly ground
　black pepper
freshly chopped parsley,
　to serve

Side suggestions:
Stroganoff is great served
with rice, pasta or potatoes.
For a low-carb side, try it
with cauliflower rice, or
cauliflower mash.

Swaps:
If you prefer, you can use
quark or fat-free natural
yogurt instead of cream
cheese, but bring to room
temperature and stir in just
before serving to prevent
splitting.

This recipe is a real Slimming Eats oldie, but one that has been loved by my readers for years. It's super-simple to make, and pairs well with a variety of sides. My family loves it served with rice or wide egg pasta, like pappardelle or tagliatelle.

1. Add the thyme to the beef stock to infuse and set aside.

2. Heat a non-stick frying pan over a high heat and spray with olive oil spray. Add the beef and season with salt and pepper. Fry for about 5 minutes until the beef starts to go golden. Remove from the pan and set aside on a plate.

3. Add the onion, garlic and mushrooms to the empty pan, along with a couple of tablespoons of the stock. As the stock reduces, keep adding more, repeating the process until only a quarter of the stock remains, and the onion and mushrooms are nicely golden and caramelized.

4. Return the beef to the pan, along with the rest of the stock and the Worcestershire sauce, balsamic vinegar, tomato purée, mustard and paprika. Simmer for a few minutes until the sauce has almost completely reduced, then stir in the cream cheese until completely melted and creamy.

5. Serve topped with some freshly chopped parsley.

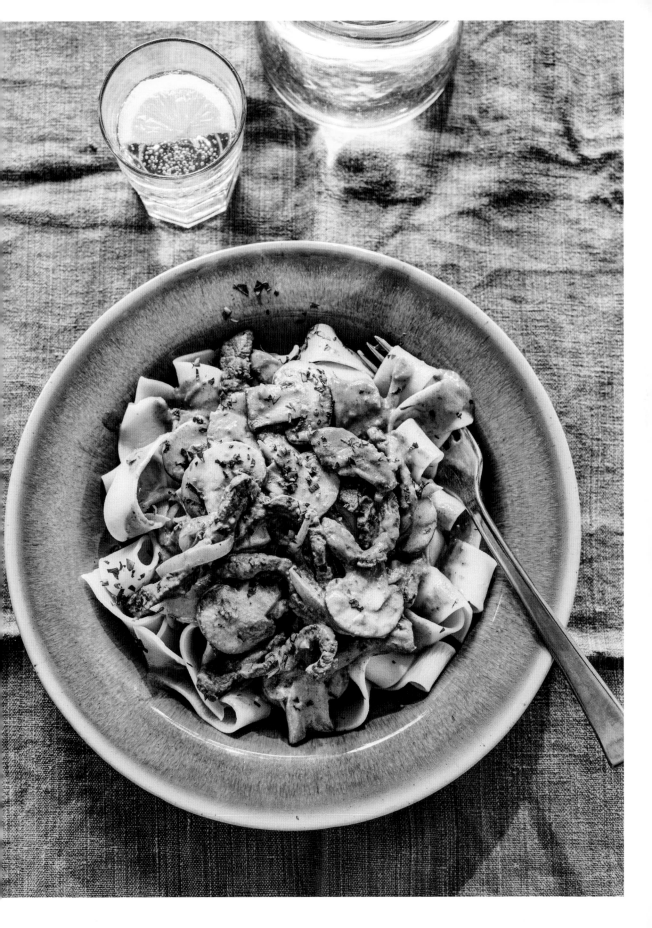

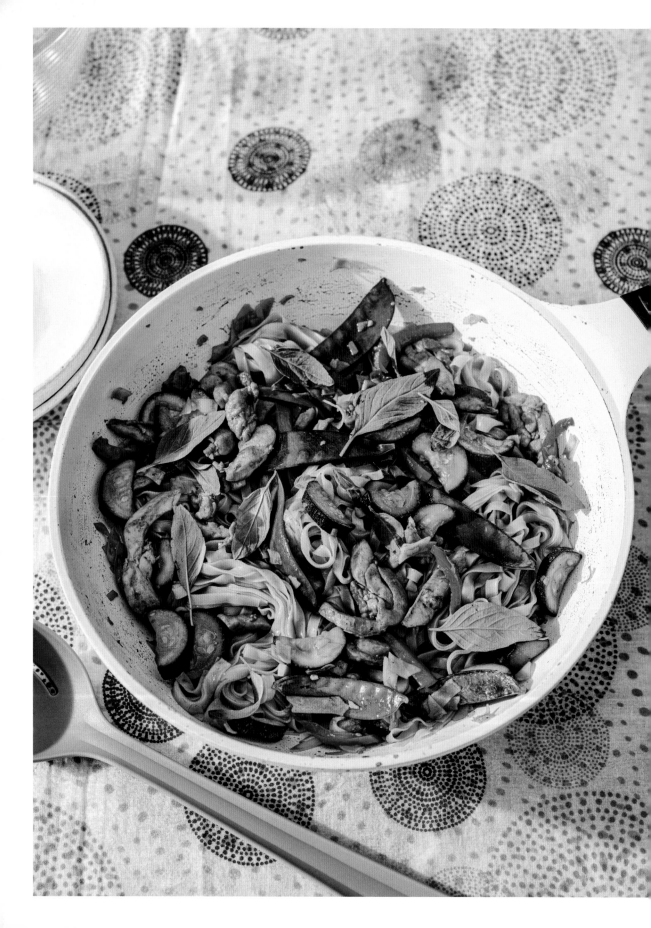

Drunken Chicken Noodles

PREP TIME: **10 MINUTES**   COOK TIME: **20 MINUTES**   SERVES: **4**

200g (7oz) dried flat
  rice noodles
olive oil spray
300g (10½oz) boneless,
  skinless chicken thighs,
  sliced into strips
1 teaspoon dark soy sauce
1 red (bell) pepper, sliced
1 courgette (zucchini), halved
  lengthways and sliced
12 mangetout (snow peas)
2 Thai red chillies, sliced
2 garlic cloves, crushed
pinch of freshly ground
  black pepper
handful of Thai basil

For the sauce:
2 tablespoons oyster sauce
1 tablespoon light soy sauce
1 tablespoon dark soy sauce
1 tablespoon maple syrup
½ tablespoon fish sauce

This is a seriously tasty treat for fans of spicy noodle dishes: tender pieces of chicken with vegetables and rice noodles, all coated in a flavoursome spicy sauce and finished off with fragrant Thai basil. It's quick, easy and packs a real punch of flavour and spice.

1. In a bowl, combine all the ingredients for the sauce with 60ml (4 tablespoons) water and set aside.

2. Cook the noodles according to the packet instructions, then drain and set aside.

3. Heat a wok or large frying pan over a medium–high heat and spray with olive oil spray. Add the chicken and soy sauce and fry for about 5 minutes until the chicken is a lovely deep golden colour. Remove from the pan and set aside on a plate.

4. Spray the empty pan with more olive oil spray and add the pepper, courgette, mangetout, chillies and garlic. Stir-fry for a couple of minutes until slightly softened.

5. Return the chicken to the pan, then pour over the sauce. Stir-fry until the chicken and vegetables are all coated in sauce. Season with a little black pepper.

6. Add the cooked noodles and Thai basil, and toss until all combined.

7. Serve and enjoy!

DF

KCALS
326

FAT
2.9g

SAT FAT
0.8g

CARBS
49.7g

SUGARS
8.5g

FIBRE
4.8g

PROTEIN
23.0g

SALT
2.68g

KCALS
401

FAT
15.6g

SAT FAT
7.7g

CARBS
28.7g

SUGARS
10.6g

FIBRE
5.1g

PROTEIN
33.9g

SALT
0.98g

Mexican Chicken Lasagne

PREP TIME: **15 MINUTES**   COOK TIME: **1 HOUR**   SERVES: **6**

olive oil spray
600g (1lb 5oz) extra-lean
   chicken or turkey mince
   (ground chicken or turkey)
1 red (bell) pepper,
   finely chopped
1 green (bell) pepper,
   finely chopped
1 onion, finely chopped
2 garlic cloves, crushed
8 tablespoons quark,
   light cream cheese or
   reduced-fat soured cream
8 dried lasagne sheets
100g (3½oz) mozzarella
120g (4¼oz) Cheddar
2 tomatoes, thinly sliced
salt and freshly ground
   black pepper
2 spring onions (scallions),
   thinly sliced, or freshly
   chopped coriander
   (cilantro) (optional)

For the spicy sauce
480g (1lb 1oz) passata
3 tablespoons tomato purée
   (paste)
1 tablespoon white wine
   vinegar
2 teaspoon mild chilli powder
2 teaspoon ground cumin
2 teaspoons paprika
1 teaspoon onion powder
½ teaspoon garlic powder
¼ teaspoon cayenne pepper
¾ tablespoon brown
   granulated sweetener

Freezing:
Freeze after step 5.

Another big hit on the Slimming Eats blog, this Mexican chicken lasagne has all the delicious flavours of Mexican food in a family-friendly lasagne recipe. It's delicious served just as it is, or paired with a simple side salad.

1. Preheat the oven to 180°C/160°C fan/350°F/gas 4.

2. To make the sauce, combine the passata, tomato purée, vinegar, spices and sweetener in a small saucepan with 240ml (8½fl oz) water. Place over a medium–high heat and bring to the boil, then reduce the heat to medium–low and simmer until the sauce reduces down and thickens slightly – this usually takes about 10 minutes, but it might vary depending on the size of your pan.

3. Heat a large frying pan over a medium–high heat and spray with olive oil spray. Add the chicken mince, peppers, onion and garlic. Cook for about 6 minutes until the chicken is browned, breaking up the mince with your spoon. Take off the heat and stir in the quark or cream cheese until all combined.

4. Spoon half of the chicken mixture into a 24 x 30cm (9.5 x 12in) ovenproof dish and spread out evenly.

5. Top with four of the lasagne sheets, then pour over half the spicy tomato sauce. Repeat to use up the rest of the chicken mixture, lasagne sheets and sauce.

6. Sprinkle over the grated mozzarella and Cheddar and top with the sliced tomato. Season with salt and pepper, then cover with foil. Bake for 20 minutes, then remove the foil and return to the oven for another 20 minutes until the cheese on top is browned. (If you like, you can place it under the grill for an extra 5 minutes at the end to really brown the top).

7. Sprinkle with the chopped spring onion or coriander (if using), then serve and enjoy!

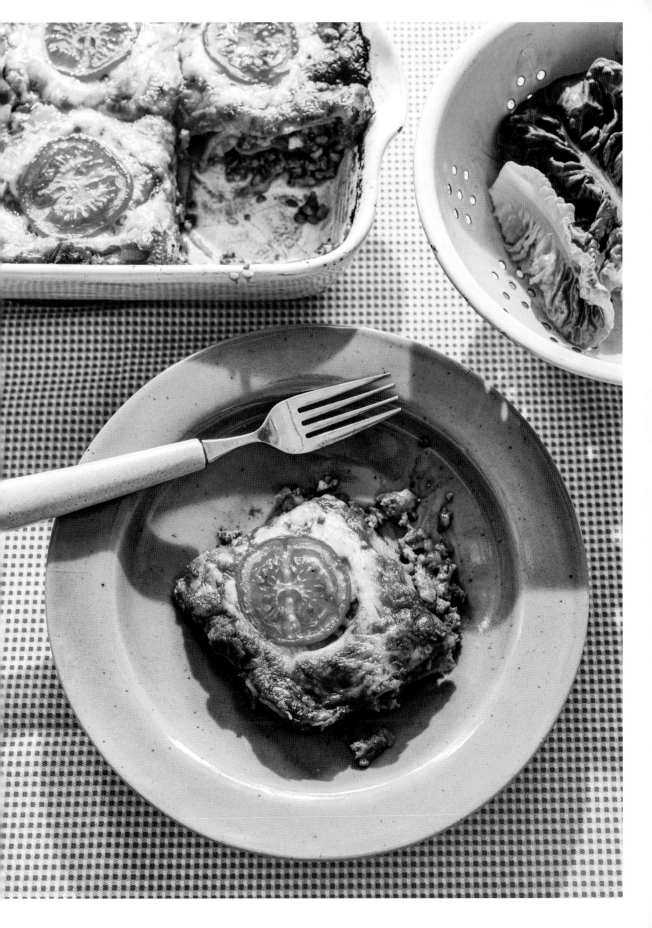

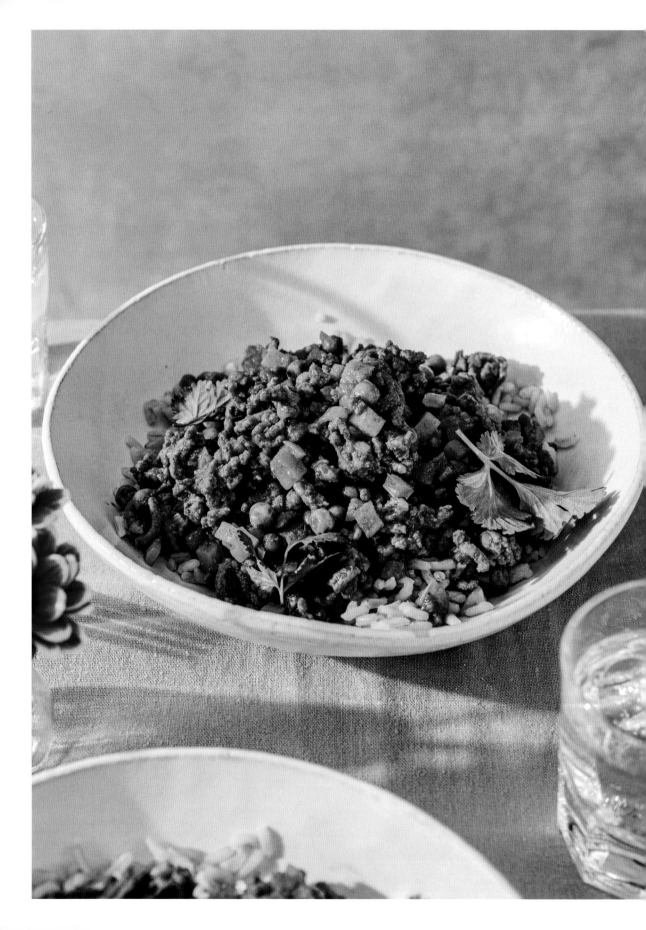

Keema Curry

PREP TIME: 10 MINUTES   **COOK TIME: 40 MINUTES**   **SERVES: 4**

low-calorie cooking oil spray
1 large onion, finely chopped
3 garlic cloves, crushed
1 large carrot, finely chopped
1 celery stalk, finely chopped
1 heaped teaspoon grated
  fresh ginger
450g (1lb) 5% fat beef mince
  (ground beef)
2 teaspoons cumin seeds
2 teaspoons ground
  coriander
1 teaspoon deggi mirch chilli
  powder (or any chilli
  powder of your choice)
1 teaspoon garam masala
1 teaspoon ground turmeric
4 tablespoons tomato purée
  (paste)
400ml (14oz) beef stock
140g (5oz) frozen peas
salt and freshly ground
  black pepper
freshly chopped coriander
  (cilantro), to serve

This easy curry is made with extra-lean beef mince and just a few store cupboard spices that mix together to create a delicious spice blend. It's perfect with basmati rice, or you can serve it with some of your other favourite homemade Indian dishes for a real feast.

1. Heat a large frying pan over a medium heat and spray with low-calorie cooking spray.

2. Add the onion, garlic, carrot, celery and ginger and cook for about 5 minutes to soften.

3. Add the beef and cook for a couple of minutes until browned, breaking up any large pieces with the back of a wooden spoon as it cooks. Stir in all the spices and tomato purée and mix to evenly coat.

4. Add the stock and bring to the boil, then reduce the heat to low and simmer for about 30 minutes until the meat is cooked through and the stock has reduced to a thicker consistency. Stir in the peas for the last few minutes.

5. Taste and season as needed with salt and pepper, then serve topped with freshly chopped coriander.

Side suggestions:
This is great served with basmati rice, or cauliflower rice if you fancy something lower in carbs. The garlic naan from page 171 would also make a great addition.

Swaps:
This can also be made with lamb, turkey or chicken mince.

242 kcals
per serving

DF

GF

KCALS
242

FAT
7.0g

SAT FAT
2.7g

CARBS
12.5g

SUGARS
8.9g

FIBRE
6.4g

PROTEIN
29.0g

SALT
0.62g

Corned Beef Hash

PREP TIME: 5 MINUTES **COOK TIME: 45 MINUTES** **SERVES: 4**

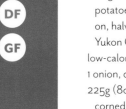

DF

GF

KCALS
251

FAT
6.7g

SAT FAT
3.3g

CARBS
26.8g

SUGARS
7.0g

FIBRE
5.4g

PROTEIN
18.4g

SALT
1.23g

600g (1lb 5oz) baby
   potatoes, skins left
   on, halved (I used
   Yukon Golds)
low-calorie cooking oil spray
1 onion, diced
225g (8oz) lean canned
   corned beef
1 green (bell) pepper, diced
1 red (bell) pepper, diced
4 spring onions (scallions),
   sliced
salt and freshly ground
   black pepper

This easy, family-friendly recipe is perfect for breakfast, lunch or dinner. It's delicious served just as it is, or with some additional sides like grilled tomatoes, fried eggs or baked beans (my kids' favourite option).

1. Preheat the oven to 200°C/180°C fan/400°F/gas 6.

2. Place the potatoes into a saucepan over a medium–high heat and cover with water. Bring to the boil, then turn off the heat and leave in the water for 5 minutes.

3. Drain well, then pat dry and place on a baking sheet. Spray with cooking oil spray and season with salt, then bake for 25–30 minutes until lightly golden. Remove from the oven and use the back of a fork to roughly flatten all the potatoes. Set aside.

4. Heat a large frying pan over a medium–high heat and spray with low-calorie cooking oil spray. Add the onion and fry for a couple of minutes until translucent, then add the corned beef and peppers and fry for a couple of minutes, breaking up the corned beef into smaller chunks with your spoon.

5. Add the potatoes and spring onions, then season with salt and pepper. Flatten down all the mixture in the pan.

6. Reduce the heat to medium and allow to brown underneath for 4–5 minutes. Finally, place under a grill, and grill until the top of the hash is golden.

7. Serve and enjoy!!

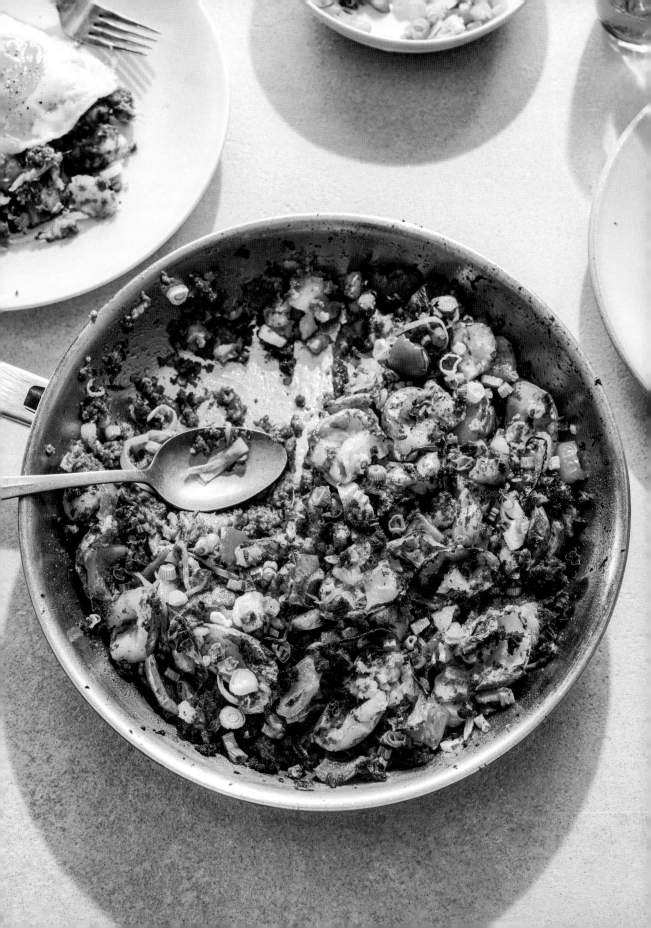

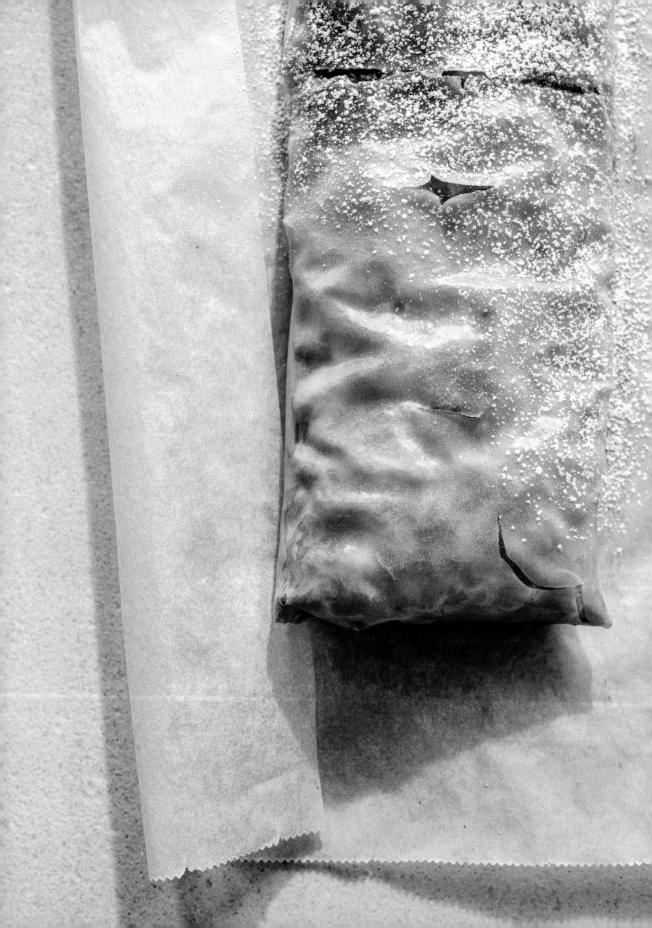

Desserts Made Simple

French Toast Casserole

PREP TIME: 5 MINUTES   **COOK TIME: 40 MINUTES**   **SERVES: 6**

4 large eggs
350ml (12fl oz) semi-skimmed milk
1 tablespoon ground cinnamon
1 teaspoon vanilla extract
4 tablespoons brown sugar sweetener
8 slices of low-calorie bread, halved diagonally (so you have 16 triangles)
2 tablespoons light brown sugar
2 tablespoons unsalted butter, melted
low-calorie cooking oil spray
1 tablespoon icing (confectioners') sugar, for dusting
150g (5½oz) frozen mixed berries, slightly defrosted, to serve

Side suggestions:
Serve with some light cream or fat-free yogurt.

If you love French toast, you will adore this easy French toast casserole, which is perfect for breakfast or dessert. It has a delicious cinnamon-sugar butter topping that is just heavenly, and it's all finished off with some mixed berries.

1. Preheat the oven to 200°C/180°C fan/400°F/gas 6.

2. In a bowl, whisk together the eggs, milk, cinnamon and vanilla with 2 tablespoons of the sweetener.

3. Layer the bread into a 20 x 25cm (10 x 8in) oven dish, arranging the slices so that they overlap. Pour the egg mixture over the top.

4. In a bowl, stir the brown sugar and remaining sweetener into the melted butter until fully dissolved, then drizzle this all over the top.

5. Spray with olive oil spray and bake for 35–40 minutes until golden.

6. Allow to cool slightly, then dust with the icing sugar and serve with the berries.

KCALS	**259**
FAT	**9.6g**
SAT FAT	**4.4g**
CARBS	**30.5g**
SUGARS	**12.3g**
FIBRE	**2.8g**
PROTEIN	**10.7g**
SALT	**0.51g**

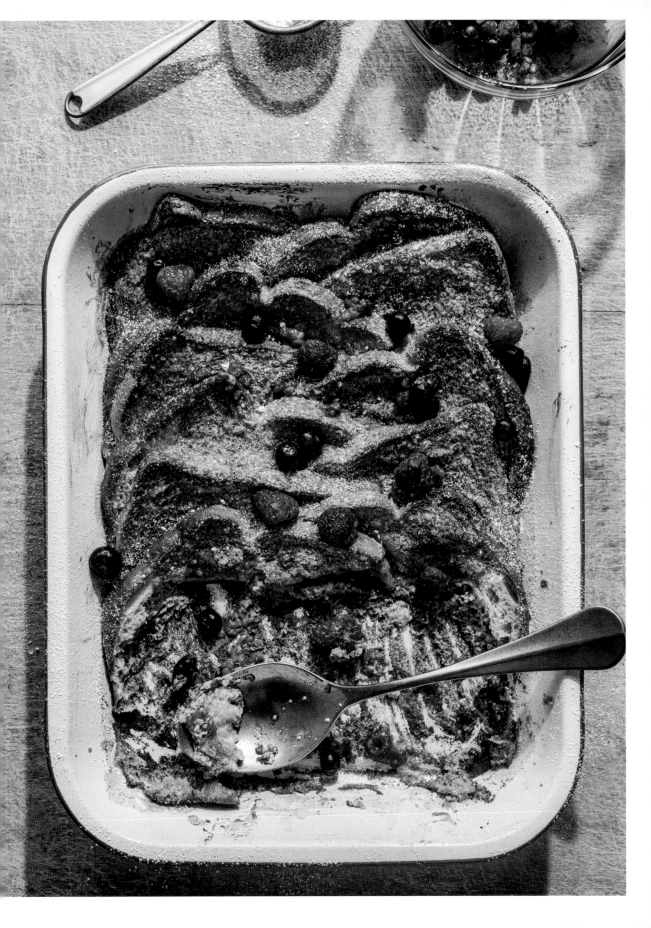

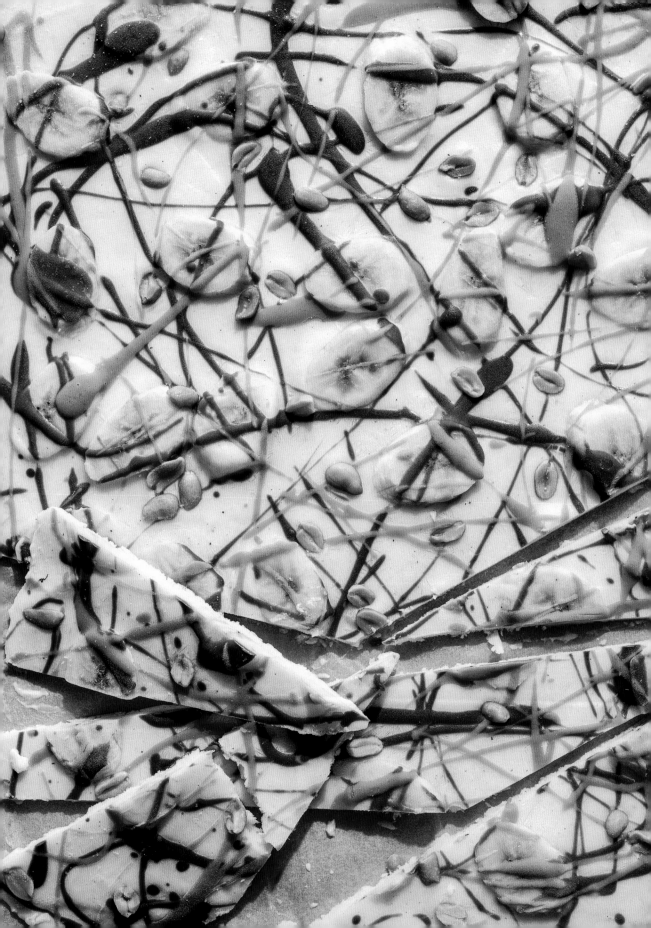

Banana, Peanut and Chocolate Yogurt Bark

PREP TIME: **5 MINUTES**   SERVES: **6**

600g (1lb 5oz) fat-free
   vanilla-flavoured
   Greek yogurt
2 small bananas, sliced
40g (1½oz) milk chocolate
   chips
20g (¾oz) peanut butter
   (smooth or crunchy)
15g (½oz) salted peanuts,
   chopped

This yogurt bark is perfect for fans of ice cream or frozen treats: delicious frozen yogurt with chunks of banana, chocolate chips and peanuts, all drizzled with milk chocolate and peanut butter.

1. Line a baking tray with baking paper.

2. Pour the Greek yogurt on to a 30 x 20cm (12 x 8 in) tray and spread it out in an even layer.

3. Scatter over the banana slices and half of the chocolate chips.

4. Melt the remaining chocolate chips in a bowl in the microwave, heating them on high in 10-second bursts until melted. Drizzle the melted chocolate over the top of the yogurt.

5. Repeat the step above with the peanut butter, melting it to a drizzling consistency and pouring it over the yogurt.

6. Finally, scatter over the salted peanuts, then place the baking tray in the freezer until the yogurt is frozen – I usually leave mine overnight. Once frozen, you can break it up into portions and store them in the freezer in a freezer bag or another container.

KCALS
165

FAT
5.4g

SAT FAT
2.1g

CARBS
17.1g

SUGARS
16.1g

FIBRE
1.2g

PROTEIN
11.4g

SALT
0.16g

Oven-baked Double Chocolate and Berry Pancakes

PREP TIME: **5 MINUTES + RESTING**   COOK TIME: **25 MINUTES**   SERVES: **3**

KCALS	**357**
FAT	**12.1g**
SAT FAT	**4.9g**
CARBS	**41.9g**
SUGARS	**14.4g**
FIBRE	**4.8g**
PROTEIN	**17.0g**
SALT	**1.05g**

low-calorie cooking oil spray
80g (2¾oz) rolled oats
1½ teaspoons baking powder
pinch of salt
20g (¾oz) cocoa powder
180g (6½oz) fat-free vanilla-flavoured Greek yogurt
2 large eggs
1 teaspoon vanilla extract
2 tablespoons granulated sweetener
125g (4½oz) mixed frozen berries
20g (¾oz) milk chocolate chips
20g (¾oz) white chocolate chips
80g (2¾oz) fresh raspberries, to serve

Side suggestion:
Serve with some fat-free yogurt.

If you love pancakes, but hate that you have to stand at the stove flipping singular pancakes for what seems like forever, then this recipe is for you: pancakes made in the oven. We use a chocolate and oat pancake mix, with milk and white chocolate chips. I serve it with berries for a pop of fresh, fruity colour and flavour.

1. Preheat the oven to 190°C/170°C fan/375°F/gas 5. Line a 23 x 33cm (9 x 13in) baking tray with baking paper and spray with low-calorie cooking oil spray.

2. Place the oats in a blender and blend until really fine.

3. Transfer to a bowl and stir in the baking powder, salt and cocoa powder.

4. Add the yogurt, eggs, vanilla and sweetener and mix until combined, then leave to sit for 10 minutes.

5. Carefully pour the rested batter into the prepared tray and gently spread it out with a silicone spatula (be careful as you do this, or the batter will sink). Scatter over the berries and milk chocolate chips and bake for 25 minutes until the batter is cooked through.

6. Remove from the oven and scatter with the white chocolate chips – they will slightly melt from the heat of the pancakes. Serve with the fresh raspberries.

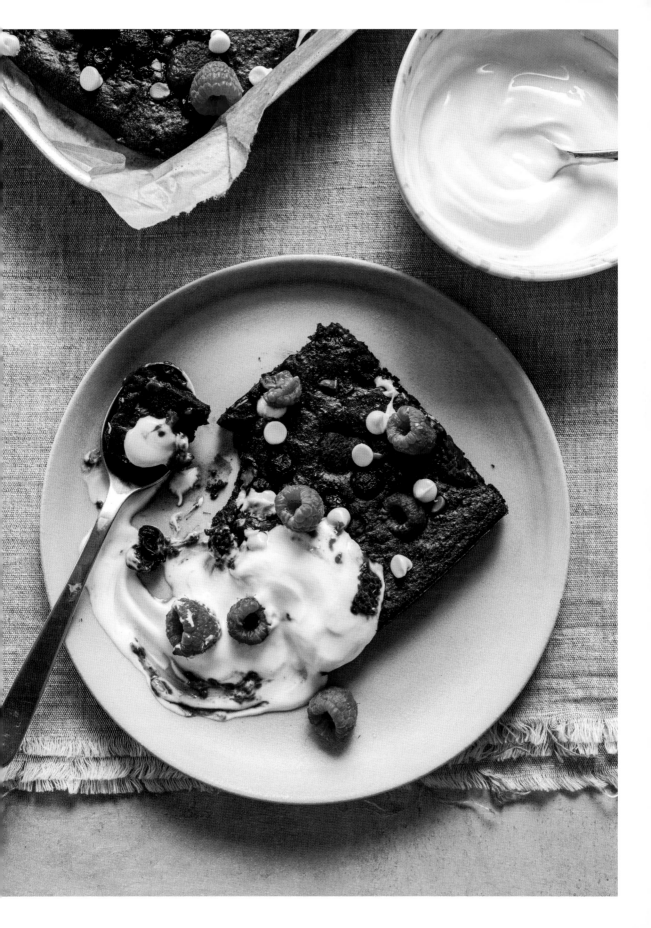

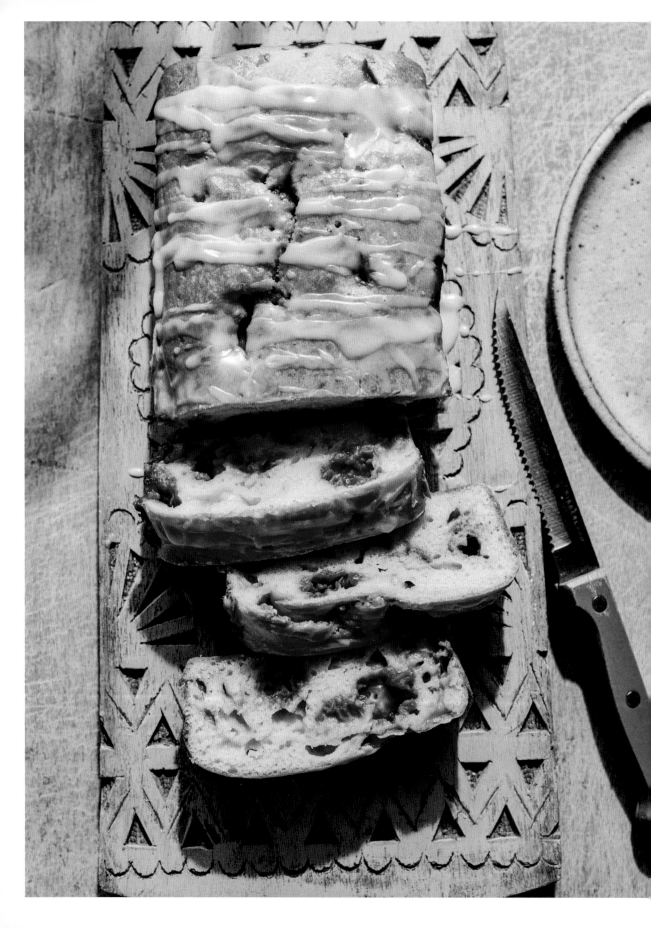

Raspberry Lemon Loaf

160 kcals
per serving

PREP TIME: 5 MINUTES   COOK TIME: **50 MINUTES**   SERVES: **10**

160g (5¾oz) plain flour
1½ teaspoons baking powder
pinch of salt
2 tablespoons unsalted
  butter
100g (3½oz) fat-free
  Greek yogurt
2 large eggs
3 tablespoons granulated
  sugar
3 tablespoons granulated
  sweetener
zest and juice of 1 lemon
100g raspberries

For the glaze
40g (1½oz) icing
  (confectioners') sugar
1 tablespoon lemon juice

Freezing:
Freeze before glazing.

Perfect for a snack or dessert, this yummy raspberry and lemon loaf cake is both moist and delicious, with beautiful flecks of colour from the raspberries and a zingy lemon glaze. A great cake you can enjoy with a cup of your favourite tea or coffee.

1. Preheat the oven to 180°C/160°C fan/350°F/gas 4 and line an 11 x 21cm (4½ x 8½in) loaf tin with baking paper.

2. In a bowl, mix together the flour, baking powder and salt.

3. In another bowl, mix together the butter, yogurt, eggs, sugar, sweetener and lemon zest and juice until well combined. Fold this into the flour mixture to create a batter and then add in the raspberries.

4. Pour the batter into the prepared tin and bake for 45–50 minutes until a skewer inserted in the centre comes out clean.

5. Remove from the oven and allow to cool slightly in the tin.

6. To make the glaze, mix together the icing sugar and lemon juice, then drizzle it over the top of the loaf.

7. Slice into 10 equal slices and serve. Store in an airtight container in a cool place. It should keep for about 4 days.

KCALS
160

FAT
3.8g

SAT FAT
2.0g

CARBS
26.6g

SUGARS
10.6g

FIBRE
0.8g

PROTEIN
4.3g

SALT
0.24g

Chocolate-drizzled Puffed Rice Bars

PREP TIME: 4 MINUTES   COOK TIME: 6 MINUTES   MAKES: 16 SQUARES

low-calorie cooking oil spray
1½ tablespoons unsalted
  butter
250g (9oz) marshmallows
120g (4¼oz) puffed rice
  cereal
15g (0½oz) white chocolate
15g (0½oz) milk chocolate

My kids love these bars, and they are so easy to make. I make up a batch regularly for them, and they are low enough in calories that I can enjoy one as a treat, too. That chewy marshmallow deliciousness, all drizzled with milk and white chocolate, is perfect when you need a sweet fix.

1. Line a 20cm (8in) square cake tin with baking paper and spray with olive oil spray.

2. Melt the butter in a saucepan over a low heat. Once melted, add the marshmallows and stir until they are melted too.

3. Once fully melted, remove from heat and add the puffed rice cereal, folding until combined. Transfer this mixture to the prepared tin and gently push down.

4. Melt the white chocolate in a bowl in the microwave, heating on high in 10-second bursts until melted. Pour the melted chocolate into a plastic food bag, then snip off one of the corners to make a piping bag. Pipe the chocolate over the puffed rice mixture. Repeat with the milk chocolate.

5. Leave to fully cool and set before slicing into 16 equal squares. These will keep for about 3 days in an airtight container in a cool place – but they never last that long with my kids around!

KCALS
101

FAT
1.8g

SAT FAT
1.1g

CARBS
20.0g

SUGARS
10.6g

FIBRE
0.1g

PROTEIN
1.2g

SALT
0.02g

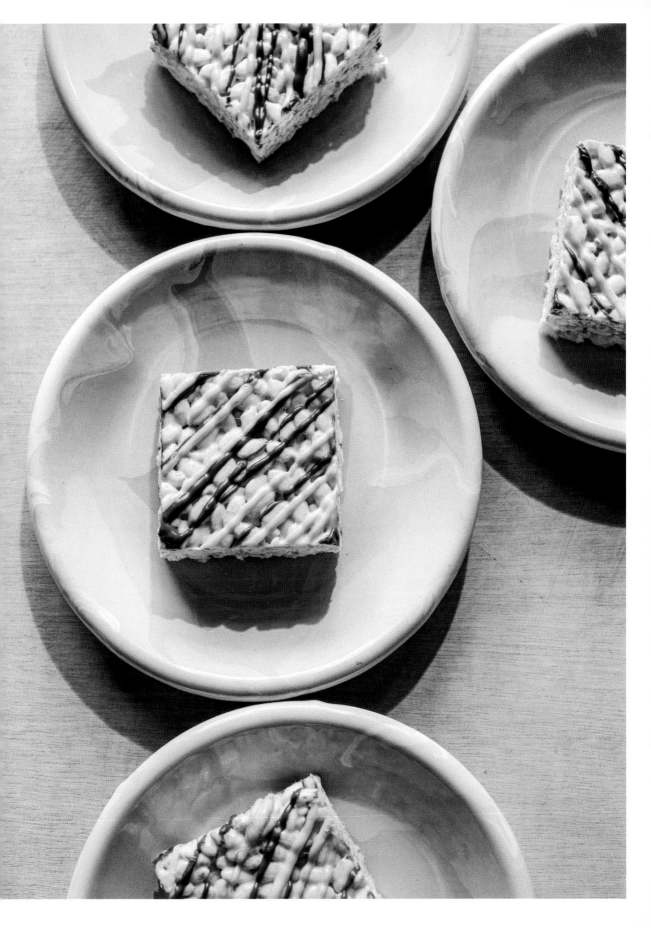

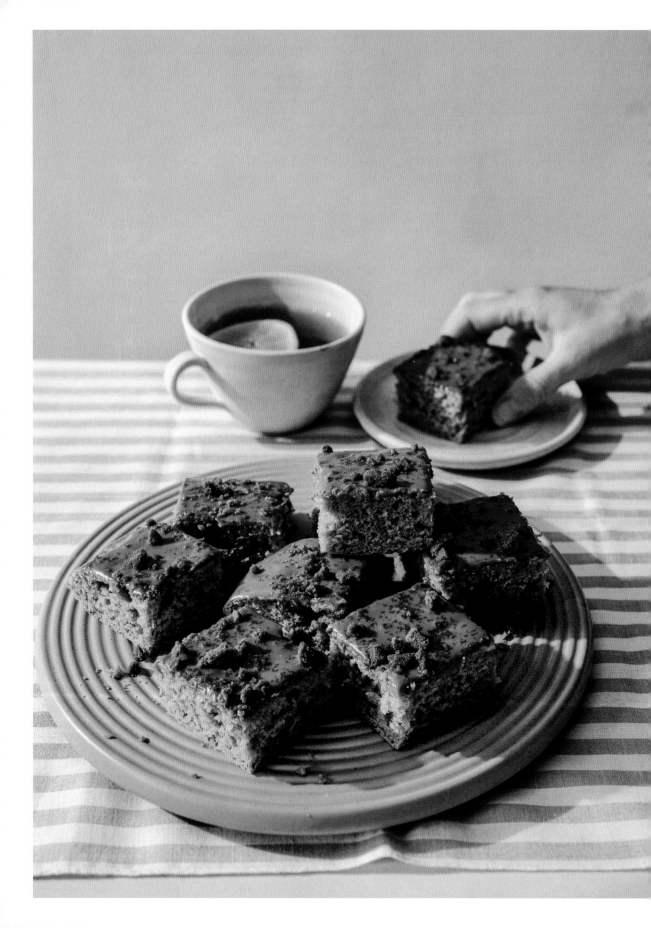

Biscoff Cake

PREP TIME: 5 MINUTES   **COOK TIME: 25 MINUTES**   **MAKES: 16 SQUARES**

low-calorie cooking oil spray
160g (5¾oz) plain flour
1½ teaspoons baking powder
pinch of salt
60g (2oz) Biscoff spread
6 tablespoons brown
   granulated sweetener
2 large eggs
1 teaspoon vanilla extract
120ml (4fl oz) oat milk

For the topping
80g (2¾oz) Biscoff spread
2 Lotus biscuits, crumbled

Note:
If you want to make a
smaller serving to avoid
the temptation to eat
more, simply halve all
the ingredients and use
a smaller cake tin.

Freezing:
Freeze before adding the
toppings.

This is the ultimate low-calorie cake for Biscoff lovers: a light Biscoff sponge cake with a decadent cookie crumb – and only 124 calories a slice! It is perfect as a snack or treat with a cuppa.

1. Preheat the oven to 180°C/160°C fan/350°F/gas 4.

2. Line a 20cm (8in) square cake tin with baking paper and spray with low-calorie cooking oil spray.

3. In a bowl, combine the flour with the baking powder and salt and mix well to combine.

4. Melt the Biscoff spread in a bowl in the microwave, heating on high in 10-second bursts until melted. Add the granulated sweetener and whisk until combined, then add the eggs, vanilla extract and oat milk and whisk until smooth.

5. Sift in the flour mixture, then fold in until combined.

6. Pour the batter into the prepared tin and bake for 25 minutes, or until a skewer inserted into the centre comes out clean.

7. Remove from the oven and allow to cool slightly.

8. To make the topping, melt the Biscoff spread in a bowl in the microwave, heating on high in 10-second bursts until runny, then pour this over the top of the cake, smoothing it all over with a spatula so you have an even layer. Sprinkle the lotus biscuit crumb over the top.

9. Slice into 16 equal squares and enjoy.

10. These will keep for about 4 days in an airtight container in a cool place; they can also be frozen once cooled if you prefer. Just place on a baking tray and place in the freezer until fully frozen, then transfer to a freezer container.

KCALS
124

FAT
4.5g

SAT FAT
1.0g

CARBS
18.0g

SUGARS
3.9g

FIBRE
0.6g

PROTEIN
2.4g

SALT
0.21g

104 kcals per serving

V

KCALS
104

FAT
1.7g

SAT FAT
0.7g

CARBS
19.7g

SUGARS
8.2g

FIBRE
0.7g

PROTEIN
2.2g

SALT
0.20g

Banana Gingerbread Cake

PREP TIME: **10 MINUTES**   COOK TIME: **25–30 MINUTES**   MAKES: **16 SQUARES**

low-calorie cooking oil spray
160g (5¾oz) plain flour
1 teaspoon baking powder
½ teaspoon bicarbonate
   of soda (baking soda)
pinch of salt
½ teaspoon ground
   cinnamon
2 teaspoons ground ginger
20g (¾oz) sultanas
   (golden raisins)
150g (5½oz) ripe bananas
1 tablespoon melted
   unsalted butter
4 tablespoons brown
   granulated sweetener
2 tablespoons maple syrup
2 tablespoons molasses
2 eggs
40g (1½oz) icing
   (confectioners') sugar

Freezing:
Freeze before adding the
icing.

This cake combines the deliciousness of banana bread with the rich heat of ginger cake, and is sure to be loved by the whole family. Delicately spiced moist banana bread with sweet sultanas and a hit of ginger, all finished off with a little icing drizzle. Whether it's for dessert or a snack, this cake is perfect – and low in calories.

1. Preheat the oven to 180°C/160°C fan/350°F/gas 4. Line a 20cm (8in) square cake tin with baking paper and spray with low-calorie cooking oil spray.

2. In a bowl, combine the flour, baking powder, bicarbonate of soda, salt, cinnamon, ginger and sultanas.

3. In a separate bowl, mash the bananas, then whisk in the melted butter, granulated sweetener, maple syrup and molasses. Now add the eggs, one at a time, whisking between each addition until well combined.

4. Sift in the flour mixture and fold in until combined.

5. Pour the batter into the prepared tin and gently tap the tin on the work surface to distribute the batter in an even layer. Bake for 25–30 minutes, or until a skewer inserted into the centre comes out clean.

6. Allow to cool slightly in tin, then transfer to a wire rack to cool completely.

7. To make the icing, put the icing sugar into a bowl and add a little drop of water at a time until you have a drizzling consistency. Be careful not to add the water too quickly, as you don't want it too runny.

8. Slice the cake into 16 equal squares and drizzle the icing over the top. Enjoy!

9. These will keep in airtight container in a cool place for about 4 days. The cake can be frozen, but I recommend freezing without the icing.

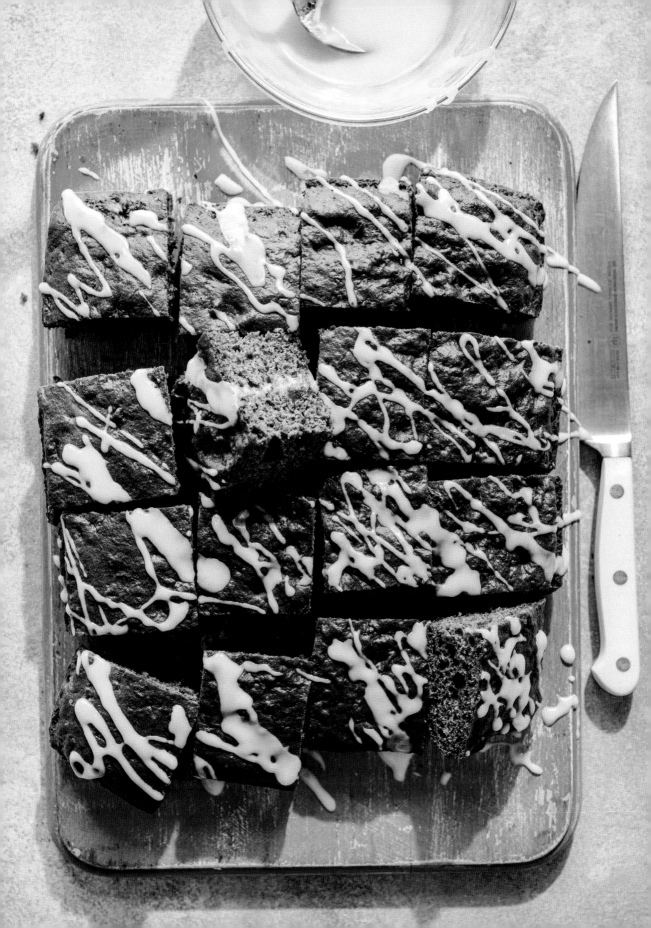

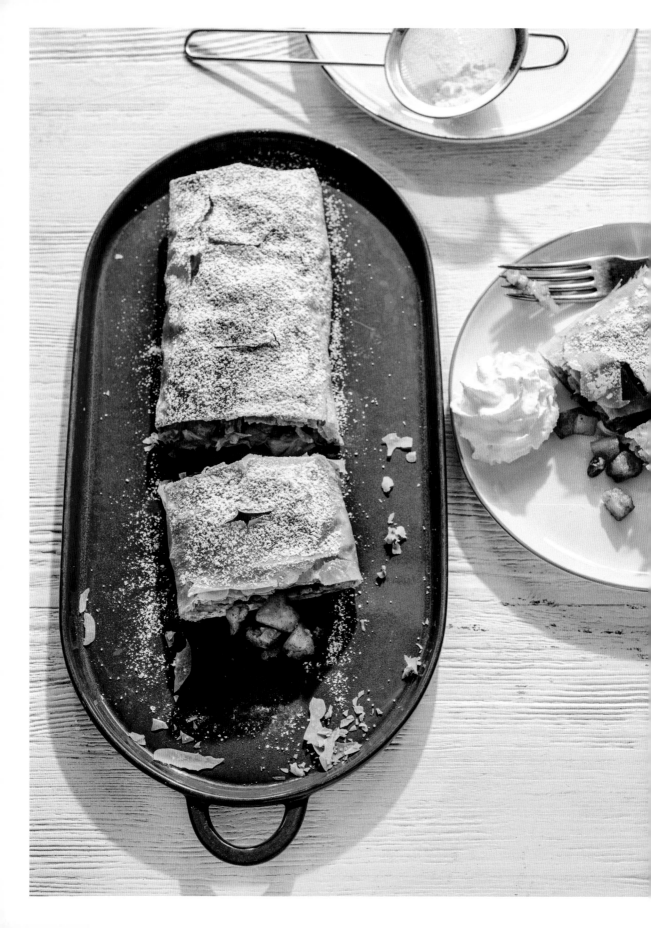

Pear and Apple Filo Strudel

PREP TIME: **15 MINUTES**   COOK TIME: **50 MINUTES**   SERVES: **4**

low-calorie cooking oil spray

180g (6½oz) apples,
  cored, peeled and diced
  (prepared weight)

20g (¾oz) sultanas
  (golden raisins)

1 tablespoon light
  brown sugar

3 tablespoons granulated
  sweetener

½ teaspoon ground
  cinnamon

180g (6½oz) ripe pears,
  peeled and diced
  (prepared weight)

2 teaspoons cornflour
  (cornstarch)

4 sheets of filo pastry

1 medium egg, beaten

1 tablespoon icing
  (confectioners') sugar

8 tablespoons light squirty
  (aerosol) cream

Freezing:

Freeze once you have
constructed the strudel,
but before brushing with
the egg. Defrost fully before
continuing with step 3.

This lighter strudel, made with filo pastry and filled with apples, pears and sultanas, is a great recipe to enjoy after dinner for a treat with the whole family. I like to serve it with a little light squirty (aerosol) cream, but it's also great with low-calorie ice cream.

1. Preheat the oven to 180°C/160°C fan/350°F/gas 4. Line a baking sheet with baking paper and spray with low-calorie cooking oil spray.

2. Combine the diced apple, sultanas, brown sugar, sweetener and cinnamon in a saucepan. Add 4 tablespoons water and cook over a medium–high heat for a few minutes until the liquid has almost completely evaporated off. Now add the diced pear and continue to cook for another few minutes until the pear and apple are just soft (you can add more water if needed). Set aside to cool. Once cooled, stir in the cornflour.

3. Spray each sheet of filo pastry with low-calorie cooking oil spray and stack them one on top of the other on the work surface. Place the apple and pear mixture in the centre of the pastry, leaving a border of about 7.5cm (3in) around the sides. Fold the shorter sides (top and bottom) over the apple and pear mixture, then fold one of the longer sides over the mixture. Repeat with the other side, tucking it underneath to seal, to create a long strudel parcel. Carefully transfer to the baking tray and brush all over with the beaten egg, then pierce a couple of holes in the top to allow steam to escape.

4. Place in the oven and bake for 35–40 minutes until golden.

5. Allow to cool for about 15 minutes, then dust with the icing sugar. Slice into 4 slices and serve with squirty cream.

6. Enjoy!

KCALS
317

FAT
7.2g

SAT FAT
3.7g

CARBS
55.5g

SUGARS
23.3g

FIBRE
3.5g

PROTEIN
5.8g

SALT
0.42g

V

Anzac-style Cookies

PREP TIME: 5 MINUTES   COOK TIME: 12 MINUTES   MAKES: 20 COOKIES

80g (2¾oz) plain
(all-purpose) flour
80g (2¾oz) rolled oats
20g (¾oz) unsweetened
shredded coconut
½ teaspoon bicarbonate
of soda (baking soda)
80g (2¾oz) unsalted butter,
melted
2 tablespoons golden syrup
4 tablespoons brown
granulated sweetener
20g (¾oz) chocolate chips
(I use mini ones)

Note:
If you want to make a smaller
batch to avoid the temptation
to eat more, then just halve
the ingredients and make
10 cookies instead of 20.

Making low-calorie cookies can sometimes seem like an impossible task; it can be so hard to replicate that yummy cookie taste without using heaps of butter and sugar. But don't despair: if you're after a lower-calorie treat, these Anzac-style cookies are a must. Kind of like a flapjack and cookie combined, and only 88 calories, they are great with a cuppa.

1. Preheat the oven to 180°C/160°C fan/350°F/gas 4 and line a large baking tray with baking paper.

2. In a large bowl, combine the flour with the oats, coconut and bicarbonate of soda.

3. In a separate bowl, mix together the butter, golden syrup and brown granulated sweetener until combined. Add this mixture to the oats and flour and mix until all combined.

4. Spoon 20 equal spoonfuls of the cookie mixture on to the prepared tray, spacing them out so they have room to spread. Add chocolate chips to each of the cookies, then flatten them slightly into cookie shapes (but not too much, as they will spread out more as they bake).

5. Bake for 10–12 minutes until lightly golden.

6. Allow to cool slightly if you can, as they will be really soft while hot.

7. Enjoy!

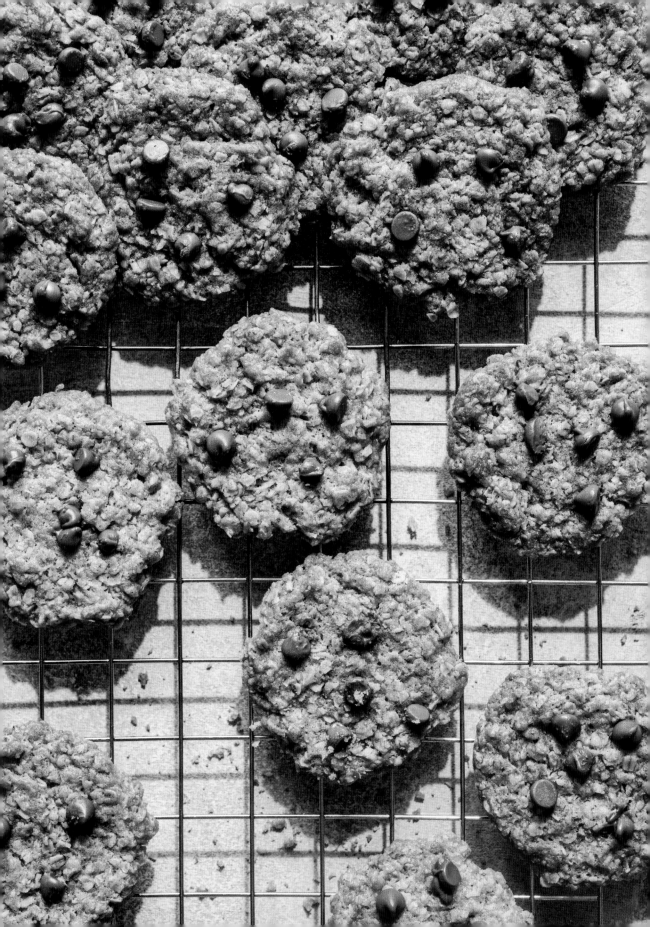

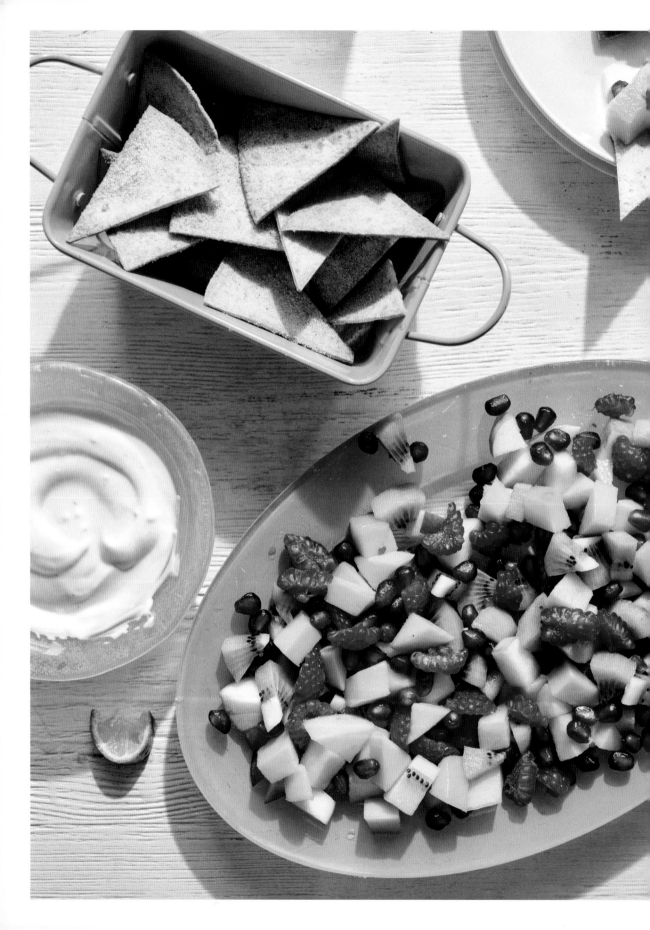

Fruit Salsa and Cheesecake Dip with Cinnamon-sugar Chips

PREP TIME: 5 MINUTES   **COOK TIME: 15 MINUTES**   **SERVES: 4**

For the fruit salsa
1 sweet crisp apple,
  diced small
2 kiwis, peeled and chopped
125g (4½oz) raspberries
1 mango, peeled and
  chopped
seeds from ½ small
  pomegranate
1 tablespoon granulated
  sweetener
½ tablespoon lime juice

For the cheesecake dip
80g (2¾oz) low-fat
  cream cheese
150g (5½oz) fat-free vanilla-
  flavoured Greek yogurt
20g (¾oz) icing
  (confectioners') sugar

For the cinnamon-sugar chips
3 low-calorie tortilla wraps
1 tablespoon unsalted
  butter, melted
1 tablespoon granulated
  sugar
1 tablespoon granulated
  sweetener
¾ teaspoon ground
  cinnamon

Variations:
I sometimes add a few chocolate chips or sprinkles to the cheesecake dip. Feel free to use any fruit you like, although a combination of crisp and soft fruit works best.

This is the perfect sharing platter for a movie night or barbecue: delicious fruit salsa with cheesecake dip and crispy cinnamon-sugar chips for dipping and scooping. My kids love this whenever I make it. I use a combination of our favourite fruit for the salsa, but you can make this with any fruit you like.

1. Preheat the oven to 200°C/180°C/400°F/gas 6 and line a baking tray with baking paper.

2. Make the fruit salsa by combining all the fruit in a bowl. Add the sweetener and lime juice and toss to coat.

3. For the cheesecake dip, whisk the cream cheese until light, then whisk in the yogurt and icing sugar until all combined.

4. For the cinnamon-sugar chips, slice each tortilla into 8 triangular wedges and brush each one with the melted butter. In a bowl, mix together the sugar, sweetener and cinnamon, then sprinkle this all over the tortilla triangles, dusting them on both sides. Spread out the tortilla triangles on the prepared baking tray and bake for 12–15 minutes until crisp and golden.

5. Serve the cinnamon-sugar chips with the fruit salsa and cream cheese dip.

308 kcals per serving

KCALS	308
FAT	6.4g
SAT FAT	3.4g
CARBS	50.1g
SUGARS	29.0g
FIBRE	5.0g
PROTEIN	10.0g
SALT	0.65g

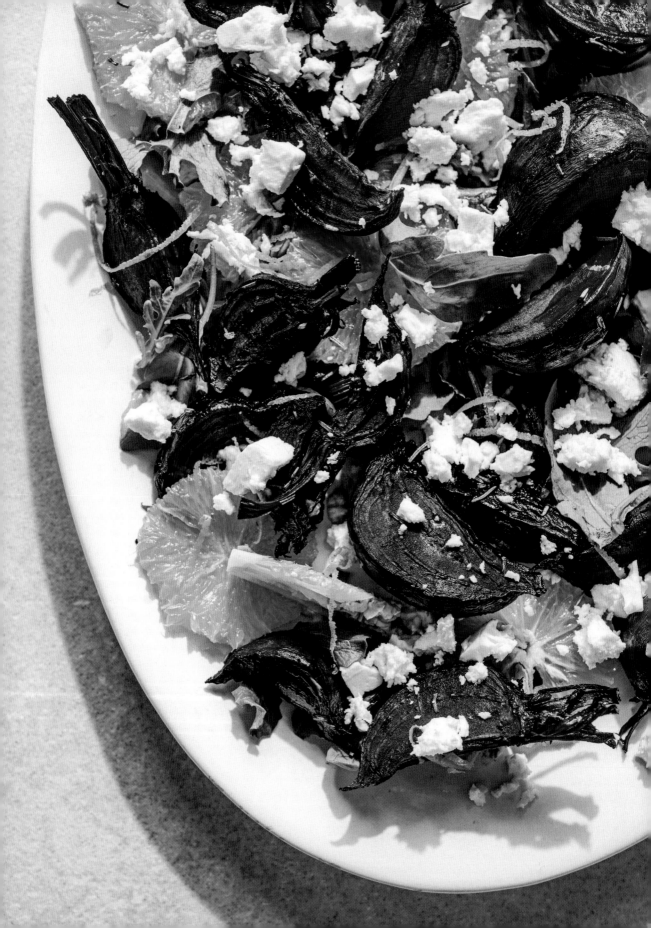

Simple Extras

KCALS
157

FAT
5.0g

SAT FAT
2.3g

CARBS
18.0g

SUGARS
16.6g

FIBRE
6.5g

PROTEIN
6.5g

SALT
0.69g

Balsamic-roasted Beetroot with Feta and Orange Salad

PREP TIME: **10 MINUTES**   COOK TIME: **60 MINUTES**   SERVES: **4**

700g (1lb 9oz) fresh
   beetroots (beets), trimmed,
   peeled and chopped
½ tablespoon extra virgin
   olive oil
2 tablespoons balsamic
   vinegar
1 tablespoon orange juice
pinch of dried rosemary
140g (5oz) baby greens
1 orange, peeled and
   thinly sliced
60g (2oz) feta, crumbled
coarse salt and freshly
   ground black pepper
orange zest, to serve

A refreshing, vibrant salad of balsamic-roasted beetroot with salty feta and citrus slices, served over a bed of baby greens. This makes a delicious side to the grilled protein of your choice.

1. Preheat the oven to 200°C/180°C fan/400°F/gas 6 and line a large baking tray with foil.

2. Place the beetroot chunks on the lined tray and drizzle over the olive oil, balsamic vinegar and orange juice. Season with a good pinch of coarse salt and black pepper, and a pinch of dried rosemary. Toss to coat and roast for 50–60 minutes until tender.

3. Arrange the baby greens on a plate or in a salad bowl and top with the roasted beetroot, along with the orange slices and crumbled feta. Serve with a little fresh orange zest grated over the top.

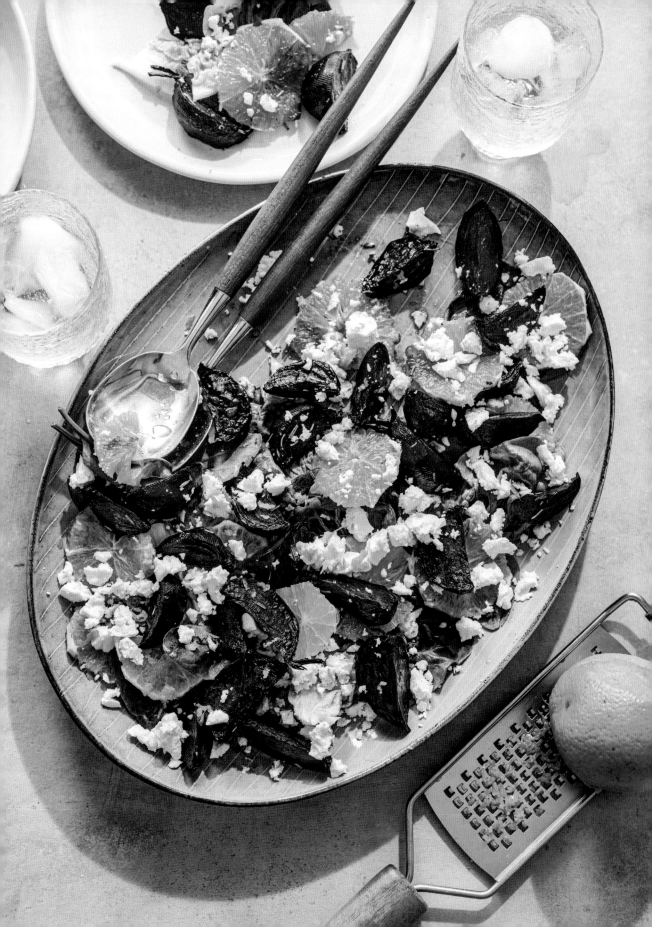

Guacamole and Salsa Two Ways

I love Mexican inspired dishes and guacamole and salsa are the perfect sides for these types of dishes. I do buy store versions occasionally when rushed for time, but there is nothing like homemade salsa and guacamole. Here are two of my favourite salsa recipes and my easy guacamole recipe, some of which are featured in the recipes in the book (see next page for photo).

Easy Guacamole

PREP TIME: **5 MINUTES**   SERVES: **4**

108 kcals
per serving

VG

DF

GF

KCAL: **108**

FAT: **9.8g**

SAT FAT: **2.1g**

CARBS: **2.3g**

SUGARS: **1.3g**

FIBRE: **2.7g**

PROTEIN: **1.2g**

SALT: **0.01g**

200g (7oz) avocado flesh, chopped
1 garlic clove, crushed
3 tablespoons finely chopped red onion
1 tablespoon fresh lime juice
½ ripe tomato, finely chopped
1½ tablespoons freshly chopped coriander
  (cilantro)
salt and freshly ground black pepper

Optional add-ins:
If you like a spicy guacamole, add a pinch of cayenne pepper.

1. In a bowl, mash together the avocado, garlic, onion and lime juice.

2. Season with salt and pepper to taste.

3. Mix in the tomato and coriander and enjoy!

Black Bean Salsa

PREP TIME: **3 MINUTES**   SERVES: **4**

150g (5½oz) canned black beans
100g (3½oz) canned sweetcorn
½ small red onion, finely diced
1 garlic clove, very finely chopped
1 ripe tomato, diced
1 jalapeño, deseeded and diced (you can
   leave the seeds in if you like the heat)
handful of coriander (cilantro), chopped
1 spring onion (scallion), chopped
juice of ½ lime
salt and freshly ground black pepper

1. Combine the ingredients in a bowl and mix to combine.

2. Season with a pinch of salt and pepper to taste.

V

DF

GF

KCAL: **73**
FAT: **0.8g**
SAT FAT: **0.1g**
CARBS: **10.6g**
SUGARS: **3.3g**
FIBRE: **4.0g**
PROTEIN: **3.8g**
SALT: **0.01g**

Pineapple Salsa

PREP TIME: **3 MINUTES**   SERVES: **4**

300g (10½oz) pineapple flesh, diced
½ small red onion, finely diced
½ red (bell) pepper, finely diced
1 small jalapeño, deseeded and diced
   (you can leave the seeds in if you
   like the heat)
2 tablespoons freshly chopped coriander
   (cilantro)
1 tablespoon lime juice
salt and freshly ground black pepper

1. Combine the ingredients in a bowl and mix to combine. Season with a pinch of salt and pepper to taste.

V

DF

GF

KCAL: **44**
FAT: **0.2g**
SAT FAT: **0.0g**
CARBS: **8.8g**
SUGARS: **8.7g**
FIBRE: **1.9g**
PROTEIN: **0.6g**
SALT: **0.01g**

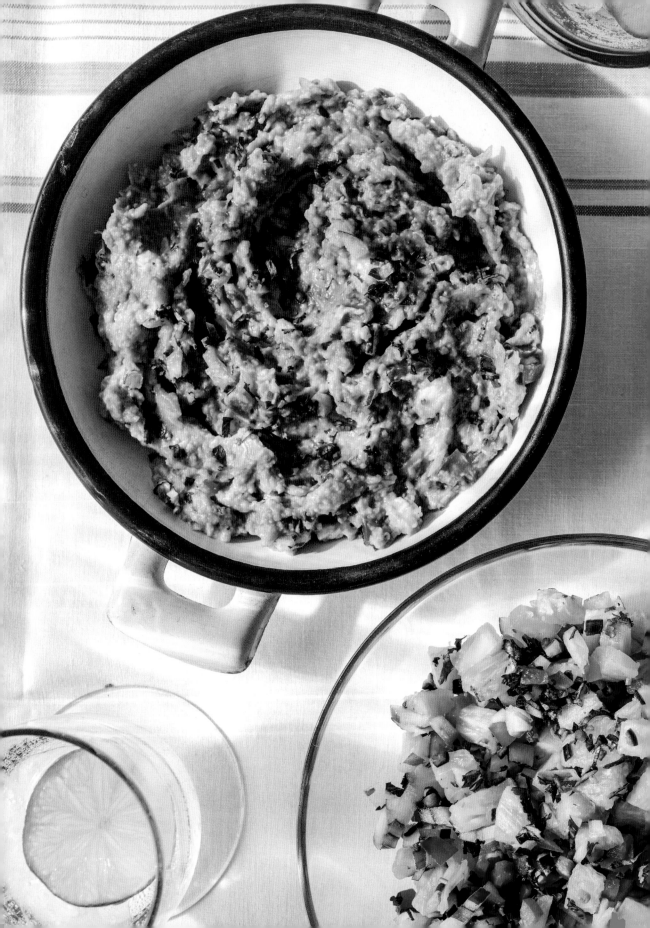

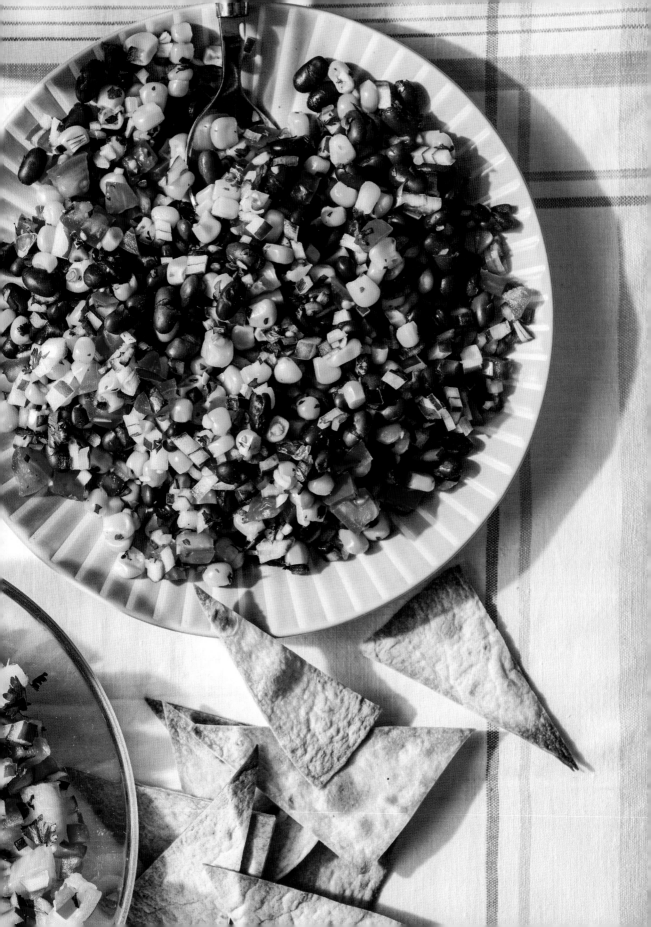

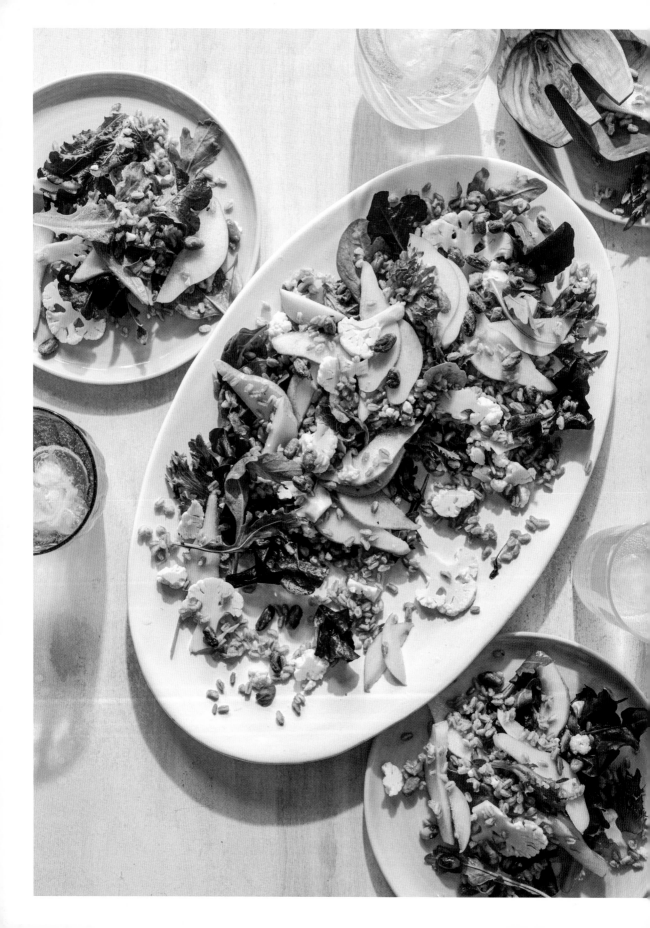

Cauliflower, Pear, Pistachio and Spelt Salad with Honey and Ginger Dressing

PREP TIME: 10 MINUTES   **COOK TIME: 15 MINUTES**   **SERVES: 4**

150g (5½oz) spelt or farro
50 shelled pistachios
olive oil spray
1 teaspoon granulated sugar
100g (3½oz) baby greens
100g (3½oz) cauliflower,
    thinly sliced with a mandolin
2 ripe pears, thinly sliced
salt and freshly ground
    black pepper

For the dressing
2 tablespoons honey
2 tablespoons apple
    cider vinegar
1 tablespoon extra virgin
    olive oil
2 teaspoons grated
    fresh ginger

Note:
I like to cook my spelt in
stock for flavour, but water
is fine too.

Swaps:
You can also swap the
spelt for quinoa or barley.
Protein like cooked chicken
or chickpeas makes a great
addition.

If you have never tried raw cauliflower, this is the salad to make. Baby greens, thin slices of raw cauliflower, cooked spelt or farro, juicy pear and candied pistachios, all combined with a simple honey and ginger dressing. It's great as it is, or with the protein of your choice. I love to serve it at barbecues.

1. Cook the spelt according to the packet instructions (see Note) and set aside to cool.

2. To make the dressing, whisk together all the ingredients in a bowl, then season with salt and pepper to your desired taste. Set aside.

3. Put the shelled pistachios into a small saucepan and spray with olive oil spray. Add the sugar, a pinch of salt and 1 tablespoon water, and heat over a medium–high heat for 4–5 minutes until the sugar and water have caramelized around the pistachios. Set aside to cool.

4. To assemble the salad, combine the greens and cauliflower in a salad bowl, then add the cooled spelt. Drizzle over the dressing and toss to coat. Taste for seasoning; I like to add a little more salt and pepper to the salad at this stage.

5. Top with the ripe pear slices and candied pistachios and enjoy!

360 kcals per serving

V

DF

KCALS
360

FAT
12.2g

SAT FAT
1.7g

CARBS
49.1g

SUGARS
20.4g

FIBRE
8.6g

PROTEIN
9.1g

SALT
0.03g

145 kcals
per serving

KCALS
145

FAT
0.5g

SAT FAT
0.1g

CARBS
28.3g

SUGARS
0.8g

FIBRE
2.7g

PROTEIN
5.2g

SALT
0.24g

Lemon and Herb Israeli Couscous

PREP TIME: **4 MINUTES**   COOK TIME: **16 MINUTES**   SERVES: **4**

olive oil spray
1 garlic clove, crushed
150g (5½oz) dried Israeli
    or pearl couscous
360ml (12fl oz) vegetable
    stock
1 tablespoon freshly
    chopped parsley
1 tablespoon freshly
    chopped mint
1 tablespoon freshly
    chopped coriander
    (cilantro)
lemon zest, to taste
1 tablespoon lemon juice
salt and freshly ground
    black pepper

Serving suggestions:
To make this delicious side
into a light meal, this is great
served with fresh cherry
or baby roma tomatoes,
cucumber and feta cheese.
Some sautéed seasoned
chickpeas or cooked lentils
are also a great addition for
some additional protein.

This fragrant Israeli couscous dish is super-quick and easy to make: just couscous, stock, fresh herbs and lemon, and you have a delicious side dish that works with a whole variety of mains. I love it as part of the Middle Eastern Lamb Bowls on page 191. You can also make this a meal in its own right by adding some feta, tomatoes and cucumber for a simple summer salad.

1. Heat a saucepan over a medium–high heat with olive oil spray. Add the garlic and fry for about 30 seconds just to release the flavour, then add the couscous and cook for a further 30 seconds.

2. Pour in the stock and bring to the boil, then cover and reduce the heat to medium–low. Simmer for 8–10 minutes until the stock is absorbed. Remove from the heat and leave with the lid on for a few minutes, just to ensure the couscous is fully cooked.

3. Spray with olive oil spray and fluff up with a fork to separate any clumps in the couscous, then add the herbs and lemon zest and juice. Mix again, then season with salt and pepper to taste.

4. Enjoy!

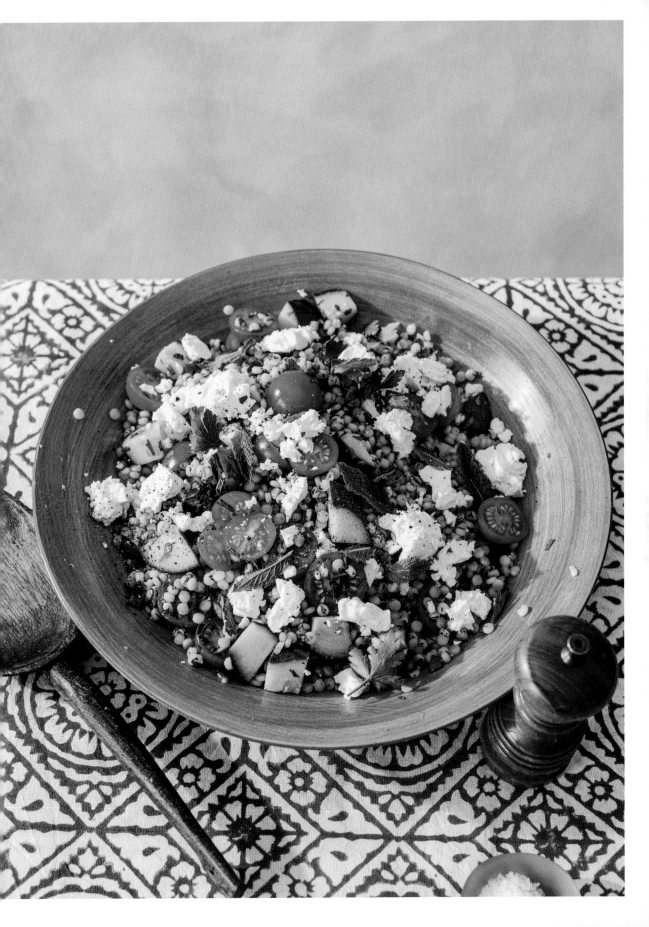

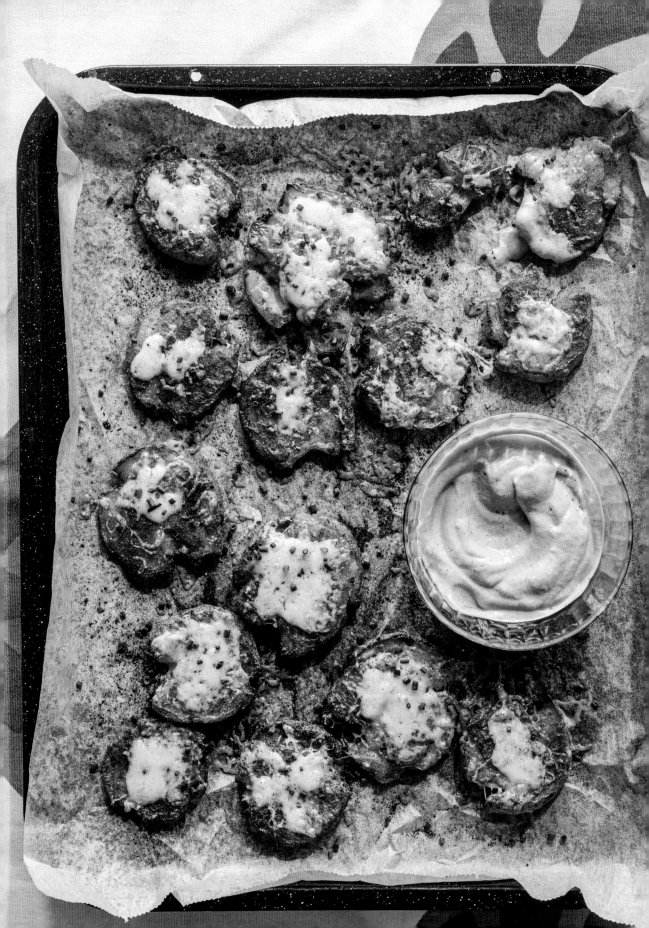

Cheddar Crushed Roast Potatoes with Special Sauce

PREP TIME: **5 MINUTES**   COOK TIME: **50 MINUTES**   SERVES: **4**

700g (1lb 9oz) baby
    potatoes (those with
    golden/yellow flesh
    are best, such as Desiree
    or Yukon Gold)
olive oil spray
½ teaspoon sweet paprika
½ teaspoon garlic powder
½ teaspoon onion powder
60g (2oz) mature Cheddar,
    finely grated
1 tablespoon fresh chives,
    chopped
salt and freshly ground
    black pepper

For the special sauce
5 tablespoons fat-free
    Greek yogurt
2 tablespoons honey
    barbecue sauce (see Note)
½ tablespoon Dijon mustard
1 teaspoon tomato purée
    (paste)

Note:
If you can't get honey barbecue
sauce, use regular barbecue
sauce and sweeten it to taste
with some granulated
sweetener, or honey or maple
syrup. Start with just a
teaspoon and increase to
your desired taste.

Swaps:
If you are not a fan of Greek
yogurt, you can swap it for
light mayonnaise (but, of
course, the calories will be
slightly higher).

Optional add-ins:
These are also delicious sprinkled
with some chopped cooked
bacon, which you can add at
the same time as the Cheddar.

This is one of my favourite sides, and so delicious that my family would gladly just eat these on their own. Boiled until just soft, then crushed, seasoned and baked until golden with melted Cheddar cheese, these little potatoes are so addictive – and made even more so by the special sauce, which is my kids' favourite dipping sauce for pretty much everything. It's delicious with potatoes, chicken, burgers and more.

1. Preheat the oven to 220°C/200°C fan/425°F/gas 7 and line a baking tray with some baking paper.

2. In a bowl, combine all the ingredients for the special sauce. Season with salt and pepper and set aside.

3. Place the potatoes in a saucepan of water over a high heat. Bring to the boil, then simmer for 12–15 minutes until just tender, but not so soft that they are falling apart. Drain the water from the saucepan and pat the potatoes dry.

4. Tip the potatoes into a large bowl. Spray with olive oil spray, then scatter over the paprika, garlic powder and onion powder. Toss to evenly coat, then transfer the potatoes to the lined tray and spread them out. Use the base of a glass to crush each potato, then spray with olive oil spray and season generously with salt and pepper.

5. Roast for 20 minutes until golden, then remove from the oven and flip the potatoes over. Spray with olive oil spray again, before returning to the oven for another 10 minutes.

6. Remove from the oven once more and sprinkle a little Cheddar over each crushed potato. Return to the oven for 5–6 minutes until the cheese is melted and golden.

7. Sprinkle with the freshly chopped chives and serve with the special sauce.

KCALS	**226**
FAT	**5.9g**
SAT FAT	**3.4g**
CARBS	**29.2g**
SUGARS	**6.3g**
FIBRE	**3.4g**
PROTEIN	**12.5g**
SALT	**0.68g**

226 kcals per serving

V

GF

122 kcals
per pancake

DF

KCALS
122

FAT
4.3g

SAT FAT
1.0g

CARBS
13.6g

SUGARS
5.3g

FIBRE
2.3g

PROTEIN
6.1g

SALT
0.71g

Mini Vegetable Okonomiyaki (Japanese Pancakes)

PREP TIME: **10 MINUTES**   COOK TIME: **15 MINUTES**   MAKES: **8**

300g (10½oz) white cabbage, thinly sliced
100g (3½oz) carrots, shredded or grated
3 spring onions (scallions), thinly sliced into strips
1 tablespoon Japanese soy sauce
pinch of sugar or granulated sweetener
80g (2¾oz) plain flour
4 large eggs, beaten
olive oil spray

For the tonkatsu sauce
1 tablespoon tomato purée (paste)
1 tablespoon soy sauce
1 tablespoon maple syrup
2 teaspoons Worcestershire sauce

For the topping
2 tablespoons light mayonnaise
1 spring onion (scallion), sliced
2.5g (half a pack) nori seaweed, sliced into thin strips (optional)
pinch of sesame seeds

This is my easy take on delicious okonomiyaki pancakes, a savoury Japanese omelette with shredded cabbage, carrots and green onions. Typically they come with various toppings, but I like to keep things simple by making them into little fritters drizzled with a quick okonomiyaki-style sauce and some light mayonnaise. The nori seaweed isn't essential: if you can get some, it adds a great burst of flavour, but they are equally delicious without. Enjoy as a side, or as a complete meal, just as they are.

1. In a bowl, combine the cabbage, carrots and spring onions. Add the soy sauce and sugar and toss to coat.

2. In a separate bowl, whisk together the flour and eggs to form a smooth batter.

3. Pour this into the bowl of shredded vegetables and toss until all combined.

4. Heat a large non-stick frying pan over a medium–high heat and spray with olive oil spray.

5. Divide the batter into two equal amounts. From one half, spoon four equal-sized pancakes into the hot frying pan. Allow to cook on one side for about 3 minutes until lightly golden, then spray with olive oil spray and flip to brown the other sides.

6. Repeat with the other half of the batter so you have 8 mini okonomiyaki pancakes.

7. In a bowl, mix together the ingredients for the tonkatsu sauce. Drizzle the sauce over the pancakes, followed by the mayonnaise (see Note). Sprinkle with the spring onion, nori seaweed and pinch of sesame seeds.

8. Enjoy!

Note:
You can loosen the tonkatsu sauce and mayo with a little water to make it easier to drizzle if needed.

Swaps:
For a spicy version, swap the tonkatsu sauce for some sriracha. You can also add some cooked protein into the pancake mix, such as bacon, prawns or chicken.

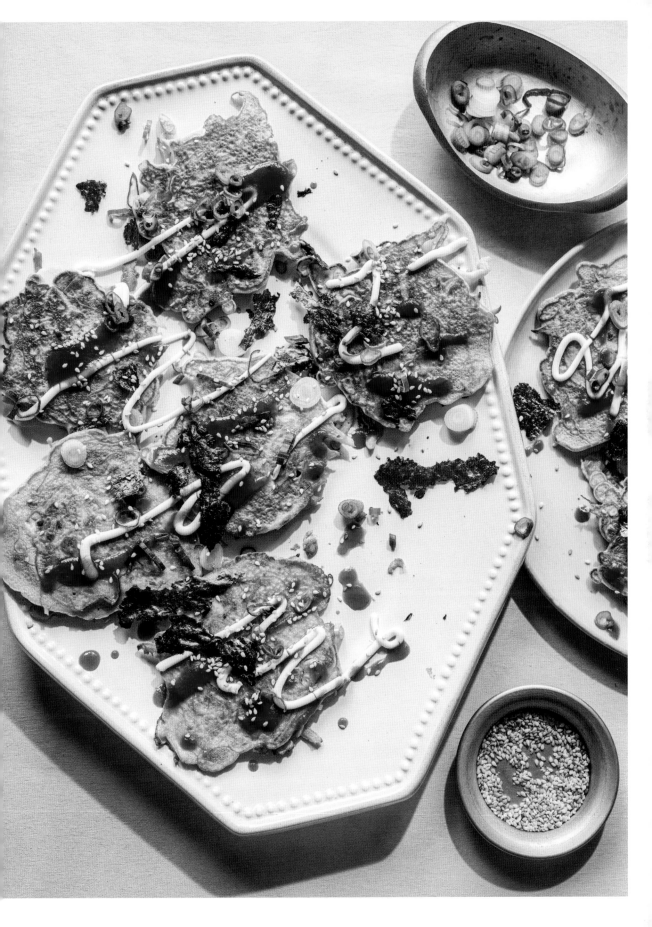

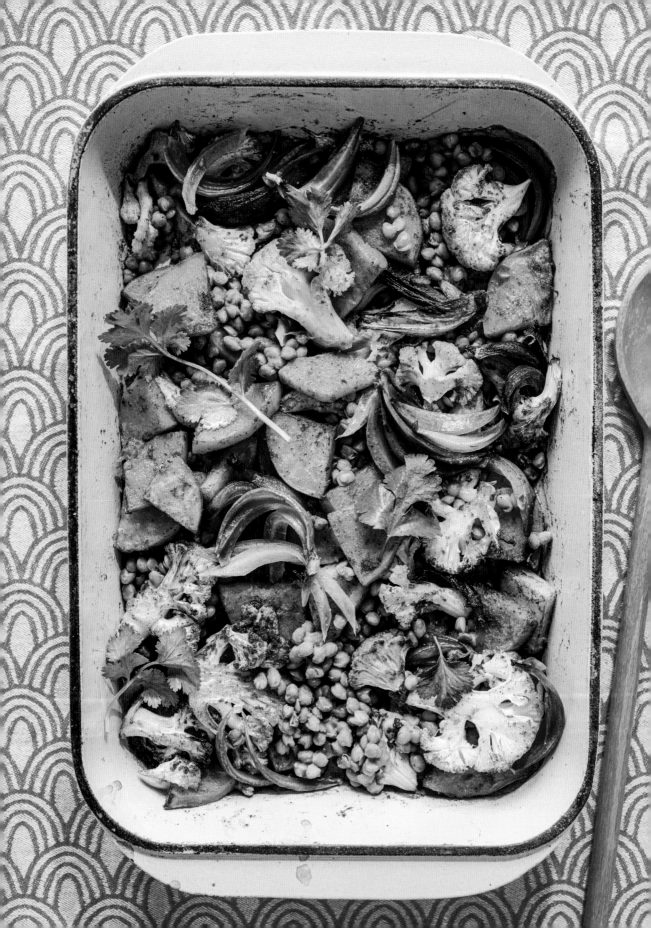

Curry Roasted Vegetables with Lentils

PREP TIME: **10 MINUTES**   COOK TIME: **45 MINUTES**   SERVES: **4**

400g (14oz) butternut
squash, peeled, quartered
lengthways and sliced
into thin quarter circles
(I use the narrow end)
200g (7oz) potatoes,
skins left on, quartered
lengthways and sliced
into thin quarter circles
½ cauliflower, sliced into
thin steaks, then broken
into florets
1 onion, quartered and sliced
2 garlic cloves, crushed
1½ tablespoons curry powder
pinch of hot chilli powder
½ tablespoon olive oil
120ml (4fl oz) vegetable
stock
200g (7oz) canned lentils,
drained (brown or green)
salt and freshly ground
black pepper
handful of freshly chopped
coriander (cilantro),
to serve

**Delicious roasted potatoes, butternut squash and cauliflower
with curry seasonings and lentils, all cooked in one tray for a
simple side dish. This is great drizzled with some natural yogurt
and lemon juice.**

1. Preheat the oven to 200°C/180°C/400°F/gas 6.

2. Combine the butternut squash, potatoes, cauliflower, onion
and garlic on a baking tray.

3. Sprinkle over the curry powder and chilli powder and season
well with salt and pepper. Drizzle with the olive oil and toss to
coat, then spread out in a thin layer across the tray.

4. Pour the stock over the vegetables, then place in the oven and
roast for 40 minutes.

5. Remove from the oven and sprinkle the lentils over the tray, then
return to the oven for 4–5 minutes, just to warm the lentils through.

6. Sprinkle with fresh coriander and serve.

Optional add-ins:
This is great with a lemony,
garlicky yogurt drizzle.
Mix 6 tablespoons fat-free
natural yogurt with
1 tablespoon lemon juice
and ½ teaspoon garlic
powder, then season with
salt. For a creamier version,
use low-fat mayonnaise
instead of yogurt.

VG
V
DF
GF

KCALS
191

FAT
2.6g

SAT FAT
0.4g

CARBS
29.1g

SUGARS
9.0g

FIBRE
10.2g

PROTEIN
7.6g

SALT
0.17g

216 kcals
per serving

German Potato Salad

PREP TIME: **10 MINUTES**   COOK TIME: **25 MINUTES**   SERVES: **4**

GF

DF

KCALS
216

FAT
5.6g

SAT FAT
2.1g

CARBS
23.8g

SUGARS
3.9g

FIBRE
4.2g

PROTEIN
15.5g

SALT
2.62g

1.3 litres (44fl oz) chicken or vegetable stock
600g (1lb 5oz) baby potatoes, halved
4 slices of lean back bacon, trimmed of visible fat and chopped
olive oil spray
1 small red onion, finely diced
2 garlic cloves, crushed
1 spring onion (scallion), chopped
½ tablespoon wholegrain mustard
2 tablespoons apple cider vinegar
1 teaspoon granulated sugar or granulated sweetener
1 tablespoon freshly chopped parsley
salt and freshly ground black pepper

If you have only ever had potato salad with eggs and mayonnaise, wait until you try this German-style version: a delicious warm potato salad with caramelized onions and golden bacon, all tossed in a vinegary mustard dressing. It's my favourite potato salad, and a great side dish for a variety of proteins, like steak or chicken. It's great to serve at a barbecue, too.

1. Set aside 120ml (4fl oz) of the stock for later, and pour the rest into a large saucepan with the potatoes. Place over a high heat and bring to the boil. Simmer for 12–15 minutes until just tender. Drain and set aside.

2. In the meantime, heat a frying pan over a medium–high heat. Add the bacon and fry for a few minutes until lightly golden, then remove from the pan and set aside on a plate.

3. Spray the empty frying pan with olive oil spray. Add the red onion and fry for a couple of minutes, then add the garlic. Gradually add the reserved stock a couple of tablespoons at time, letting each addition reduce before adding more, until the onions are really softened and caramelized – this will take 8–10 minutes.

4. Add the potatoes to the frying pan and spray with some more olive oil spray. Fry for 1 minute just to coat with all the flavour.

5. Return the bacon to the pan, along with the spring onion, mustard, vinegar and sugar, and toss to coat.

6. Transfer to a serving bowl and sprinkle with the parsley. Season with salt and pepper and toss again in the bowl.

7. This is best served warm, but it can be enjoyed cold.

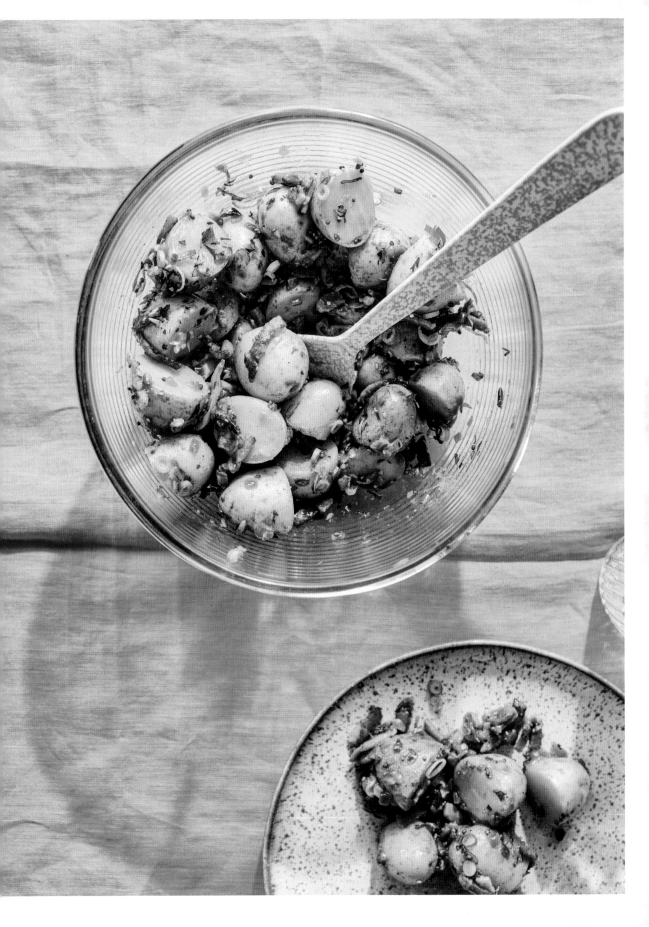

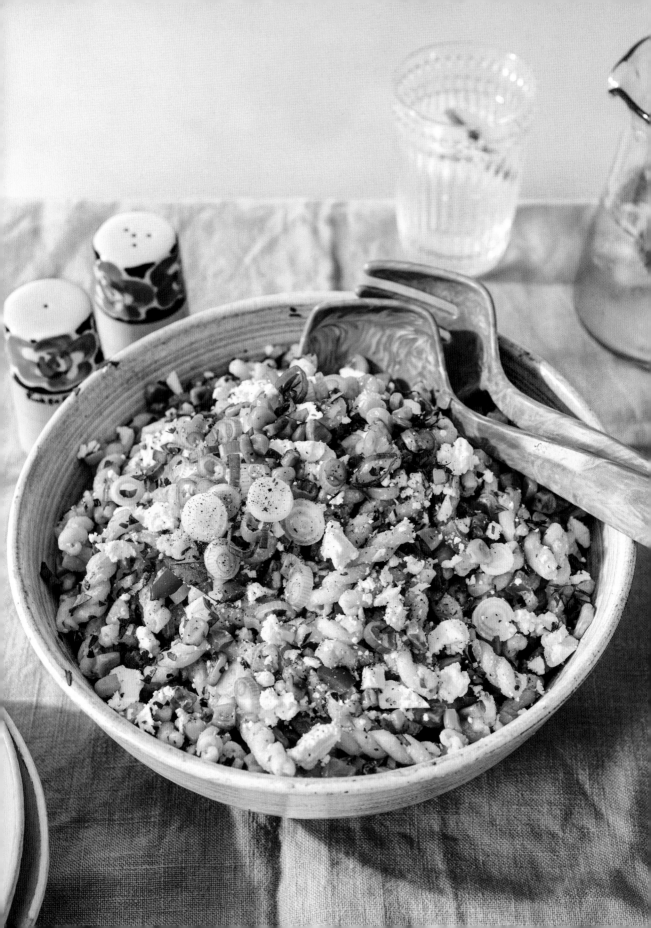

Mexican Street Corn Pasta Salad

PREP TIME: 5 MINUTES   **COOK TIME: 15 MINUTES**   **SERVES: 4 (OR 6 AS A SIDE)**

180g (6½oz) dried pasta
(I used gemelli)
olive oil spray
350g (12oz) frozen or
canned sweetcorn
½ small red onion,
finely diced
2 spring onions (scallions),
finely chopped
½ small red (bell) pepper,
finely diced
1 jalapeñño, deseeded
and finely chopped
handful of coriander
(cilantro), chopped
juice of ½ lime
½ teaspoon paprika
½ teaspoon garlic powder
pinch of cayenne pepper
50g (1¾oz) feta, crumbled
20g (¾oz) Parmesan or
vegetarian Italian-style
hard cheese, grated
2 tablespoons light
mayonnaise
100g (3½oz) fat-free
plain Greek yogurt
salt and freshly ground
black pepper

Optional add-in:
This is also great with some
diced avocado mixed in.

Elote is a popular and delicious Mexican street food consisting of charred corn on the cob, coated in mayonnaise, seasonings and cotija cheese. That is the inspiration for this yummy pasta salad. I make it every summer, and it's great served alongside grilled meats or as part of a barbecue. Instead of the cotija, which can be sometimes hard to source, I use crumbly, salty feta and Parmesan, which is more readily available.

1. Cook the pasta according to the packet instructions, then drain and set aside to cool slightly.

2. Heat a frying pan over a high heat and spray with olive oil spray. Once hot, add the corn and let it get really charred (but not burned) on one side, then toss in the pan to char it on the other side. This will take a couple of minutes.

3. Add to a large bowl with the pasta and the remaining ingredients. Season with salt and pepper and gently toss to combine everything

4. Enjoy!

KCALS
290

FAT
7.4g

SAT FAT
3.0g

CARBS
38.3g

SUGARS
5.7g

FIBRE
5.6g

PROTEIN
14.6g

SALT
0.43g

206 kcals
per serving

V

GF

KCALS
206

FAT
2.5g

SAT FAT
1.1g

CARBS
39.6g

SUGARS
5.6g

FIBRE
3.8g

PROTEIN
4.3g

SALT
0.35g

Seasoned Rice

PREP TIME: **5 MINUTES**   COOK TIME: **25 MINUTES**   SERVES: **4**

½ tablespoon salted butter
1 onion, finely diced
1 small carrot, finely diced
½ red (bell) pepper,
    finely diced
2 garlic cloves, crushed
1 tablespoon dried parsley
1 teaspoon paprika
½ teaspoon onion powder
½ teaspoon garlic powder
pinch of red chilli flakes or
    cayenne pepper (optional)
160g (5¾oz) long-grain rice
475ml (16fl oz) vegetable
    stock
salt and freshly ground
    black pepper

Freezing:
Make sure you reheat the
rice safely.

Plain rice can sometimes be a bit boring as a side dish, especially if it's a recipe that doesn't have much sauce. So I often make up a pan of this easy seasoned rice, which my family loves. It makes a great rice side dish for a variety of mains like the Bourbon Chicken with Vegetables on page 94 or the Honey Chipotle Chicken on page 146.

1. Melt the butter in a large frying pan over a medium–high heat. Add the onion, carrot, red pepper and garlic and fry for about 5 minutes until softened.

2. Add the parsley, paprika, onion powder and garlic powder, and season with salt and pepper. (If you like a bit of spiciness in your rice, add the cayenne or chilli flakes at this point.)

3. Add the rice and fry for a couple of minutes until translucent, then pour in the stock. Bring to the boil, then reduce the heat to medium. Cover and simmer for about 12 minutes until the stock is absorbed, then turn off the heat and leave with the lid on for 10–12 minutes to finish cooking perfectly.

4. Fluff up the rice with a fork and enjoy.

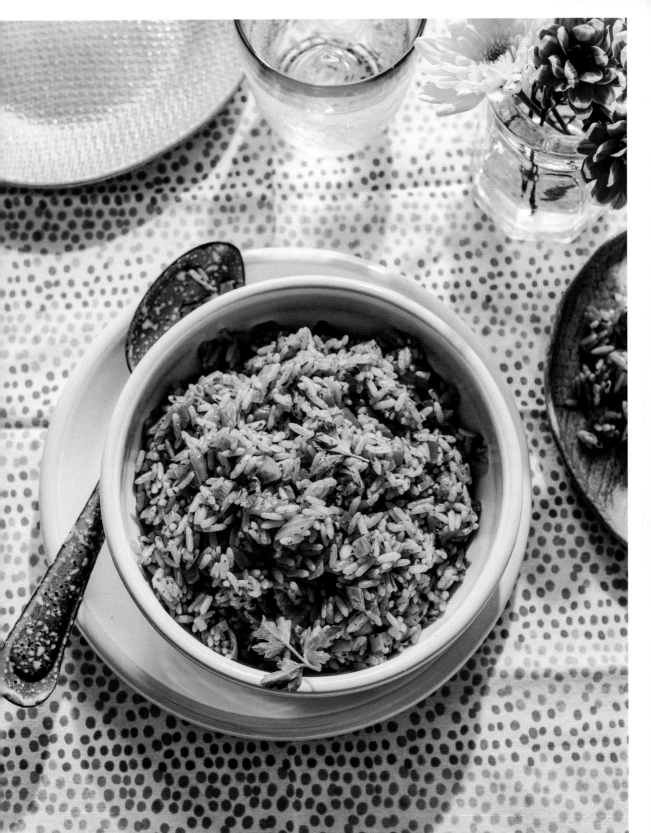

Moroccan Seasoning

KCAL: **7**

FAT: **0.4g**

SAT FAT: **0.1g**

CARBS: **0.2g**

SUGARS: **0.1g**

FIBRE: **0.7g**

PROTEIN: **0.4g**

SALT: **0.65g**

Garlic and Herb

KCAL: **7**

FAT: **0.1g**

SAT FAT: **0.0g**

CARBS: **0.8g**

SUGARS: **0.1g**

FIBRE: **0.6g**

PROTEIN: **0.4g**

SALT: **0.78g**

All-purpose Seasoning

KCAL: **6**

FAT: **0.2g**

SAT FAT: **0.0g**

CARBS: **0.5g**

SUGARS: **0.1g**

FIBRE: **0.5g**

PROTEIN: **0.3g**

SALT: **0.95g**

Ranch Seasoning

KCAL: **6**

FAT: **0.0g**

SAT FAT: **0.0g**

CARBS: **1.0g**

SUGARS: **0.1g**

FIBRE: **0.3g**

PROTEIN: **0.3g**

SALT: **0.82g**

Spice Mixes

I love making my own spice mixes. Seasoning is super-important for creating delicious flavour in your meals. Here are some of my most-used spice mixes. Mix up batches of your favourites and keep in jars so you always have them on hand. They feature in some of the recipes in this book, but they are also great for seasoning vegetables or protein when creating your own meals.

Moroccan Seasoning

2 tablespoons sweet paprika

1½ tablespoons ground cumin

1 tablespoon ground turmeric

1 tablespoon ground coriander

1 tablespoon sea salt

2 teaspoons dried rosemary,

1½ teaspoons garlic powder

1 teaspoon oregano

1 teaspoon ground cinnamon

½ teaspoon ground ginger

½ teaspoon ground cloves

½ teaspoon cayenne pepper

Garlic and Herb

1½ tablespoons garlic powder

1½ tablespoons onion powder

1 tablespoon sea salt

1 tablespoon sweet paprika

1 tablespoon dried basil

1 tablespoon dried parsley

1 teaspoon dried thyme

1 teaspoon freshly ground black pepper

1 teaspoon ground coriander

All-purpose Seasoning

2 tablespoons sweet paprika

2 tablespoons sea salt

1½ tablespoons garlic powder

1½ tablespoons onion powder

1 tablespoon mild chilli powder

1 tablespoon dried parsley

½ tablespoon dried basil

1 teaspoon ground cumin

½ tablespoon black pepper

1 teaspoon ground coriander

* For a spicy version, add
   ¾ tablespoon cayenne pepper

Ranch Seasoning

¾ teaspoon garlic powder

¾ teaspoon onion powder

½ teaspoon dried dill

½ teaspoon dried parsley

½ teaspoon dried chives

½ teaspoon coarse salt

pinch of freshly ground black pepper

* For Ranch Dressing, mix this with 180g (6½oz)
   fat free Greek yogurt, 4 tablespoons
   semi-skimmed milk, 2 teaspoons lemon juice
   and 1 teaspoon maple syrup.

Piri Piri Seasoning

2½ tablespoons sweet paprika
1½ tablespoons onion powder
1½ tablespoons garlic powder
1 tablespoon hot smoked paprika
1 tablespoon salt
1 tablespoon dried parsley
2 teaspoons dried oregano
1½ teaspoons ground ginger
1 teaspoon dried basil
1 teaspoon freshly ground black pepper
1 teaspoon ground green cardamom.

Kansas Barbecue Rub

3 tablespoons sweet paprika
2 tablespoon light brown sugar
1 tablespoon smoked paprika
1½ tablespoon garlic powder
1½ tablespoons onion powder
1 tablespoon celery salt
1 tablespoon salt
2 teaspoons coarse black pepper
1 teaspoon mustard powder
½ tablespoon dried thyme
½ tablespoon dried rosemary
¾ teaspoon cayenne pepper

Cajun Seasoning

4 tablespoons paprika
1½ tablespoons garlic powder
1½ tablespoons onion powder,
1 tablespoon dried oregano
1 tablespoon dried thyme
¾ tablespoon freshly ground black pepper
2 tablespoons salt
¾ tablespoon cayenne pepper

Taco Seasoning

2 tablespoons mild chilli powder
1½ tablespoons paprika
1 tablespoon ground cumin
½ tablespoon dried oregano
1 teaspoon garlic powder
1 teaspoon onion powder
½ tablespoon salt
1 teaspoon freshly ground black pepper

**Piri Piri
Seasoning**
KCAL: **6**
FAT: **0.2g**
SAT FAT: **0.0g**
CARBS: **0.6g**
SUGARS: **0.2g**
FIBRE: **0.6g**
PROTEIN: **0.3g**
SALT: **0.50g**

**Kansas Barbecue
Rub**
KCAL: **9**
FAT: **0.2g**
SAT FAT: **0.0g**
CARBS: **1.4g**
SUGARS: **1.1g**
FIBRE: **0.5g**
PROTEIN: **0.3g**
SALT: **0.58g**

Cajun Seasoning
KCAL: **6**
FAT: **0.2g**
SAT FAT: **0.0g**
CARBS: **0.5g**
SUGARS: **0.1g**
FIBRE: **0.5g**
PROTEIN: **0.3g**
SALT: **0.74g**

Taco Seasoning
KCAL: **6**
FAT: **0.3g**
SAT FAT: **0.0g**
CARBS: **0.1g**
SUGARS: **0.2g**
FIBRE: **0.7g**
PROTEIN: **0.4g**
SALT: **0.46g**

Index

A

all-purpose seasoning 280
allergens 23
Anzac-style cookies 252
apples: caramel apple pie overnight
    oats 176
    pear and apple filo strudel 251
arroz con albondigas bowls 192
artichokes: one-pot spinach and
    artichoke risotto 123
aubergines (eggplant) 24
    one-pot Moroccan-style lamb pilaf 50
    ratatouille lasagne 111
avocados: fish tacos with avocado
    sauce 61
    guacamole 260

B

bacon: bacon, Cheddar, red pepper and
    spring onion frittata muffins 124
    barbecue chicken, bacon and ranch
    loaded fries 86
    German potato salad 274
baked bean cheesy potato-topped pie 211
baking trays 11
balsamic-roasted beetroot with feta
    and orange salad 258
bananas: banana gingerbread cake 248
    banana, peanut and chocolate yogurt
    bark 239
    chocolate peanut banana overnight
    oats 177
    tropical overnight oats 175
bang bang chicken pasta 208
barbecue chicken, bacon and ranch
loaded fries 86
barbecue marinade 81
barbecue salmon cauliflower
    rice bowl 183
barbecue sauce 86
beans 24
    see also **black beans, butter beans** *etc*
beansprouts 19
    bibimbap bowls 188
bechamel sauce 111
beef: beef stroganoff 224
    bibimbap bowls 188
    cheesy bolognese gnocchi bake 207
    corned beef hash 232
    easy cheat's beef pho bowls 184
    harissa meatballs 108
    keema curry 231
    lasagne soup with cheesy ricotta
    balls 149
    Marmite minced beef and
    vegetable filo pie 119
    one-pot cheeseburger pasta 204
    one-pot French onion beef pasta 46
    one-pot taco beef rice skillet 219
    salsa meatloaves 97
    Shanghai-style beef 172
    slow cooker Japanese beef curry 154
    slow cooker pot roast 150
    slow cooker ropa vieja 157

Southwestern beef potato traybake 82
    steak salad bowl 199
beetroot: balsamic-roasted beetroot
with feta and orange salad 258
berries: French toast casserole 236
    oven-baked double chocolate
    and berry pancakes 240
bibimbap bowls 188
Biscoff cake 247
black beans: black bean salsa 261
    butternut squash and black bean
enchilada casserole 104
    slow cooker bean and sweet
    potato chilli 158
    Southwestern beef potato traybake 82
blenders 10
Bourbon chicken with vegetables 94
bread: crispy oven-baked toast 69
    French toast casserole 236
    garlic naan bread 171
    grilled cheese bites 85
    substitutes for 19
breakfast quesadillas 74
broccoli 19
    Bourbon chicken with vegetables 94
Brussels sprouts: harvest chicken
    quinoa bowl 179
    lemon and garlic Brussels 90
buffalo chicken pasta bake 220
burgers, teriyaki turkey 57
butter beans: Mediterranean cod 132
butternut squash: butternut squash
    and black bean enchilada
    casserole 104
    creamy mushroom and vegetable
    barley soup 187
    curry roasted vegetables with
    lentils 273
    harvest chicken quinoa bowl 179
    slow cooker chickpea and vegetable
    korma 162

C

cabbage: chicken vegetable yaki udon 54
    gochujang cabbage wedges 81
    mini vegetable okonomiyaki 270
    slaw 57
    slow cooker pork with cabbage and
    white beans 153
Cajun dressing 199
Cajun spice mix 281
cakes: banana gingerbread cake 248
    Biscoff cake 247
    raspberry lemon loaf 243
cannellini beans: slow cooker pork
    with cabbage and white beans 153
caramel apple pie overnight oats 176
carrots: roasted vegetable soup 85
cauliflower: barbecue salmon
    cauliflower rice bowl 183
    cauliflower mash 18
    cauliflower, pear, pistachio and spelt
    salad 265
    cauliflower rice 18

egg-fried cauliflower rice 172
ham, leek and cauliflower pie 131
herby vegetable toad-in-the-hole 135
maple turmeric chicken traybake 70
cheese 24
    bacon, Cheddar, red pepper and
    spring onion frittata muffins 124
    baked bean cheesy potato-topped
    pie 211
    balsamic-roasted beetroot with feta
    and orange salad 258
    bechamel sauce 111
    buffalo chicken pasta bake 220
    Cheddar crushed roast potatoes 269
    cheesy bolognese gnocchi bake 207
    cheesy jalapeno chicken bake 107
    cheesy potato topping 131
    cheesy ricotta balls 149
    dairy-free cheese 23
    feta, spinach and sweet potato
    frittata muffins 124
    Greek chicken tray bake 89
    grilled cheese bites 85
    Mexican chicken lasagne 228
    one-pot cheeseburger pasta 204
    one-pot spicy and cheesy Korean
    macaroni 38
    one-pot taco beef rice skillet 219
    paneer in spicy tomato sauce 42
    panko-Parmesan pork loin chops 90
    pesto Caprese chicken bake 120
    piri piri halloumi traybake 73
    pizza spaghetti pie 127
    smothered garlic chicken 216
    whipped feta 108
cheesecake dip 255
chicken: baked chicken pathia 115
    bang bang chicken pasta 208
    barbecue chicken, bacon and ranch
    loaded fries 86
    Bourbon chicken with vegetables 94
    buffalo chicken pasta bake 220
    cheesy jalapeno chicken bake 107
    chicken, vegetable and gnocchi
    traybake 77
    chicken vegetable yaki udon 54
    creamy honey mustard chicken 212
    drunken chicken noodles 227
    fajita chicken pasta 215
    Greek chicken tray bake 89
    harvest chicken quinoa bowl 179
    honey chipotle chicken 146
    Jamaican chicken stew 116
    kung pao chicken 145
    maple turmeric chicken traybake 70
    Mexican chicken lasagne 228
    one-pot chicken Cordon Bleu pasta 49
    one-pot chicken Riesling pasta 58
    one-pot New Orleans dirty rice 41
    peanut chicken rice bake 128
    pesto Caprese chicken bake 120
    slow cooker chicken and mango
    curry 165
    smothered garlic chicken 216

spiced chicken salad bowls 195
spicy ginger chicken 223
chickpeas: freezing 22
harissa meatballs 108
lemon, orzo and chickpea soup 142
slow cooker chickpea and vegetable korma 162
chillies: kung pao chicken 145
slow cooker bean and sweet potato chilli 158
chipotle paste: honey chipotle chicken 146
chocolate: banana, peanut and chocolate yogurt bark 239
chocolate-drizzled puffed rice bars 244
chocolate peanut banana overnight oats 177
oven-baked double chocolate and berry pancakes 240
choppers 10
chopping boards 9
chorizo and prawn Israeli couscous 45
cinnamon-sugar chips 255
coconut: Anzac-style cookies 252
coconut milk, oven-baked poached fish in 112
cod, Mediterranean 132
containers 11, 22
cookies, Anzac-style 252
corned beef hash 232
cornflake halibut with garlic potatoes 98
courgettes (zucchini): garlic butter prawns and vegetables 37
Greek chicken tray bake 89
minty leeks, courgette and peas 98
ratatouille lasagne 111
couscous: lemon and herb Israeli couscous 266
one-pot chorizo and prawn Israeli couscous 45
cream cheese 15
beef stroganoff 224
buffalo chicken pasta bake 220
cheesecake dip 255
creamy honey mustard chicken 212
Mexican chicken lasagne 228
cucumber: sticky sriracha tofu bowls 196
curry: baked chicken pathia 115
curry roasted vegetables with lentils 273
keema curry 231
one-pot Thai red prawn and vegetable rice 53
slow cooker chicken and mango curry 165
slow cooker chickpea and vegetable korma 162
slow cooker Japanese beef curry 154
spiced chicken salad bowls 195

D
dairy products 15–16
defrosting meals 22
dietary requirements 23

dips 101
drunken chicken noodles 227

E
easy cheat's beef pho bowls 184
eggs 24
breakfast quesadillas 74
easy shakshuka with crispy oven-baked toast 69
egg-fried cauliflower rice 172
egg-in-a-hole 93
frittata muffins 124
poached eggs 123
enchilada sauce 104
equipment 9–11
exercise 26

F
fajita chicken pasta 215
fennel: sausage and fennel hot pot 141
fish: cornflake halibut 98
fish tacos with avocado sauce 61
oven-baked poached fish 112
see also **cod**, **salmon** *etc*
flours, gluten-free 23
food diaries 25
food processors 10
freezing 22
French toast casserole 236
fries: ranch loaded fries 86
sweet potato fries 199
veggie fries/cubes 18–19
frittata muffins 124
fruit salsa and cheesecake dip 255
frying pans 10, 20

G
garlic: freezing 22
garlic and herb spice mix 280
garlic butter prawns and vegetables 37
garlic mayo 30
garlic naan bread 171
garlic potatoes 98
lemon and garlic Brussels 90
smothered garlic chicken 216
German potato salad 274
ginger: banana gingerbread cake 248
freezing 22
gluten-free ingredients 23
gnocchi: cheesy bolognese gnocchi bake 207
chicken, vegetable and gnocchi traybake 77
creamy sun-dried tomato gnocchi 33
gochujang cabbage wedges 81
gravy, onion 135
Greek chicken tray bake 89
green beans, salsa meatloaves with 97
guacamole 260

H
ham: egg-in-a-hole 93
ham, leek and cauliflower pie 131
haricot beans: sun-dried tomato, bean and lentil soup 168

harissa meatballs 108
harvest chicken quinoa bowl 179
healthy eating 25–6
herbs 13
herby vegetable toad-in-the-hole 135
hobbies, non-food 26
hoisin pork tenderloin 66
honey Cajun salmon with succotash 78
honey chipotle chicken 146
hot pot, sausage and fennel 141

I
ingredients 12–13

J
Jamaican chicken stew 116

K
Kansas barbecue rub 281
keema curry 231
kidney beans: slow cooker bean and sweet potato chilli 158
knives 9
Korean barbecue pork 81
kung pao chicken 145

L
lamb: Middle Eastern-style lamb bowls 191
one-pot Moroccan-style lamb pilaf 50
slow cooker lamb and mint casserole 161
lasagne: lasagne soup 149
Mexican chicken lasagne 228
ratatouille 111
leeks: ham, leek and cauliflower pie 131
minty leeks, courgette and peas 98
lemon: lemon and garlic Brussels 90
lemon and herb Israeli couscous 266
lemon dill dip 101
lemon, orzo and chickpea soup 142
raspberry lemon loaf 243
lentils 24
curry roasted vegetables with lentils 273
lentil quinoa shawarma pittas 30
sun-dried tomato, bean and lentil soup 168
sweet potato lentil dhal bowl 171

M
macaroni, one-pot spicy and cheesy Korean 38
mangoes: mint and mango raita 195
slow cooker chicken and mango curry 165
maple turmeric chicken traybake 70
marinades 81
Marmite minced beef and vegetable filo pie 119
marshmallows: chocolate-drizzled puffed rice bars 244
mayonnaise: garlic mayo 30
lemon dill dip 101
measuring equipment 9

meat 15
  substitutes 24
  thermometers 9
  see also beef, pork etc
meatballs: arroz con albondigas
    bowls 192
  harissa meatballs 108
meatloaves, salsa 97
Mediterranean cod 132
Mexican chicken lasagne 228
Mexican street corn pasta salad 277
Middle Eastern-style lamb bowls 191
milk 16
  dairy-free milks 23
mint: mint and mango raita 195
  mint sauce 161
Moroccan seasoning 280
muffins, frittata 124
mushrooms: beef stroganoff 224
  bibimbap bowls 188
  chicken vegetable yaki udon 54
  creamy mushroom and vegetable
barley soup 187
  creamy sun-dried tomato gnocchi 33
  egg-in-a-hole with balsamic
    mushrooms 93
  Marmite minced beef and vegetable
    filo pie 119
  one-pot chicken Riesling pasta 58
  smothered garlic chicken 216

N
naan bread 171
noodles: chicken vegetable yaki udon 54
  drunken chicken noodles 227
  easy cheat's beef pho bowls 184
  pork potsticker noodle bowl 180
nuts 24

O
oats: Anzac-style cookies 252
  caramel apple pie overnight oats 176
  chocolate peanut banana overnight
    oats 177
  tropical overnight oats 175
oil sprays 15
okonomiyaki, mini vegetable 270
olives: Greek chicken tray bake 89
  slow cooker ropa vieja 157
one-pot meals 20
onions: one-pot French onion beef
pasta 46
  onion gravy 135
  pickled onions 138
oranges: balsamic-roasted beetroot
    with feta and orange salad 258
oven-baked double chocolate and
  berry pancakes 240
oven-baked poached fish 112
oven temperatures 17

P
pak choi: oven-baked poached fish 112
pancakes: mini vegetable okonomiyaki
    270
  oven-baked double chocolate and
    berry pancakes 240

paneer in spicy tomato sauce 42
panko-Parmesan pork loin chops 90
pasta 20
  bang bang chicken pasta 208
  buffalo chicken pasta bake 220
  fajita chicken pasta 215
  gluten-free pasta 23
  high-protein pastas 24
  lasagne soup with cheesy ricotta
    balls 149
  lemon, orzo and chickpea soup 142
  Mexican chicken lasagne 228
  Mexican street corn pasta salad 277
  one-pot cheeseburger pasta 204
  one-pot chicken Cordon Bleu pasta 49
  one-pot chicken Riesling pasta 58
  one-pot French onion beef pasta 46
  one-pot smoky paprika sausage
    penne 62
  one-pot spicy and cheesy Korean
    macaroni 38
  pizza spaghetti pie 127
  ratatouille lasagne 111
patties, salmon 101
peanut butter: banana, peanut and
    chocolate yogurt bark 239
  chocolate peanut banana overnight
    oats 177
  peanut chicken rice bake 128
pears: barbecue marinade 81
  cauliflower, pear, pistachio and
    spelt salad 265
  pear and apple filo strudel 251
peas: keema curry 231
  minty leeks, courgette and peas 98
pepper 16
peppers: arroz con albondigas bowls 192
  bacon, Cheddar, red pepper and
    spring onion frittata muffins 124
  chicken, vegetable and gnocchi
    traybake 77
  corned beef hash 232
  fajita chicken pasta 215
  garlic butter prawns and vegetables 37
  honey Cajun salmon with succotash 78
  Jamaican chicken stew 116
  kung pao chicken 145
  Mediterranean cod 132
  Mexican chicken lasagne 228
  one-pot chorizo and prawn Israeli
    couscous 45
  one-pot New Orleans dirty rice 41
  one-pot smoky paprika sausage
    penne 62
  one-pot Thai red prawn and vegetable
    rice 53
  piri piri halloumi traybake 73
  pork and pineapple stir-fry 34
  ratatouille lasagne 111
  salmon patties 101
  sausage and fennel hot pot 141
  slow cooker ropa vieja 157
  Southwestern beef potato traybake 82
  spicy red pepper dip 101
pesto: pesto Caprese chicken bake 120
  tomato and pesto frittata muffins 124
pickled onions 138

pies: ham, leek and cauliflower pie 131
  Marmite minced beef and vegetable
    filo pie 119
pilaf, one-pot Moroccan-style lamb 50
pineapple: pineapple salsa 261
  pork and pineapple stir-fry 34
  tropical overnight oats 175
pinto beans: slow cooker bean and
    sweet potato chilli 158
piri piri halloumi traybake 73
piri piri spice mix 281
pistachios: cauliflower, pear, pistachio
    and spelt salad 265
pittas, lentil quinoa shawarma 30
pizza spaghetti pie 127
planning meals 25
pork: hoisin pork tenderloin 66
  Korean barbecue pork 81
  one-pot New Orleans dirty rice 41
  panko-Parmesan pork loin chops 90
  pork and pineapple stir-fry 34
  pork potsticker noodle bowl 180
  slow cooker pork 153
  Yucatan-style pulled pork 138
  zuppa toscana soup bowls 200
planning meals 25
portion sizes 15
pot roast, slow cooker 150
potatoes: baked bean cheesy potato-
    topped pie 211
  barbecue chicken, bacon and ranch
    loaded fries 86
  Cheddar crushed roast potatoes 269
  cheesy potato topping 131
  corned beef hash 232
  curry roasted vegetables with
    lentils 273
  garlic potatoes 98
  German potato salad 274
  Greek chicken tray bake 89
  slow cooker Japanese beef curry 154
  slow cooker pot roast 150
  Southwestern beef potato traybake 82
  zuppa toscana soup bowls 200
prawns (**shrimp**): garlic butter prawns
    and vegetables 37
  one-pot chorizo and prawn Israeli
    couscous 45
  one-pot Thai red prawn and vegetable
    rice 53
protein 20, 21
puffed rice bars, chocolate-drizzled 244

Q
quesadillas, breakfast 74
quinoa 24
  harvest chicken quinoa bowl 179
  lentil quinoa shawarma pittas 30

R
raita, mint and mango 195
ranch seasoning 280
raspberry lemon loaf 243
ratatouille lasagne 111
rice 20
  arroz con albondigas bowls 192
  bibimbap bowls 188

freezing 22
hoisin pork tenderloin with special fried rice 66
one-pot Moroccan-style lamb pilaf 50
one-pot New Orleans dirty rice 41
one-pot spinach and artichoke risotto 123
one-pot taco beef rice skillet 219
one-pot Thai red prawn and vegetable rice 53
peanut chicken rice bake 128
seasoned rice 278
sticky sriracha tofu bowls 196
risotto, one-pot spinach and artichoke 123
roasted vegetables 18
root vegetables: veggie mash 18
see also carrots, potatoes *etc*
ropa vieja, slow cooker 157

S
salads 19
balsamic-roasted beetroot with feta and orange salad 258
cauliflower, pear, pistachio and spelt salad 265
German potato salad 274
Mexican street corn pasta salad 277
steak salad bowl 199
salmon: barbecue salmon cauliflower rice bowl 183
honey Cajun salmon with succotash 78
salmon patties with two dips 101
salsa: black bean salsa 261
fruit salsa 255
pineapple salsa 261
salsa meatloaves 97
salt 16
saucepans 10
sauces, thickening 17
sausages: breakfast quesadillas 74
one-pot smoky paprika sausage penne 62
sausage and fennel hot pot 141
zuppa toscana soup bowls 200
scales 9
scaling recipes down 14–15
seasonings 16, 20, 21
shakshuka with crispy oven-baked toast 69
Shanghai-style beef 172
sheet-pan meals 21
shopping 14
shredded vegetables 19
shrimp *see* **prawns**
sides 18
slaw 57
slow cookers 11
smothered garlic chicken 216
snacks 25–6
social media 26
soups: creamy mushroom and vegetable barley soup 187
lasagne soup with cheesy ricotta balls 149
lemon, orzo and chickpea soup 142
roasted vegetable soup 85

sun-dried tomato, bean and lentil soup 168
zuppa toscana soup bowls 200
Southwestern beef potato traybake 82
soy sauce 23
barbecue marinade 81
spaghetti: bang bang chicken pasta 208
one-pot chicken Riesling pasta 58
pizza spaghetti pie 127
spelt: cauliflower, pear, pistachio and spelt salad 265
spice mixes 280–1
spices 13
spinach: creamy sun-dried tomato gnocchi 33
feta, spinach and sweet potato frittata muffins 124
one-pot spinach and artichoke risotto 123
spiralized vegetables 10, 18
sriracha tofu bowls 196
stalks 19
steak salad bowl 199
stews: butternut squash and black bean enchilada casserole 104
Jamaican chicken stew 116
slow cooker lamb and mint casserole 161
slow cooker ropa vieja 157
stock 16
strudel, pear and apple filo 251
succotash, honey Cajun salmon with 78
sun-dried tomato, bean and lentil soup 168
sweet potatoes: barbecue salmon cauliflower rice bowl 183
creamy sun-dried tomato gnocchi 33
feta, spinach and sweet potato frittata muffins 124
piri piri halloumi traybake 73
roasted vegetable soup 85
salsa meatloaves with green beans and sweet potato 97
slow cooker bean and sweet potato chilli 158
sweet potato fries 199
sweet potato lentil dhal bowl 171
sweetcorn: Mexican street corn pasta salad 277
one-pot taco beef rice skillet 219
sweeteners 16–17

T
taco seasoning 219
taco spice mix 281
tacos, fish 61
temperatures 17
teriyaki turkey burgers 57
thermometers 9
thickening sauces 17
toad-in-the-hole: egg-in-a-hole 93
herby vegetable toad-in-the-hole 135
toast, crispy oven-baked 69
tofu: sticky sriracha tofu bowls 196
tomatoes: baked chicken pathia 115
barbecue sauce 86
buffalo chicken pasta bake 220

butternut squash and black bean enchilada casserole 104
cheesy bolognese gnocchi bake 207
creamy sun-dried tomato gnocchi 33
easy shakshuka with crispy oven-baked toast 69
egg-in-a-hole with tomatoes 93
Greek chicken tray bake 89
harissa meatballs 108
honey chipotle chicken 146
lasagne soup 149
Mediterranean cod 132
one-pot smoky paprika sausage penne 62
paneer in spicy tomato sauce 42
pesto Caprese chicken bake 120
pizza sauce 127
ratatouille lasagne 111
sausage and fennel hot pot 141
slow cooker ropa vieja 157
spicy sauce 228
sun-dried tomato, bean and lentil soup 168
tomato and pesto frittata muffins 124
tonkatsu sauce 270
tortillas: breakfast quesadillas 74
butternut squash and black bean enchilada casserole 104
cinnamon-sugar chips 255
fish tacos with avocado sauce 61
tropical overnight oats 175
turkey: arroz con albondigas bowls 192
teriyaki turkey burgers 57

U
utensils 9
vegetables: meat substitutes 24
one-pot meals 20
sheet-pan meals 21
sides 18–19
see also potatoes, tomatoes *etc*
vegetarian swaps 24

W
white beans: sausage and fennel hot pot 141

Y
yogurt 15–16
banana, peanut and chocolate yogurt bark 239
caramel apple pie overnight oats 176
cheesecake dip 255
chocolate peanut banana overnight oats 177
lemon dill dip 101
mint and mango raita 195
oven-baked double chocolate and berry pancakes 240
spicy red pepper dip 101
tropical overnight oats 175
Yucatan-style pulled pork 138

Z
zucchini *see* **courgettes**
zuppa toscana soup bowls 200

Recipe Index

Simple Stovetop

Lentil Quinoa Shawarma Pittas 30
Creamy Sun-dried Tomato Gnocchi with Spinach, Mushrooms and Sweet Potato 33
Pork and Pineapple Stir-fry 34
Garlic Butter Prawns and Vegetables 37
One-pot Spicy and Cheesy Korean Macaroni 38
One-pot New Orleans Dirty Rice 41
Paneer in Spicy Tomato Sauce 42
One-pot Chorizo and Prawn Israeli Couscous 45
One-pot French Onion Beef Pasta 46
One-pot Chicken Cordon Bleu Pasta 49
One-pot Moroccan-style Lamb Pilaf 50
One-pot Thai Red Prawn and Vegetable Rice 53
Chicken Vegetable Yaki Udon 54
Teriyaki Turkey Burgers with Slaw and Sriracha Mayo 57
One-pot Chicken Riesling Pasta 58
Fish Tacos with Avocado Sauce 61
One-pot Smoky Paprika Sausage Penne 62

Sheet-pan Meals Made Simple

Hoisin Pork Tenderloin with Special Fried Rice 66
Easy Shakshuka with Crispy Oven-baked Toast 69
Maple Turmeric Chicken Traybake 70
Piri Piri Halloumi Traybake 73
Breakfast Quesadillas 74
Chicken, Vegetable and Gnocchi Traybake 77
Honey Cajun Salmon with Succotash 78
Korean Barbecue Pork with Spicy Gochujang Cabbage Wedges 81
Southwestern Beef Potato Traybake 82
Roasted Vegetable Soup with Grilled Cheese Bites 85
Barbecue Chicken, Bacon and Ranch Loaded Fries 86
Greek Chicken Tray Bake 89
Panko-Parmesan Pork Loin Chops with Lemon and Garlic Shredded Brussels 90
Egg-in-a-Hole with Balsamic Mushrooms and Tomatoes 93
Bourbon Chicken with Vegetables 94
Salsa Meatloaves with Green Beans and Sweet Potato 97
Cornflake Halibut with Garlic Potatoes, Leeks, Courgette and Peas 98
Salmon Patties with Two Dips 101

Made Simple in the Oven

Butternut Squash and Black Bean Enchilada Casserole 104
Cheesy Jalapeño Chicken Bake 107
Harissa Meatballs with Whipped Feta 108

Ratatouille Lasagne 111
Oven-baked Poached Fish in Coconut Milk 112
Baked Chicken Pathia 115
Jamaican Chicken Stew 116
Marmite Minced Beef and Vegetable Filo Pie 119
Pesto Caprese Chicken Bake 120
Oven-baked Spinach and Artichoke Risotto with Poached Eggs 123
Frittata Muffins – Three Ways 124
Pizza Spaghetti Pie 127
Peanut Chicken Rice Bake 128
Ham, Leek and Cauliflower Pie with Rustic Cheesy Potato Topping 131
Mediterranean Cod 132
Herby Vegetable Toad-in-the-Hole with Onion Gravy 135

Slow Cooker Recipes

Yucatan-style Pulled Pork 138
Sausage and Fennel Hot Pot 141
Lemon, Orzo and Chickpea Soup 142
Kung Pao Chicken 145
Honey Chipotle Chicken 146
Lasagne Soup with Cheesy Ricotta Balls 149
Slow Cooker Pot Roast 150
Slow Cooker Pork with Cabbage and White Beans 153
Slow Cooker Japanese Beef Curry 154
Slow Cooker Ropa Vieja 157
Slow Cooker Bean and Sweet Potato Chilli 158
Slow Cooker Lamb and Mint Casserole 161
Slow Cooker Chickpea and Vegetable Korma 162
Slow Cooker Chicken and Mango Curry 165

Delicious Bowls

Sun-dried Tomato, Bean and Lentil Soup 168
Sweet Potato Lentil Dhal Bowl with Garlic Naan 171
Shanghai-style Beef with Egg-fried Cauliflower Rice 172
Overnight Oats Bowls – Three Ways 175
Harvest Chicken Quinoa Bowl 179
Pork Potsticker Noodle Bowl 180
Barbecue Salmon Cauliflower Rice Bowl 183
Easy Cheat's Beef Pho Bowls 184
Creamy Mushroom and Vegetable Barley Soup 187
Bibimbap Bowls 188
Middle Eastern-style Lamb Bowls 191
Arroz Con Albondigas Bowls 192
Spiced Chicken Salad Bowls 195
Sticky Sriracha Tofu Bowls 196
Steak Salad Bowl with Sweet Potato Fries and Creamy Cajun Dressing 199
Zuppa Toscana Soup Bowls 200

Blog Favourites

One-pot Cheeseburger Pasta 204
Cheesy Bolognese Gnocchi Bake 207
Bang Bang Chicken Pasta 208
Baked Bean Cheesy Potato-topped Pie 211
Creamy Honey Mustard Chicken 212
Fajita Chicken Pasta 215
Smothered Garlic Chicken 216
One-pot Taco Beef Rice Skillet 219
Buffalo Chicken Pasta Bake 220
Spicy Ginger Chicken 223
Beef Stroganoff 224
Drunken Chicken Noodles 227
Mexican Chicken Lasagne 228
Keema Curry 231
Corned Beef Hash 232

Desserts Made Simple

French Toast Casserole 236
Banana, Peanut and Chocolate Yogurt Bark 239
Oven-baked Double Chocolate and Berry Pancakes 240
Raspberry Lemon Loaf 243
Chocolate-drizzled Puffed Rice Bars 244
Biscoff Cake 247
Banana Gingerbread Cake 248
Pear and Apple Filo Strudel 251
Anzac-style Cookies 252
Fruit Salsa and Cheesecake Dip with Cinnamon-sugar Chips 255

Simple Extras

Balsamic-roasted Beetroot with Feta and Orange Salad 258
Guacamole and Salsa Two Ways 260
Cauliflower, Pear, Pistachio and Spelt Salad with Honey and Ginger Dressing 265
Lemon and Herb Israeli Couscous 266
Cheddar Crushed Roast Potatoes with Special Sauce 269
Mini Vegetable Okonomiyaki (Japanese Pancakes) 270
Curry Roasted Vegetables with Lentils 273
German Potato Salad 274
Mexican Street Corn Pasta Salad 277
Seasoned Rice 278
Spice Mixes 280

Acknowledgements

There are so many people who have made this book possible and worked tirelessly behind the scenes to make this book another great success.

Firstly, the amazing and wonderful support of my family. At times, when I doubt myself or I am incredibly stressed due to deadlines or deep in the mess of my kitchen after a day of recipe testing, they are always there encouraging me in every way possible. My husband Gavin is the behind the scenes supporter – and to whom without his support I may possibly have not survived the process of writing this book. You have been there both emotionally and technically, always believing in me and convincing me I can do this, as well as managing all the technical side of things like my website and social media, ensuring they run smoothly while I am busy in the kitchen and working on this book. To my amazing children, Isaac and Felicity, for always being my little taste testers and making me smile and laugh whenever it's needed.

To my Dad – thank you for encouraging me with my love for cooking and introducing me to so many different cuisines from a young age. I know you are super proud of what Slimming Eats has become today and are constantly sharing my book and recipes with your friends and acquaintances.

Kathy, my amazing friend and neighbour, thank you for those days out shopping or a long chat over a cup of tea or coffee when I need a break from the crazy of my kitchen. To Kerry and Clare, for always supporting me through this exciting and sometimes crazy ride of writing a cookbook.

And the rest of my friends and family who have been incredibly supportive on this amazing journey of publishing a book.

To the amazing team at Yellow Kite, Hodder and Stoughton and Mobius for believing in Slimming Eats and helping create this cookbook, especially Lauren Whelan, Nicky Ross, Isabel Gonzalez-Prendergast and Liv Nightingall. The amazing team of photographers, food stylists, prop stylists and nutritionists – Liz and Max Haarala Hamilton, Jen Kay, Rosie Reynolds, Troy Willis and Kerry Torrens. Nathan Burton for the beautiful designs and layout of the book. Tara O'Sullivan for all the copy editing and turning my rambles into readable text.

Thank you to Moira, Claire, Andra and Steph for continuing to be an extra set of eyes and support in the Facebook group community.

Finally, thanks to my readers, without you, this book wouldn't be possible in the first place. Your continued support, with photos and stories of your progress is what keeps me going. Above all else, providing recipes that helps people with their own journey means more to me than anything else. Being able to make a difference in someone else's life, however big or small, is the ultimate reward for my work and makes it all worthwhile.

I do hope you enjoy these recipes and that they find a regular place in your meal planning and heart.

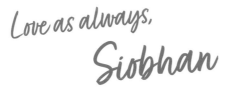

Love as always,

Siobhan

First published in Great Britain in 2022 by Yellow Kite
An imprint of Hodder & Stoughton
An Hachette UK company

1

Hardback ISBN 978 1 399 70824 1
eBook ISBN 978 1 399 70825 8

Associate Publisher: Lauren Whelan
Editorial Director: Nicky Ross
Project Editor: Isabel Gonzalez-Prendergast
Assistant Editor: Liv Nightingall
Designer: Nathan Burton
Photography: Liz & Max Haarala Hamilton
Food Stylists: Rosie Reynolds & Troy Willis
Props Stylist: Jen Kay
Senior Production Controller: Rachel Southey

Colour origination by Alta Image London
Printed and bound in Germany by Mohn Media

Hodder & Stoughton policy is to use papers that are natural, renewable and recyclable products
and made from wood grown in sustainable forests. The logging and manufacturing processes
are expected to conform to the environmental regulations of the country of origin.

Yellow Kite
Hodder & Stoughton Ltd
Carmelite House
50 Victoria Embankment
London
EC4Y 0DZ

www.yellowkitebooks.co.uk
www.hodder.co.uk

Notes

The information and references contained herein are for informational purposes only. They are designed to support,
not replace, any ongoing medical advice given by a healthcare professional and should not be construed as the giving
of medical advice nor relied upon as a basis for any decision or action. Readers should consult their doctor before
altering their diet, particularly if they are on a set diet prescribed by their doctor or dietician.
The calorie count for each recipe is an estimate only and may vary depending on the brand of ingredients used, and due to the natural
biological variations in the composition of foods such as meat, fish, fruit and vegetables. It does not include the nutritional content
of garnishes or any optional accompaniments recommended for taste/serving in the ingredients list.